Recent Results
in Cancer Research

189

Managing Editors
P.M. Schlag, Berlin   H.-J. Senn, St. Gallen

Associate Editors
P. Kleihues, Zürich   F. Stiefel, Lausanne
B. Groner, Frankfurt   A. Wallgren, Göteborg

Founding Editor
P. Rentchnik, Geneva

Andrea Tannapfel

(Editor)

Malignant Mesothelioma

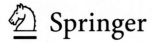
Springer

Editor
Prof. Andrea Tannapfel
Institut für Pathologie
Ruhr-Universität Bochum
BG Kliniken Bergmannsheil
Bürke-de-la-Camp Platz 1
44789 Bochum, Germany
andrea.tannapfel@ruhr-uni-bochum.de

ISBN 978-3-642-10861-7   e-ISBN 978-3-642-10862-4
DOI 10.1007/978-3-642-10862-4
Springer Heidelberg Dordrecht London New York

Library of Congress Control Number: 2011923338

Cover design: estudioCalamar Figueres/Berlin

Printed on acid-free paper

Springer is part of Springer Science + Business Media (www.springer.com)

Preface

Malignant mesothelioma is a rare and aggressive tumor arising from the mesothelium. Pleural, peritoneal, and pericardial mesothelioma are possible entities according to the site of origin.

Diffuse malignant mesothelioma is strongly associated with exposure to asbestos and was first referred by Selikoff in 1965 as a "signal tumor" because of its close association with occupational and environmental exposure to asbestos.

There is a clear positive correlation between historical asbestos exposure and deaths caused by mesothelioma. Approximately, 2500 patients in the United States of America and 1000 patients in Germany annually are diagnosed with malignant mesothelioma. The incidence peak of mesothelioma will be reached in the next 10–20 years due to the extended latency period of about 30–40 years or more after exposure.

This issue of "Recent Results in Cancer Research" – Malignant Mesothelioma – is a comprehensive compilation of all topics related to asbestos and mesothelioma, written by well-known experts in their fields.

We intend to provide a broad overview of mineralogy of asbestos, analysis for lung tissue fiber content, and epidemiology of this disease.

The book also refers to all new diagnostic pathways like imaging, pathohistological as well as molecular approaches, genetic and molecular biological characteristics, and potential use of biomarkers for screening of mesothelioma.

Recent developments and novel approaches in surgery, chemotherapy, and radiotherapy of malignant mesothelioma are outlined by experts in this field.

The chapter about mineralogy of asbestos emphasizes the pivotal role of different physicochemical and biological features of chrysotile and amphibole asbestos for understanding the different hazards of exposure.

An outstanding team of international leading experts have contributed to this book. It is addressed to oncologists, radiologists, thoracic surgeons, pathologists, and pulmonologists with the intention to provide a scientific-based up-to-date view on mesothelioma research, diagnosis, and therapy strategies. A comprehensive understanding of all aspects of this disease will be the foundation to perform successful future laboratory research and clinical studies.

Andrea Tannapfel
Volker Neumann

Contents

10   Early Stages of Mesothelioma, Screening and Biomarkers.   169
Sonja Klebe and Douglas W. Henderson

Mineralogy of Asbestos

1

Thomas A. Sporn

Abstract The term asbestos collectively refers to a group of naturally occurring fibrous minerals which have been exploited in numerous commercial and industrial settings and applications dating to antiquity. Its myriad uses as a "miracle mineral" owe to its remarkable properties of extreme resistance to thermal and chemical breakdown, tensile strength, and fibrous habit which allows it to be spun and woven into textiles. Abundant in nature, it has been mined considerably, and in all continents save Antarctica. The nomenclature concerning asbestos and its related species is complex, owing to the interest held therein by scientific disciplines such as geology, mineralogy and medicine, as well as legal and regulatory authorities. As fibrous silicates, asbestos minerals are broadly classified into the *serpentine* (chrysotile) and *amphibole* (crocidolite, amosite, tremolite, anthophyllite, actinolite) groups, both of which may also contain allied but nonfibrous forms of similar or even identical chemical composition, nonpathogenic to humans. Recently, fibrous amphiboles, not historically classified or regulated as asbestos (winchite, richterite), have been implicated in the causation of serious disease due to their profusion as natural contaminants of vermiculite, a commercially useful and nonfibrous silicate mineral. Although generally grouped, classified, and regulated collectively as asbestos, the serpentine and amphibole groups have different geologic occurrences and, more importantly, significant differences in crystalline structures and chemical compositions. These in turn impart differences in fiber structure and dimension, as well as biopersistence, leading to marked differences in relative potency for causing disease in humans for the group of minerals known as asbestos.

1.1
Introduction and Historical Background

Minerals are naturally occurring, inorganic compounds of specific chemical composition and crystal structure. Their nomenclature typically stems as an honorific, to indicate a pertinent geographic area or to highlight a distinctive characteristic of the compound. Derived from the Greek asbestos ("unquenchable" or "indestructible"), asbestos is the collective term for a family of naturally occurring fibrous silicates that exist in metamorphic, altered basic, or ultra

T.A. Sporn
Department of Pathology,
Duke University Medical Center,
200 Trent Drive, Durham, NC 27710, USA
e-mail: sporn001@mc.duke.edu

A. Tannapfel (ed.), *Malignant Mesothelioma*, Recent Results in Cancer Research 189,
DOI: 10.1007/978-3-642-10862-4_1, © Springer-Verlag Berlin Heidelberg 2011

basic igneous rock. Asbestos and asbestiform minerals are narrowly defined and classified, as will be discussed below. The asbestos minerals have found much utility owing to their common properties of thermochemical and electrical resistance, high tensile strength, and flexibility. Insoluble in water and organic solvents, its fine fibers may be spun and woven into textiles and incorporated into many other types of materials, asbestos has seen literally thousands of industrial applications. The usage of asbestos dates, through fact and fable, to thousands of years ago. Once believed to have almost magical capabilities, first descriptions document its usage in the manufacture of pottery in Finland ca. 2500 BC. Additional historical attributions for early asbestos usage include cremation garments for royalty and for embalming the pharaohs of ancient Egypt, and the emperor Charlemagne reportedly astonished his guests at a feast by throwing table cloths made from asbestos into a fire from which the garments would be removed clean and unharmed. Medieval alchemists termed the mineral "salamander stone" referring to a mythical fireproof animal, and during these times asbestos was used in suits of armor [1]. Deposits of asbestos in the Ural Mountains led to the development of factories producing asbestos textiles in 1720. In the seventeenth century, fibrous minerals discovered in Germany termed Bergflachs or Bergleder likely contained amphibole asbestos, and by the mid-nineteenth century, some 20 asbestos mines were operating in Europe [19]. In colonial America, asbestos deposits were discovered in Pennsylvania and New England, where it was woven into textiles, and chrysotile was discovered in Quebec, Canada in 1860 [19]. Significant commercial usage of asbestos did not occur until the latter part of the nineteenth century, with the development of the demand for insulation for the burgeoning steam technology. At the turn of the twentieth century, additional applications for the useful minerals had been developed, deposits of amphibole asbestos species had been discovered in South Africa,

and asbestos was once more being mined in the Urals, this time in large quantities. Commercial exploitation of asbestos was now global and full-blown, and by 1980 over 100 million tons of asbestos had been mined worldwide [19], accompanied by the development of serious health concerns related to its usage. It is the purpose of this chapter to describe what asbestos is from a mineralogic perspective, where it is to be found, and what are the important distinctions that allow relative differences within members of the asbestos group to have differing potencies on the basis of such differences in terms of inducing injury and producing disease following inhalation. It is well known from animal models that the oncogenic potential of fibrous dust increases following reductions in fiber diameter, and decreases with reduction in fiber length, and these considerations are generally more important than the chemical composition of the fibers themselves [5, 6, 16, 21]. The longer fibers have more potency to induce cell injury, proliferation, oxidant release, and inflammation. It is also the durability of the fibrous dust that confers biopersistence, and the potential to induce malignant disease following deposition of fibers in the peripheral airways and migration of fibers to the serosal membrane. Contemporary usage of asbestos has been curtailed following its wide recognition as a most dangerous substance; it is noteworthy that the health hazards of asbestos date to antiquity as well. Pliny the Elder cautioned against the purchase of quarry slaves from asbestos mines, noting that they tended to die young [1].

1.2
Geologic and Mineralogic Features

Asbestos is properly considered a commercial and legal rather than a mineralogic term for a group of fibrous silicate minerals with crystalline structure and by definition have lengths >5 μm and aspect (length: diameter) ratios of

3 or greater. In the USA, the nomenclature as defined by the Environmental Protection Agency encompasses six unique mineral species, conventionally divided into two distinct groups, the amphiboles and the serpentines [22]. Chrysotile is the sole member of the latter group, and as of the year 2000, accounted for virtually 100% of the asbestos used commercially. Historically, at least 90% of commercially used asbestos has been chrysotile. The amphibole group contains grunerite-cummingtonite (amosite, *vide infra*), crocidolite (a fibrous variant of riebeckite), tremolite, actinolite, and anthophyllite. The name amosite is derived from the acronym AMOSA – Asbestos Mines of South Africa –giving reference to the company in the Transvaal Province of South Africa, the sole mine producing the mineral. As such, amosite, too, is a commercial, rather than a true mineralogic term, but by convention, amosite is used synonymously for the fibrous forms of grunerite-cummingtonite, just as crocidolite for the fibrous form of riebeckite. Among the amphiboles, only crocidolite and amosite have undergone significant commercial exploitation in industrialized countries, and collectively account for less than 10% of asbestos utilized in the last century. Large amounts of amosite were imported into the USA during World War II for

usage in warship and merchant vessel insulation. The so-called noncommercial amphiboles, actinolite, tremolite, and anthophyllite, are common mineral species with wide distribution. They are relevant insofar as they are contaminants of other commercially useful mineral species such as talc and vermiculite, as well as chrysotile, and have been implicated in the induction of disease in humans. The asbestos minerals have nonpathogenic, nonasbestiform mineral counterparts of identical chemical composition. The noncommercial species of amphiboles all require the word "asbestos" after their mineral name for the purpose of distinguishing them from the nonasbestos forms. This is not necessary for crocidolite, amosite, and chrysotile as the nonasbestos forms have different names as discussed above (see Fig. 1.1).

Asbestos minerals owe their fibrous habit to the parallel growth of very fine and elongate crystals, producing bundles. The amphiboles may also occur as nonfibrous, chunky, acicular and shard-like forms. Nonfibrous serpentine minerals include antigorite and lizardite. The nonfibrous forms of both serpentine and amphibole minerals are more common and widespread than the asbestiform species.

Deposits of commercial asbestos are to be found in four types of rocks: the banded

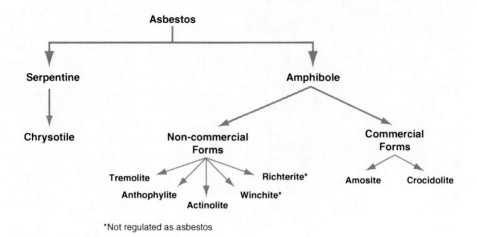

Fig. 1.1 Classification of asbestos and asbestiform silicates

ironstones, containing amosite and crocidolite; the alpine-type ultramafic rocks, containing chrysotile, anthophyllite, and tremolite; stratiform ultramafic inclusions, containing chrysotile and tremolite; and serpentinized limestone (chrysotile) [19].

1.3
Distribution and Physicochemical Properties of Chrysotile

Chrysotile is a common serpentine mineral with worldwide distribution, and the only one of this series mined as asbestos. The type 1 (alpine type, ultramafic rock) deposits are the most important sources of chrysotile asbestos, with principal localities occurring in the Ural Mountains of Russia and the Appalachian Mountains of the Canadian province of Quebec and the state of Vermont in the USA, as well as the state of California. Chrysotile has also been mined in the Italian Alps, Cypress, Zimbabwe, and the People's Republic of China [19] (Table 1.1). Commercially useful chrysotile is prepared from chrysotile ore in the milling process, with extracted long fiber

Table 1.1 Geographic distribution of asbestos species

Asbestos mineral	Geographic distribution
Chrysotile	Canada (Quebec), USA (Vermont, California), Russia, China
Crocidolite	South Africa (NW Cape Province, Transvaal), Western Australia
Amosite	South Africa
Tremolite	Turkey, Cyprus, Greece
Anthophyllite	Finland, USA
Actinolite	South Africa (Cape Province)
Winchite/Richterite[a]	USA (Montana)

[a]Asbestiform amphibole species, not classified as asbestos

chrysotile finding usage in textiles, and shorter fibers used in construction materials such as joint compound. Among the commercially exploited seams of the mineral, geographic variations are to be expected, both in terms of physical characteristics of the fibers, type, as well as proximity to fibrous species of noncommercial amphiboles. For example, the rich chrysotile ores quarried at the Coalinga, California yield fibers almost exclusively less than 5 µm [9]. There is also variance in the presence of other potentially dangerous minerals even within neighboring seams. McDonald et al attributed the difference in reported deaths due to mesothelioma among workers in several different mines within the province of Quebec to be attributable to local variances in the amount of tremolite contamination known to exist within the various mines [12]. The topic of chrysotile purity following milling, and the potential contamination by noncommercial species, is frequently argued in the ongoing asbestos litigation in the USA.

Silicates may be classified on the basis of the polymerization type of the silicate ions and the variance in crystalline structure that occurs through association of various cations. Chrysotile is a hydrated (approximately 13% water as a crystal), phyllosilicate (sheet silicate) with chemical composition $Mg_3Si_2O_5(OH)_4$, containing the $(Si_2O_5)n^{-2}$ building block typical of the serpentine group of minerals [4] (Fig. 1.2). Whereas other serpentines and other layered silicates (clays, mica) form flat sheets, spatial imbalances between magnesium and silica ions within the tetrahedral and octahedral sheets of chrysotile cause the layers to roll to form concentric hollow cylinders. Chrysotile fibers will thus appear scroll-like when viewed end on (Fig. 1.3), containing a central capillary with 2–4.5 nm in diameter. The milling of chrysotile ore yields bundles of fibers of variable length, and some fibers may exceed 100 µm. The fibers may be curvilinear ("serpentine"), often with splayed ends due to the separation of fibers into individual and smaller fibrillar units (Fig. 1.4).

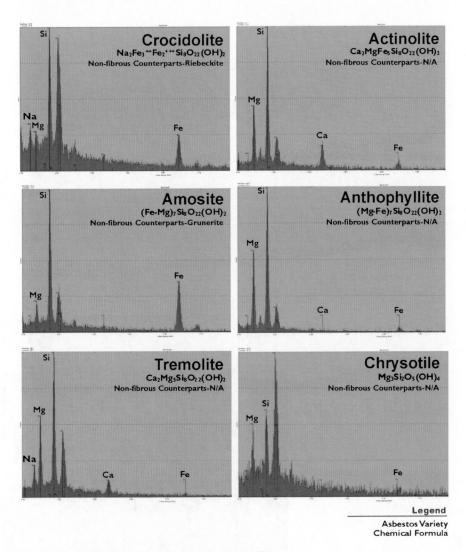

Fig. 1.2 Chemical composition and elemental spectra of asbestos

Some very long chrysotile fibers may be quite thin, but the diameter of chrysotile fibers tends to increase with increasing fiber length. Magnesium is an important constituent of both chrysotile and the amphiboles; the presence of soluble magnesium molecules on the outside of the curled chrysotile structure permits its leaching at the surface, facilitating the breakdown of fibers, within lung tissue, into successively smaller, fragile fibrils, which are then readily cleared from the body. Loss of magnesium changes the surface charge from positive to negative, which diminishes the oncogenic potential [16]. The clearance halftime of inhaled chrysotile within the lower respiratory tract is measured in only weeks, and may be much less. For example, with a clearance halftime measured in hours, the Calidria chrysotile from California is among

1

Fig. 1.3 Crystalline structure of chrysotile (Schematic diagram modified from [18])

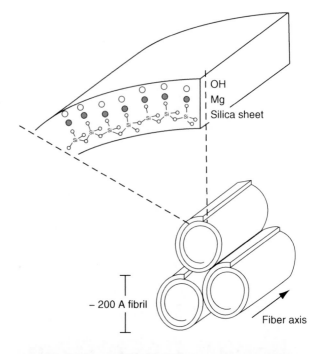

Fig. 1.4 Chrysotile asbestos fibers, scanning electron photomicrograph. Note long fibers of variable thickness and curvilinear "serpentine" morphology

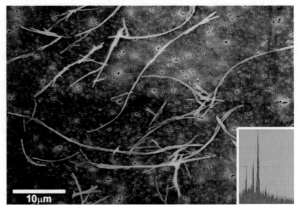

the mineral fibers with the most rapid clearance from the lung. Other chrysotile may have biopersistence similar to the range reported for glass and stone wools [3]. Thermoresistant to a degree, 70% of the chrysotile structure is lost at 575°C, with complete loss of the structure occurring at 650°C [10]. Such high temperatures may be observed in the automotive braking process, causing pyrolysis and conversion to the nonfibrous, nonpathogenic silicate mineral forsterite [10]. Due to its physicochemical characteristics, chrysotile has a greatly reduced biopersistence in contrast to the amphibole species, and those features as described above provide a likely explanation for the reported reductions in oncogenicity for this species in humans in contrast to the amphiboles [2, 17], and for the epidemiologic studies that conclude that motor vehicle mechanics performing brake repair are not at increased risk for developing mesothelioma [8].

1.4
Distribution and Physicochemical Properties of the Amphibole Species

The amphibole asbestos minerals crocidolite, amosite, anthophyllite, tremolite, and actionolite are inosilicates, or chain silicates. Tremolite, actinolite, and anthophyllite are grouped together with chrysotile as "white asbestos" and classified under the United Nations chemical identification schema as UN2590. Amosite "brown asbestos" and crocidolite "blue asbestos" are classified as UN2212. Amphiboles typically occur when veins of the mineral are created when cracks form in rocks during movement of the earth. These conditions help provide the environment necessary for massive amphibole crystallization and transformation to the fibrous form. The amphibole minerals are common, but their occurrence as exploitable forms is limited to certain locations where they obtain the proper physicochemical characteristics and abundance to be used as commercial asbestos. The major deposits of commercial amphiboles have generally been limited to the banded ironstones of Western Australia and the Transvaal and Cape Provinces of South Africa. Alpine-type and stratiform ultramafic rock are sources of chrysotile, as well as the noncommercial amphiboles tremolite, actinolite, and anthophyllite, the major source for the latter occurring in Finland with smaller deposits in rocky outcrops of the USA [19]. Another source of asbestiform amphiboles is to be found in the area around Libby, Montana, USA. Libby is the site of the largest mined deposit of vermiculite in the world, and the alkaline-ultramafic rock is rich in amphiboles, chiefly richterite and winchite (sodic-calcic tremolite), all of which can exist in asbestiform or fibrous habit [15, 23]. The latter species are not listed in the US Federal Regulations governing asbestos, but their recognition is important in view of the abnormally high number of asbestos-related diseases and deaths in former vermiculite miners and millers and residents of this area, and the potency of the Libby amphibole in terms of inducing mesothelioma is reported to be similar to crocidolite [7, 13, 14]. Anthophyllite, tremolite, and actinolite are common constituents of the earth's crust, but have not been exploited commercially in industrialized countries, and are frequently associated with serpentine minerals, vermiculite, and talc. The noncommercial amphiboles may assume a variety of forms, including nonfibrous forms.

The chemical and crystalline structures of the amphiboles are highly similar, and generally may be distinguished only on the basis of chemical composition, and in specific the cation constituents (Fig. 1.2). Crystalline amphibole minerals demonstrate perfect prismatic cleavage, with direction of the cleavage parallel to the length of the silicate chains [20]. The silicate chains are formed by linear arrays of SiO_4 tetrahedra linked by octagonal groups of cations, and may be of significant length (Fig. 1.5). The crystalline amphibole fibers are substantially more brittle than chrysotile, limiting their potential for fabrication. These mineralogic attributes confer the potential for great fiber length, and accordingly, significant pathogenicity following deposition in the lung (Figs. 1.6–1.9). As their straight, broad fibers are resistant to fiber fragmentation and chemical degradation in the body, the biopersistence of the amphiboles is much greater than chrysotile, and their clearance halftime is generally measured in decades. The crystalline structure of the amphiboles also contains less water than chrysotile, and there is greater resistance to pyrolysis. Amphibole fibers are less flexible than chrysotile, permitting greater friability with potential to release respirable particles.

1

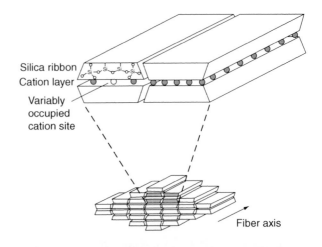

Silica ribbon
Cation layer

Variably
occupied
cation site

Fiber axis

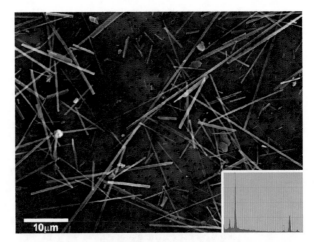

Fig. 1.6 Amphibole asbestos fibers,
scanning electron photomicrograph.
Note long, straight, and slender fiber
morphology

10μm

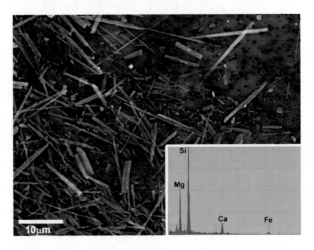

Fig. 1.7 Libby asbestiform amphibole
asbestos fibers, scanning electron
photomicrograph. Note varying fiber
morphologies, with thick, thin, short,
and long fibers all represented

10μm

Fig. 1.8 Amosite asbestos body. Note longitudinal cleavage of long, slender fiber

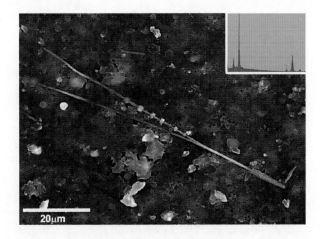

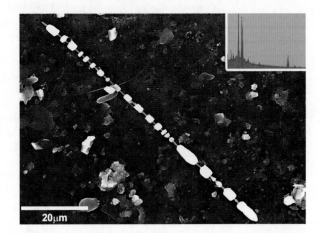

Fig. 1.9 Crocidolite asbestos body. Note characteristic, long, slender fiber undergoing ferrugination

1.5 Identification and Characterization of Asbestos

Several techniques are available for the identification of asbestos fibers, making use of the morphologic, chemical composition, and crystallogic features of the mineral [18]. The techniques include phase-contrast microscopy, polarizing microscopy with dispersion staining, infra-red spectroscopy, x-ray and electron diffraction, and analytic electron microscopy. Each technique has its own advantages and disadvantages, and it is beyond the scope of this chapter to offer a detailed comparison. In brief, phase-contrast microscopy is used to demonstrate the morphologic features of fibers such as size, shape, and aspect ratio, but is seldom used owing to the limits of the resolution of light microscopy, its inability to distinguish asbestos fibers from non-asbestos mineral fibers, or provide information regarding the chemical composition of fibers. Polarizing microscopy provides information pertaining to the crystallinity of fibers, and may be used to distinguish among the various asbestos fiber species and to make the distinction between asbestos and nonasbestos fibers.

This technique is also limited by the resolution of light microscopy. Infrared spectrophotometry is a bulk analytical technique unable to examine individual fibers, and is used to identify the characteristic spectra of the asbestos minerals. It is not generally used to identify asbestos in tissue or environmental samples. The x-ray diffraction is also a bulk analytical technique which identifies diffraction patterns produced as x-rays pass through various crystalline materials [11]. It is generally considered a qualitative technique to measure the quantity of asbestos within a sample.

Most investigators prefer some form of analytic electron microscopy for the identification of asbestos [18]. AEM has the ability to provide high resolution images of the details of the smallest of fibers, and to provide crystallographic compositional data for individual fibers through selected area electron diffraction, and elemental composition information through energy dispersive spectrometry (EDS). EDS focuses an electron beam on individual particles, and observes the x-ray spectra produced by the beam and the atoms within the particle. The spectra so produced consist of peaks distributed according to the energies of the x-rays, which are in turn related to the elemental composition of the fiber or particle being studied. Such spectra may be then compared to standards for confirmation of identification (Fig. 1.2). Analytic scanning electron microscopy (SEM) and transmission electron microscopy (TEM) are both useful, albeit expensive and time consuming. TEM generally offers superior resolution, but the preparatory techniques are more complicated.

References

1. Barbalance RC (Oct 2004) A brief history of asbestos use and associated health risks. EnvironmentalChemistry.com. http://Environ-mentalChemsitry.com/yogi/environmental/asbestoshistory2004.html Accessed 1 Aug 2010
2. Berman DW, Crump KS (2008) A meta-analysis of asbestos-related cancer risk that addressed fiber size and mineral type. Crit Rev Toxicol 38(S1):49–73
3. Bernstein DM (2005) Understanding chrysotile asbestos: a new perspective based upon current data. In: Proceedings of the IOHA 2005, vol J3, Pilanesberg, pp 1–10
4. Craighead JE, Gibbs A, Pooley F (2008) Mineralogy of asbestos. In: Craighead JE, Gibbs A (eds) Asbestos and its diseases. Oxford University Press, New York, pp 23–38, Ch. 2
5. Davis JMG (1989) Mineral fibre carcinogenesis: experimental data relating to the importance of fiber types, size, deposition, dissolution and migration. In: Bignon J, Peto J, Saracci R (eds) Non-occupational exposure to mineral fibres, IARC Scientific Publication no. 90. IARC, Lyon, pp 33–45
6. Davis JMG, Jones A (1988) Comparison of the pathogenicity of long and short chrysotile asbestos in rats. Br J Exp Pathol 69:717–737
7. Gibbs GW, Berry G (2008) Mesothelioma and asbestos. Regul Toxicol Pharmacol 52:s223–s231
8. Goodman M, Teta MJ, Hessel PA, Garabrant DH et al (2004) Mesothelioma and lung cancer among motor vehicle mechanics: a meta-analysis. Ann Occup Hyg 48(4):309–326
9. Ilgren E (2008) The fiber length of Coalinga chrysotile: enhanced clearance due to its short nature in aqueous solution with a brief critique on "short fiber toxicity". Indoor Built Environ 17(1):5–26
10. Langer AM (2003) Reduction of the biological potential of chrysotile asbestos arising from conditions of service on brake pads. Regul Toxicol Pharmacol 38:71–77
11. Langer AM, Mackler AD, Pooley FD (1974) Electron microscopical investigation of asbestos fibers. Environ Health Perspect 9:63–80
12. McDonald AD, Case BW, Churg A, Dufresne A, Gibbs GW, Sebastien P, McDonald JC (1997) Mesothelioma in Quebec chrysotile mines and millers: epidemiology and etiology. Ann Occup Hyg 41(6):707–719
13. McDonald JC, Harris J, Armstron B (2002) Cohort mortality study of vermiculite miners exposed to fibrous talc: an update. Ann Occup Hyg 46(suppl 1):93–94

14. McDonald JC, Harris J, Armstrong B (2004) Mortality in a cohort of miners exposed to fibrous amphibole in Libby Montana. Occup Environ Med 61:363–366

15. Meeker GP, Bern AM, Brownfield IK, Lowers HA et al (2003) The composition and morphologies of amphiboles from the Rainy Creek Complex near Libby, Montana. Am Mineralog 88:1955–1969

16. Mossman BT, Churg A (1998) Mechanisms in the pathogenesis of asbestosis and silicosis. Am J Respir Crit Care Med 157:1666–1680

17. Pierce JS, McKinely MA, Paustenbach DJ, Finely BL (2008) An evaluation of reported no-effect chrysotile exposures for lung cancer and mesothelioma. Crit Rev Toxicol 38:191–214

18. Roggli VL, Coin PC (2004) Mineralogy of asbestos. In: Roggli VL, Oury TD, Sporn TA (eds) Pathology of asbestos associated diseases. Springer, New York, pp 1–16, Ch. 1

19. Ross M (1981) The geologic occurrences and health hazards of amphibole and serpentine asbestos. In: Veblen DR (ed) Amphiboles and other hydrous pyriboles, reviews in mineralogy, vol 9A. Mineralogical Society of America, Washington, DC, pp 279–323, Ch. 6

20. Skinner HCW et al (1988) Fibrous minerals and synthetic fibers. In: Skinner HCW, Ross M, Frondel C (eds) Asbestos and other fibrous materials: mineralogy, crystal chemistry and health effects. Oxford University Press, New York, pp 20–94, Ch. 2

21. Stanton MF, Wrench C (1972) Mechanisms of mesothelioma induction with asbestos and fibrous glass. J Natl Cancer Inst 48: 797–821

22. US Department of Health and Human Services (2001) Asbestos, chemical and physical information, Agency for Toxic Substances and Disease Registry. US Department of Health and Human Services, Atlanta

23. Wylie AG, Verkouteren JR (2000) Amphibole asbestos from Libby, Montana. Am Mineralog 85:1540–1542

Epidemiology of Mesothelioma and Historical Background

2

J.E. Craighead

Abstract Mesothelioma is a "new" malignant disease strongly associated with exposure to amphibole asbestos exposure (amosite and crocidolite) environmentally and in the work place. Nonetheless, in recent years, we have learned that many cases of mesothelioma are idiopathic, while some are caused by therapeutic irradiation or chronic inflammation in body cavities. This paper reviews the key epidemiological features of the malignancy in the context of the biological and mineralogical factors that influence mesothelioma development. These tumors challenge the diagnostic pathologist's acumen, the epidemiologist's skill in devising meaningful and definitive studies, the industrial hygienist's knowledge of environmental hazards in diverse occupational settings, and the clinician's skill in managing an intrepid and uniformly fatal malignancy.

Many, if not most, of the major life-threatening diseases afflicting humankind were recognized well before the Christian era. In that context,

malignant mesothelioma is a "new" disease with its diagnostic features and natural history having been known to medical science for less than a century. It is my charge in this brief overview to trace the development of our knowledge of mesotheliomas as clinical and pathological entities, relating the occurrence of this malignancy to exposure to a unique family of fibrous minerals that gives rise to the majority of cases of mesothelioma. In doing so, we now are obliged to recognize the occasional patient with idiopathic disease and as of yet unidentified genetic or environmental parameters of disease susceptibility as mesotheliomas are studied critically.

As I sat at the breakfast table this morning, the now inevitable television advertisement appeared announcing the availability of skilled litigants in nationally prominent law firms who will make themselves available to asbestos "victims" whose suffering, they argue, deserves a substantial monetary award. Similarly, vivid advertisements soliciting the afflicted are plastered on the sides of municipal buses and in subways in major cities in America. Clearly, the search for the rare unfortunate few who suffer from mesothelioma has become big business for lawyers in the USA. The ultimate outcome is ligation that has already bankrupted countless

J.E. Craighead
Department of Pathology, University of Vermont, Burlington, VT 05405, USA
e-mail: john.craighead@theibcinc.com

A. Tannapfel (ed.), *Malignant Mesothelioma*, Recent Results in Cancer Research 189,
DOI: 10.1007/978-3-642-10862-4_2, © Springer-Verlag Berlin Heidelberg 2011

American businesses as plaintiffs seek redress for the presumptive, subtle injury patients unknowingly suffered as a result of the supposed callous disregard of insensitive industrialists. Will advertisement focused on the general public bring to the attention of medical science "new" etiologies for these unique cancers? Or, will these cases redefine the epidemiological features of the disease and its etiological relationship to low-dose asbestos exposure? Can subtle unrecognized exposures result in the malignant disease? Only time will tell. Unfortunately today's juries, rather than scientists, are obliged to draw conclusions based on incomplete evidence presented by advocates in the courtroom.

It is difficult to be certain when mesothelioma became a recognizable clinical and pathological entity, given its rarity in the general population and the ability of these tumors to mimic common neoplasms involving the pleural and peritoneal cavities [54]. E. Wagner [79], a German pathologist, is generally accorded credit for the initial description of a tumor believed to be the prototype of the modern day mesothelioma. In the past, these malignant lesions often simulated the clinical picture of pleural tuberculosis, a condition that was not uncommon centuries ago. Sensitive diagnostic tools, electron microscopy [22, 75], and immunocytochemistry [18], now make it possible for the pathologist to recognize these tumors with a high degree of certainty when, so often, skilled clinicians demure. It has only been during the last 3 decades that newer diagnostic tools have allowed the epidemiologist the luxury of carrying out analyses using dependable patient data.

Even the term mesothelioma has been a matter of uncertainty for those who seek an orderly nomenclature. Thus, in the first few decades of the last century some 30 different names were used when referring to tumors having at least some of the morphological features of the malignant lesions now recognized as mesotheliomas, the most common of which was "endothelioma," a convenient designation attesting to the vague

resemblance of the tumor cells to vascular endothelial cells. Finally, in the early 1930s, Klemperer and Rabin [41] proposed the designation "mesothelioma" in describing a clinical/pathological entity that commonly exhibited both sarcomatous and carcinomatous histological features, either exclusively or as a random mixture of the two. But even as late 1957, an occasional "doubting Thomas" questioned the existence of such tumors. For example, in a case report published in the widely read *New England Journal of Medicine*, the renowned diagnostic pathologist and Harvard professor Benjamin Castleman announced to the medical community that a case under discussion in a clinical/pathological conference was the first mesothelioma he had been comfortable in diagnosing.

This was merely 2 years before Christopher Wagner (a pathologist) and his colleagues, the tuberculosis specialist Kit Sleggs and Paul Marchand [81], a chest physician, described in a landmark publication an epidemic of mesothelioma consequent to environmental exposure to crocidolite asbestos. It was Sleggs who prophetically identified a cadre of unique patients believed to have tuberculous pleuritis but who failed to respond to the customarily effective management of tuberculosis at the time. It was Marchand [48] who helped recognize the common occurrence of this disease among members of the indigenous population who were believed to have a most unusual form of lung cancer. However, at the time, senior South African pathologists, including Ian Webster [82], had little difficulty diagnosing the unique tumors which Wagner (at the time a junior level pathologist) brought to their attention, for they were already aware of similar lesions occurring elsewhere in the amphibole asbestos mining districts of South Africa [80]. But who among the pathologists in the Northern Hemisphere paid much heed to an apparent epidemic of an unheard of malignancy occurring in the native population of an obscure corner of southern Africa, particularly when the mining industry was more than anxious to suppress knowledge of a suspect industry-associated cancer? At the time, everyone knew that, in general, cancer was a sporadically occurring condition, not one that manifested itself as an epidemic in both women and men, and on occasion, teenagers. To me, as a practicing pathologist in a major Boston teaching hospital in the early 1960s, mesothelioma was rarely a consideration in the differential diagnosis of a chest tumor.

Diagnostic uncertainty, nonetheless, continued to plague the histopathologist for years thereafter when these rare entities came to their attention. Recognizing this conundrum in the mid-1960s, leaders in the world community of pathology established review panels in Europe and North America to evaluate pathological material from individual suspect cases [39]. These experts then tendered a specific diagnosis or arbitrarily expressed either uncertainty or frank disagreement as to the identity of the tumor among the members of the assembled panel. Clearly, clinical case surveys and epidemiological studies would have proven fruitless in the absence of a concrete diagnostic identification of the tumors. But, improvements in the tools available to the pathologist were forthcoming. As noted above, it was not until the 1970s that electron microscopy was introduced, imperfect as it was, and in the 1980s immunohistochemistry came into vogue as a diagnostic crutch. To this date, new markers of malignant mesothelial cells continue to be introduced in an effort to confront the ambiguities of diagnostic pathology, allowing a more precise diagnosis. Nonetheless, an occasional case generates controversy even among experienced pathologists.

Prior to the 1960s, a case of mesothelioma was a "rare bird" perhaps coming to the attention of the hospital pathologist once or twice in a professional lifetime. Often as a sporadic malignancy of childhood and adolescence, they were idiopathic curiosities too uncommon to warrant serious research (asbestos-related mesotheliomas have not been found to develop in those younger than 35 years despite an occasional claim to the contrary) [33]. There is every reason to believe that many obscure thoracic neoplasms of unknown etiology in women were either classified in the past as breast cancer believed to have metastasized to the pleura, or ovarian cancer spreading unabated throughout the abdominal cavity, implanting on the peritoneal wall. And then there are the anatomic variants, some simulating sarcomas or a complex obscure tumor such as a synovial sarcoma [40]. All too often, mesotheliomas mimicked adenocarcinomas of bronchogenic origin developing at the periphery of the lung and invading the pleural cavity, the so-called pseudomesotheliomatous adenocarcinoma.

Although asbestosis as a clinical and pathological entity among textile workers was recognized in the UK and the USA and was considered a potential cause of lung disease before 1900 [57], many millers died of asbestosis after a period of dust exposure of no longer than a decade. Accordingly, because of its relatively long latency period, it is the writer's belief that mesotheliomas failed to appear before patients had died because of asbestosis or left the work force. It was not until after the First World War that public health authorities recognized what was believed to be an increase in lung cancer among tradesmen without clinical evidence of asbestosis, but a history of work in an industry where asbestos was liberally used [25, 57]. Most probably, some of these cases were mesotheliomas, but who would know in the absence of autopsies and a clear idea of the diverse pathological features of these tumors? Who could imagine sarcomas developing in anatomic concert with malignant epithelial cells (the so-called biphasic tumors)? It was not until the Second World War that industry-related mesotheliomas were recognized to be occurring in Europe. Alas, these early cases were reported in the wartime German literature as "pleural cancer" in publications [83, 84], out of the reach of most American and British physicians at the

2

for better
dispersion
add amosite

Amosite added to asbestos cement
has a dispersive action giving
uniform fibre distribution leading
to greater strength and
improved surface texture.
Full technical advisory service
available to reinforced cement and
insulation material manufacturers
from the world's leading
producers of amphibole fibres.

Cape Asbestos Fibres Limited
114 Park Street London W1 · England · Telex 23759
North American Asbestos Corporation
200 South Michigan Ave · Chicago · Illinois 60604 · USA
Telephone: (312) 922-7435
(Members of the Cape Asbestos Group of Companies)   TW2640

for
fibre length
-amosite

Amosite is naturally longer than other
types of asbestos fibre. Length plus
resilience makes Amosite the ideal fibre
for high temperature and acoustic
insulations and for lightweight fire
resistant products.
Full technical advisory service available
to reinforced cement and insulation
material manufacturers from the world's
leading producers of amphibole fibres.

Cape Asbestos Fibres Limited
114 Park Street London W1 · England · Telex 23759
North American Asbestos Corporation
200 South Michigan Ave · Chicago · Illinois 60604 · USA
Telephone: (312) 922-7435
(Members of the Cape Asbestos Group of Companies)   TW2760

Fig. 2.1 Examples of promotional advertisements published in trade journals in the past

time (but apparently known and ignored by the Allied intelligence community).

Prior to that time, more specifically in 1934, the passenger vessel *SS Morro Castle* was destroyed at sea by fire, a tragedy that prompted an inquiry by the US Congress into the apparent ineffectual fireproofing of American registered ships including naval vessels. It was already known that amosite asbestos was resistant to the degrading effects of sea water and could provide excellent insulation protection per unit of weight. Accordingly, by 1940 the US Navy specifications for new ships and those undergoing reconditioning and repair dictated the routine insulation of a vessel's interior with amosite and to a variable extent, chrysotile. Most commercial shippers (i.e., the merchant marine) soon abided by these regulatory criteria, precautions that no doubt saved ships and the lives of many sailors during the war, but has resulted in much suffering thereafter. With the mobilization for the Second World War, amosite was routinely incorporated into the insulation of some 3,000 newly launched merchant vessels and navy warships, resulting in the gross contamination of a vessel's interior compartments, particularly the engine rooms (Fig. 2.1). For example, a recent evaluation of a mothballed World War II Navy destroyer demonstrated roughly 25 t of asbestos insulation still intact in the bowels of the vessel.

It would be rank speculation to attempt to estimate the numbers of Navy personnel and merchant mariners who were heavily exposed aboard ship while serving their country, and to the best of the writer's knowledge, no serious attempt has ever been made by governments in Europe or North America to estimate the exposures sustained by wartime servicemen and the outcome in the form of disease. Not surprisingly, shipyards were also heavily contaminated by friable asbestos and millions (because of a high turnover rate of shipyard workers in the Allied countries and occupied Europe) were heavily exposed to crocidolite and amosite as well as large amounts of chrysotile asbestos during the late 1930s and 1940s. Who knows how they fared.

Responsibly, the US Navy commissioned a study during the waning years of the Second World War to assess the possible adverse effects of asbestos on personnel, focusing on the disease asbestosis [30]. Unfortunately, the observation period was much too short because the latency of asbestosis is variable but often a matter of decades, even with heavy exposure, and mesothelioma rarely becomes evident before an elapsed period of some 20 years from the time of initial exposure. Drs. Fleisher and Drinker, who conducted the above study, may have been competent in their trade but they failed as historians. Either they ignored or were not aware of the European experience with asbestos malignancies. Importation of crocidolite and amosite into Germany and Britain began in the early 1900s. Clearly, mesotheliomas were erupting among industrial workers and naval personnel throughout the 1920s and 1930s. But, alas, at the time many mesotheliomas were believed to be traditional lung cancers [67].

A recently completed, unpublished evaluation of case material in my laboratory strongly suggests that exposures in the 1940s during the war may give rise to mesotheliomas diagnosed some 40–60 years later (the duration of latency is thought by many authorities to be inversely related to the intensity of exposure). However, since the latency period of most mesotheliomas ranges from 20 to 40 years, it was not until the 1960s that mesotheliomas attributable to wartime exposure began to appear in large numbers in Great Britain [26, 34, 68, 74, 85] and Germany [9]. Soon, an increasingly large number of cases were diagnosed among American shipyard workers who were then engaged in other forms of employment [76]. But as noted above, it was not until 1960 that the first compelling report relating environmental crocidolite exposure to mesothelioma was published, and it was 1971 when amosite was also considered a likely cause, if not the major culprit, in industrialized societies by knowledgeable members of the public health community. In the USA, credit must be accorded Dr. Irving Selikoff, a chest physician, who recognized the impending disaster as mesotheliomas came to his attention among workers at the Union Asbestos and Rubber Company (UNARCO) in New Jersey where Unibestos

amosite insulation for newly constructed ships was manufactured. Interestingly enough, the initial cases identified by Dr. Selikoff were peritoneal mesotheliomas, attesting to the heavy exposures these workers had sustained.

It was then that the pathfinding physicians, Drs. Irving Selikoff and Christopher Wagner organized a landmark conference under the auspices of the New York Academy of Sciences to consider the accumulating scientific observations associating asbestos exposure with malignant and nonmalignant diseases, including the common types of lung cancer and both peritoneal and pleural mesotheliomas.

At this juncture, a pause seems appropriate to summarize briefly what clinicians and epidemiologists have learned over the past half century regarding this fascinating malignancy and its relationship to asbestos exposure. As we all know, mesotheliomas usually develop unilaterally in the pleural cavities, and to a more limited extent in the abdomen. But they also develop on rare occasions in the pericardium, the spermatic cords, and both the male and female gonads. Because these highly malignant lesions are shrouded in body cavities, they generally are widespread and incurable when clinicians finally are obliged to search for the cause of subtle chest or abdominal discomfort accompanied by a unilateral pleural effusion or ascites. Despite the current availability of potent chemotherapy (as discussed elsewhere in this symposium) and the increasingly common extrapleural pneumonectomies (carried out by intrepid thoracic surgeons in an all too often futile attempt to eliminate or control the spread of the neoplasm) the prognosis is grim and most patients are dead within a period of 3 years from the time of diagnosis. As noted above, the vast majority of mesotheliomas develop in the chest cavities where they gradually invade the chest wall and mediastinum and not infrequently metastasize to the contralateral lung, the spinal vertebrae, and the peritoneal cavity. In the abdomen they trigger the accumulation of massive

2

ascites while spreading widely to implant on the surfaces of the peritoneal wall and major organs, only occasionally metastasizing to the chest.

The pathogenesis of mesotheliomas in a population of occupationally exposed men or women is largely dependent upon mineralogical type and the fiber dimension as well as the severity of exposure. On occasion, the incidence of abdominal tumors is as great as 20% of a heavily exposed worker population whereas in most situations it is lower. However, in Great Britain, Coggon et al. [16] discovered a greater than sixfold occurrence of peritoneal tumors in comparison to pleural malignant lesions among construction workers. Carpenters seem to be at exceptional risk for mesotheliomas in the UK, most probably because of the widespread use of composition asbestos boards in the past.

As noted above, the latency of these lesions from the time of first exposure until the onset of symptoms is unpredictable. Almost invariably, it is greater than 20 years but at times it can be as long as 50 or 60 years. Who knows what disease processes lurk in body cavities before the malignancy is sufficiently large to cause symptoms? Of interest has been the reported substantially shorter latency period among a few environmentally exposed patients in the crocidolite mining district of Western Australia [2, 3]. It is generally agreed that peritoneal mesotheliomas develop as a result of heavier and more prolonged exposures, but comparative quantitative thresholds have never been established for any asbestos type because of the profound difficulties of conducting comprehensive long-term studies on a rare disease sometimes caused by exceedingly low dosages of a toxic substance. But the lack of evidence is not evidence for a lack of a threshold since many members of the general population have asbestos particles in their lungs in the absence of disease [23]. The classical nonmalignant stigmata of exposure, that is, pleural plaques, bilaterally symmetrical pleural thickening, and asbestosis are surrogate measures of relatively heavy exposure to an amphibole. They occur more frequently in those with peritoneal rather than pleural malignant disease, suggesting that a heavier exposure is required to initiate these lesions in the abdominal cavity. Too little epidemiological information on spermatic cord and gonadal lesions exists to allow conclusions regarding causation and latency since it is likely that many of these tumors are idiopathic and not caused by asbestos exposure. It has been the author's experience that some peritoneal mesotheliomas present clinically for the first time as tumorous masses in the spermatic cord simulating hernias. Anecdotally, it has been hypothesized that talc particles and asbestos accumulations on or around ovaries may play a causative role in the genesis of ovarian mesothelioma, a hypothesis that now dictates the nonuse of talc on surgical gloves.

Are all mesotheliomas caused by exposure to asbestos? Of course not! According to the comprehensive studies of Spirtas et al. [70], overall the attributable risk for exposure to asbestos is 88% for men, but in only 58% of male cases could asbestos exposure be implicated in a patient's abdominal tumor. In women, the attributable risk proved to be 23% for pleural and peritoneal mesotheliomas combined. (Unfortunately, these epidemiologists were dealing with numbers and not detailed case information; thus, it is impossible to determine the validity of a claim of asbestos exposure, and the type(s) involved). But as William Blake has told us: "to generalize is to be an idiot!" Overstated? Yes, since all too often subtle, brief but heavy exposures to asbestos in a patient's distant past can on occasion be linked causatively to the disease. The writer is aware of several cases of mesotheliomas in white collar, middle aged men whose only known exposure was summertime employment in industry while attending college.

To an extent, the information briefly summarized above represents events occurring in another time frame of history when preliminary information on environmental asbestos exposure was

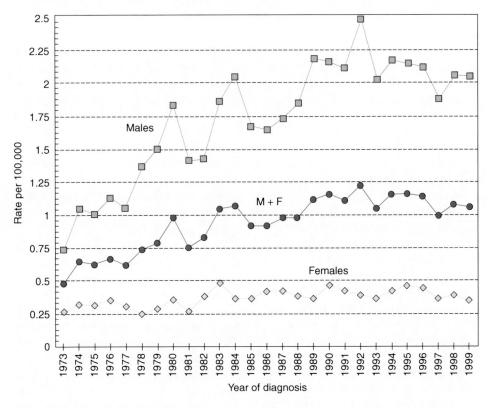

Fig. 2.2 Age-adjusted incidence of mesothelioma in the USA from 1973 to 1999 (Data from the Surveillance Epidemiology and End Results registry [SEER])

accumulating and risks were poorly defined. More recently, accumulating data suggests the likelihood of a new pattern of disease in younger members of the population, more specifically, men and women entering the workforce since the 1980s. The writer has evaluated the occupational background of some 35 men younger than 45 years who suffered from abdominal mesotheliomas but had no known history of vocational or avocational exposure to asbestos. Similarly, countless numbers of idiopathic thoracic mesotheliomas are now being diagnosed in the USA. These patients display none of the traditional markers of exposure and have no compelling history of exposure. Burdorf et al. [14] noted in the Netherlands and Sweden a consistent low

incidence of mesotheliomas among women, an observation that has also been documented in the USA (Fig. 2.2). If there truly exists a background incidence of mesotheliomas that are not caused by asbestos, pathologists have yet to recognize unique morphological features of the disease that would allow the identification of idiopathic mesotheliomas. There may be exceptions to this claim, however, that is, the so-called well-differentiated papillary mesothelioma, which occurs on rare occasions in the abdominal cavity of young women who have no history of exposure to asbestos. These tumors fail to exhibit invasive characteristics and on occasion resolve without treatment. And, the writer has observed only glandulopapillary features in the idiopathic abdominal mesotheliomas he has discovered in young men.

Indirect passive exposures of spouses and children in the household to the clothes of asbestos workers were believed in the past to occasionally result in pleural plaques and/or mesothelioma, but all too often the conclusions were anecdotal and presumptive rather than based on proof. Only a limited number of fiber burden analyses have been carried out on the lung tissue of household members of an asbestos worker substantiating the claim of indirect, inadvertent exposure. Hillerdal [36] has reported the development of mesothelioma in a housewife believed to have been exposed to approximately 1 fiber/mL for 2 h, once per week for a period of 5 years. Ferrante and his colleagues [28] documented 18 cases of mesothelioma in homemakers who laundered the work clothes of their husbands, all cement factory workers, over a 20 year period [60].

Exposures of residents in a community surrounding an industrial source of asbestos were recently alleged by Maule and her colleagues [50]. Those living near an asbestos cement plant had a relative risk of 10.5. In Japan, Kurumatani and Kumagai [42] documented a standardized mortality rate of 14 among men and 41 for women who occupied homes located within a radius of 300 m of an asbestos cement pipe plant that used both chrysotile and crocidolite. In an unpublished report, public health epidemiologists, in the state of New Jersey, reported an odds ratio of 31.7 in the community of Manville located near a large asbestos manufacturing plant that is no longer operative.

By the mid-1960s the news was "out of the bag" and investigators on several continents scurried to gather experimental and epidemiological evidence, which would elucidate the enormous gaps in our knowledge. A flurry of laboratory studies soon demonstrated that asbestos causes neoplasm to develop in rodents and subhuman primates when massive amounts of the fibrous minerals are injected by artificial means into the animals' pleural and peritoneal cavities [19]. Insightful experimental work by Stanton and Wrench [71] using a modification of this approach showed that relatively long, thin fibers triggered the development of malignant mesotheliomas in rodents, a concept now found to be relevant to human disease based on epidemiological studies. These studies have distinct limitations because of their artificiality, particularly the introduction of asbestos directly into the body cavity, thus bypassing the cleansing apparatus of the respiratory tract. Inhalation studies using rats have yielded quite different results (Table 2.1).

Of note are the studies [8, 10, 13] which showed that smooth-surfaced materials such as plastic sheets of various configurations induce sarcomas in rats when implanted subcutaneously, an observation suggesting a possible model for asbestos-induced mesothelioma in which the vast surface area of long and thin fibers (surface area = $\pi r^2 \times$ length), such as with crocidolite, triggers malignant transformation by mechanisms discussed in more detail below.

Experimental modeling in animals and casts of the human respiratory tract by Timbrell [77]

Table 2.1 Summary data for inhalation experiments in rats conducted by Davis and Coworkers (Adapted from [6])

Fiber type	Description	Dosage[a]	# Tumors/ # tested
Chrysotile	UICC-A	0.4	1/42
Chrysotile	UICC-A	2.0	0/42
Chrysotile	Long	5.5	3/40
Chrysotile	Short	1.2	1/40
Amosite	Long	2.1	3/40
Amosite	Short	0.07	1/42
Crocidolite	UICC	0.4	1/43
Crocidolite	UICC	0.9	0/40
Tremolite	Korean	1.6	2/39
Control		0	0/228

PCM Phase contrast microscopy: fibers/mL $\times 10^3$
[a]Exposure 7 h/day, 5 days/week for 1 year

showed that the depth of a fiber's penetration into the lung is roughly the inverse of its diameter. Fiber length does not prove to be an impediment to the transport of a thin fiber down the branching tubular network of the tracheobronchial tree to finally deposit it at the level of the pleura. Importantly, fiber length is most probably a critical factor in arousing a luxuriant alveolar macrophage response near the mesothelial cells of the pleura, where oxidant chemicals and proteases are generated as a product of the scavenger cells that attempt to imbibe the long indigestible fibers, an event that is most probably catalyzed by the amphibole fiber's iron concentration. Additionally, biochemical and molecular studies have provided plausible insights into the mechanisms of carcinogenesis, work that strongly implicated oxygen and nitrogen free radicals generated by macrophages in mutagenesis by means of direct DNA damage [35, 58]. Other studies have explored the possible effects of factors generated by experimentally exposed cells in vitro on the growth of tumors in vivo [12, 20, 21].

Alas, there still remain gaps in our knowledge of the biological basis for the diverse morphological features of mesotheliomas and their constituent cells. However, we might reflect on the original findings of the renowned experimental histologist Maximow [52, 53], who demonstrated in vitro spontaneous transformation of one cell type to another, quite independent of asbestos or other foreign materials, an observation expanded upon more recently by Stout and Murray [73]. Among the products that might be elicited by mesothelioma cells are cell differentiation factors that could account for the morphological variability in individual tumors and between tumors in different cases. We might also consider the relevance of our rapidly evolving knowledge of the pluripotential properties of newly discovered lines of stem cell that have the capacity to differentiate into a variety of cell types when experimentally introduced into host animals. In a recent report,

McQualter et al. [55] described a population of multipotential epithelial stem/progenitor cells in the mouse lung, which they claimed have the capacity for self-renewal and possibly remodeling as well as regeneration and repair. At this time we have no compelling experimental or epidemiological evidence to account for the various routes of differentiation manifest by mesothelial cells as they undergo malignant transformation. More simply stated, why are some tumors sarcomatoid and others epitheloid and still others a mixture of the two? [45].

Quite independent of the experimental work concerned with mechanism of tumorigenesis, epidemiological studies during the past 50 years have provided science with a vast body of meaningful insights which have helped dictate the scope of governmental regulations designed to control exposure and the uses of asbestos by industry. It has now been clearly shown that friable amphiboles (crocidolite, amosite, and tremolite) are the major cause of mesothelioma worldwide, with crocidolite being the most potent carcinogen (most probably because the fibers tend to be exceptionally long and thin) but amosite by far the commonest cause worldwide. This is not startling new information for it emanates from work accomplished before the 1970s, but despite much effort we have yet to establish scientifically defensible threshold levels for regulatory purposes. It is clear that these three types of amphiboles are biologically similar, only differing in relative pathogenicity, whereas the orphan anthophyllite (comprised of relatively thick and blunt fibers) either lacks the capacity to cause mesotheliomas or does so rarely, even though anthophyllite induces the formation of pleural plaques in humans with alacrity [6]. Unfortunately, chrysotile, which worldwide was the major commercially used asbestos in the past, has yielded the most vexing epidemiological data and considerable regulatory controversy. Indeed, there have been countless opinions published which allude to the possibility, rather than the probability, that chrysotile causes mesothelioma while many other

2

carefully conducted and comprehensive epidemiological surveys in Canada indicate that pure, friable chrysotile is blameless [5, 15, 17, 37, 54, 67]. Indeed, the most recently acquired information from studies of South African miner populations [61] supports the notion that the relatively obscure contaminant, tremolite, is causatively responsible for the occasional mesothelioma developing in Canadian miners and millers of crude chrysotile ore. Hodgson and Darnton [38] recently supplemented their 2000 report referenced above with an evaluation of a comparative meta-analysis conducted by Loomis et al. [44] which shows different mesothelioma rates for chrysotile miners and textile millers. The data further supports the evidence exonerating chrysotile as a cause of this neoplasm.

Of major concern and a subject of controversy is the capacity of asbestos to cause mesotheliomas in the family members of asbestos workers [27, 32]. Anecdotal observations convincingly argue that such cases occur as a result of indirect exposure, but again there is insufficient data to calculate a threshold. Obviously, the definition of a threshold for those indirectly exposed in the home due to the laundering of a family member's work clothes or re-entrainment of subtle asbestos accumulations in the home setting is beyond the capabilities of modern epidemiology. Despite arguments to the contrary, the most obvious occurrences of this type have been in households where a family member has worked in a shipyard, an asbestos production plant, or as a plumber/pipefitter. Roggli et al. [65] has published some of the more detailed information on this topic including the results of fiber burden analyses on lung tissue of diseased family members. Interestingly enough, 9 of the 34 homemakers in his study had pleural plaques and three had abdominal mesotheliomas, an incidence approaching ten percent! As might be expected, a substantial proportion of these patients had increased concentrations of amphiboles in their lung tissue.

Environmental exposures (occurring outside of the occupational setting and the home) resulting in mesotheliomas are also an issue [29, 60]. There is now abundant evidence to indicate that crocidolite causes malignant disease in the community setting with "outbreaks" documented in residents of North America, Africa, Australia, and Asia [2, 3, 18, 43]. But what about members of the general public? Environmental monitoring of urban air (and potable water) has shown that the ambient air in major cities contains minute amounts of asbestos, primarily chrysotile fibers. Some would argue that cases of idiopathic mesothelioma are, in fact, a reflection of lifelong low-level exposures to ambient asbestos even though evidence supporting such conjecture is limited. Recently, Goldberg et al. [31] published data suggesting that the distribution of cases of mesotheliomas believed to be "idiopathic" in French communities was similar to the geographic distribution of patients with asbestos-related tumors, suggesting that subtle asbestos exposure was also the cause of these so-called idiopathic cases.

Why is mesothelioma such a relatively rare neoplasm, even among workers heavily exposed to asbestos? Certainly, the prolonged latency periods of this malignancy influences the outcome, since many potential "victims" fail to live long enough to develop a mesothelioma, succumbing to other more common diseases unrelated to asbestos exposure. But the answer could also lie in the crypts of our individual genetic makeup. Thus, the occurrence of the malignancy might well be based on biological factors that predispose to susceptibility (or resistance) to the carcinogenic effects of asbestos [11]. In experimental studies, we found differences in the incidence of malignant disease in mice of several different inbred strains after intraperitoneal introduction of asbestos, an observation suggesting genetic influences on latency and overall susceptibility [20, 21]. Rare, sporadic, "family" outbreaks of mesotheliomas are consistent with this observation [7, 46, 49, 64]. And, in the genetically mediated disease of humans known as Mediterranean Fever, the characteristic chronic serositis, which occurs in the body cavities of these patients, is associated with the sporadic, uncommon appearance of mesothelioma in mid-life [43, 63]. Perhaps this is a reflection of the apparent role of smoldering inflammation in the pathogenesis of mesothelioma, as has been proposed for the infrequent development of mesotheliomas in those afflicted with chronic tuberculosis [57, 66]. In Turkey, the relatively common appearance of mesotheliomas among members of isolated population groups who are exposed to erionite, a volcanic fibrous zeolite mineral, has again raised the possible role of genetic factors in carcinogenesis for consideration [4, 24]. Could inheritance be responsible for the development of mesothelioma in patients years after they received therapeutic irradiation for neoplastic disease [1, 51, 72]? Clearly, we are only now acquiring insights into possible predisposing factors that might ultimately influence the development of this unique malignancy. The interplay between environmental and host factors, to a large extent, remains to be defined [76].

References

1. Anderson KA et al (1985) Malignant pleural mesothelioma following radiotherapy in a 16-year-old boy. Cancer 56:273
2. Armstrong BK et al (1984) Epidemiology of malignant mesothelioma in Western Australia. Med J Aust 141:86
3. Armstrong BK et al (1988) Mortality in miners and millers of crocidolite in Western Australia. Br J Ind Med 45:5–13
4. Artvinli M, Baris YI (1979) Malignant mesotheliomas in a small village in the Anatolian region of Turkey: an epidemiologic study. J Natl Cancer Inst 63:17
5. Berman DW, Crump KS (2008) Technical support document for a protocol to assess asbestos-related risk. US Environmental Protection Agency publication. US Environmental Protection Agency, Washington, DC

6. Berman DW et al (1995) The sizes, shapes, and mineralogy of asbestos structures that induce lung tumors or mesothelioma in AF/HAN rats following inhalation. Risk Anal 15:181–195
7. Bianchi C et al (1993) Asbestos-related familial mesothelioma. Eur J Cancer Prevent 2: 247–250
8. Bischoff F, Bryson G (1964) Carcinogenesis through solid state surfaces. Prog Exp Tumor Res 5:65
9. Bohlig H et al (1970) Epidemiology of malignant mesothelioma in Hamburg. Environ Res 3:365
10. Bolen JW, Thorning D (1980) Mesotheliomas: a light and electronmicroscopical study concerning histogenetic relationships between the epithelial and the mesenchymal variants. Am J Surg Pathol 4:451
11. Brain JD (1989) The susceptible individual: an overview. In: Utell M (ed) Susceptibility to inhaled pollutants, ASTM Special Technical Publication. ASTM, Philadelphia
12. Brody AR, Overby LH (1989) Incorporation of tritiated thymidine by epithelial and interstitial cells in bronchiolar-alveolar regions of asbestos-exposed rats. Am J Pathol 134:133–140
13. Buoen LC et al (1975) Foreign body tumorigenesis: in vitro isolation and expansion of preneoplastaic clonal cell populations. J Natl Cancer Inst 55:721
14. Burdorf A et al (2007) Asbestos exposure and differences in occurrences of peritoneal mesothelioma between men and women across countries. Occup Environ Med 64:839–842
15. Chanhinian AP, Pass HI (2000) Malignant mesothelioma. In: Holland JC, Frei E (eds) Cancer medicine, 5th edn. BC Decker, Hamilton
16. Coggon D et al (1995) Differences in occupational mortality from pleural cancer, peritoneal cancer and asbestosis. Occup Environ Med 52:775–777
17. Craighead JE (1987) Current pathogenetic concepts of diffuse malignant mesothelioma. Hum Pathol 18:544–557
18. Craighead JE, Gibbs AR (2008) Asbestos and its diseases. Oxford University Press, New York
19. Craighead J et al (1987) Biologic characteristics of asbestos-induced malignant mesothelioma in rats. Chest 91S:12–13
20. Craighead JE et al (1993) Genetic factors influence malignant mesothelioma development in mice. Eur Respir Rev 3:118–120

21. Craighead JE et al (1993) The pathogenetic role of growth factors in human and rat malignant mesotheliomas. Eur Respir Rev 3(11):159–160

22. Dionne GP, Wang NS (1977) A scanning electron microscopic study of diffuse mesothelioma and some lung carcinomas. Cancer 40:707

23. Dodson RF et al (2005) Asbestos burden in cases of mesothelioma from individuals from various regions of the United States. Ultrastruct Pathol 29:415–433

24. Dogan AU et al (2006) Genetic predisposition to fiber carcinogenesis causes a mesothelioma epidemic in Turkey. Cancer Res 66:5063–5068

25. Dreessen WC et al. (1938) A study of asbestosis in the asbestos textile industry. Public Health Bulletin 241. US Treasury Department, Public Health Service

26. Edge JR (1976) Asbestos related disease in Barrow-in-Furness. Environ Res 11:244–247

27. Enterline PE (1983) Cancer produced by non-occupational asbestos exposure in the United States. J Air Pollut Control Assoc 33:318–322

28. Ferrante D et al (2007) Cancer mortality and incidence of mesothelioma in a cohort of wives of asbestos workers in Casale Monferranto, Italy. Environ Health Perspect 115:1401–1405

29. Fischbein A, Rohl AN (1985) Pleural mesothelioma and neighborhood asbestos exposure. JAMA 252:86

30. Fleischer WE et al (1946) A health survey of pipe covering operations in constructing naval vessels. J Ind Hyg Toxicol 28:9

31. Goldberg S, Rey G, Luce D et al (2010) Possible effect of environmental exposure to asbestos on geographical variation in mesothelioma rates. Occup Environ Med 67(6):417–421

32. Greenberg M, Davies TA (1974) Mesothelioma register 1967–1968. Br J Ind Med 31:91

33. Grundy GW, Miller RW (1972) Malignant mesothelioma in childhood. Cancer 30:1216

34. Haries PG (1976) Experience with asbestos disease and its control in Great Britain's naval dockyards. Environ Res 11:261–267

35. Heintz NH et al (2010) Asbestos, lung cancers, and mesotheliomas: from molecular approaches to targeting tumor survival pathways. Am J Respir Cell Mol Biol 42:133–139

36. Hillerdal G (1999) Mesothelioma: cases associated with non-occupational and low dose exposures. Occup Environ Med 56:505–513

37. Hodgson JT, Darnton A (2000) The quantitative risks of mesothelioma and lung cancer in relation to asbestos exposure. Ann Occup Hyg 44:565–601

38. Hodgson JT, Darnton A (2010) Mesothelioma risk from chrysotile. Occup Environ Med 67:432

39. Kannerstein M, Churg J (1979) Functions of mesothelioma panels. Ann NY Acad Sci 330:433

40. Karn CM et al (1994) Cardiac synovial sarcoma with translocation (X; 18) associated with asbestos exposure. Cancer 73:74–78

41. Klemperer P, Rabin CB (1931) Primary neoplasms of the pleura. A report of five cases. Arch Pathol 11:385

42. Kurumatani N, Kumagai S (2008) Mapping the risk of mesothelioma due to neighborhood asbestos exposure. Am J Respir Crit Care Med 178:624–629

43. Lidar M et al (2002) Thoracic and lung involvement in familial Mediterranean fever (FMF). Clin Chest Med 23:505–511

44. Loomis D et al (2009) Lung cancer mortality and fibre exposures among North Carolina asbestos textile workers. Occup Environ Med 66:535–542

45. Luo S et al (2003) Asbestos related diseases from environmental exposure to crocidolite in Da-yao, China. I. Review of exposure and epidemiological data. Occup Environ Med 60:35–42

46. Lynch HT et al (1985) Familial mesothelioma: review and family study. Cancer Genet Cytogenet 15:25

47. Mack TM (1995) Sarcomas and other malignancies of soft tissue, retroperitoneum, peritoneum, pleura, heart, mediastinum, and spleen. Cancer 75:211–244

48. Marchand PE (1991) The discovery of mesothelioma in the Northwestern Cape Province in the Republic of South Africa. Am J Ind Med 19:241–246

49. Martensson G et al (1984) Malignant mesothelioma in two pairs of siblings: is there a hereditary predisposing factor? Eur J Respir Dis 65:179

50. Maule MM et al (2007) Modeling mesothelioma risk associated with environmental asbestos exposure. Environ Health Perspect 115:1066–1071

51. Maurer R, Egloff B (1975) Malignant peritoneal mesothelioma after cholangiography with thorotrast. Cancer 36:1381

52. Maximow A (1927) Morphology of the mesenchymal reactions. Arch Pathol 4:557–606

53. Maximow A (1927) Uber das mesothel (deck-zellen der serosen haute) und die zellen der serosen exsudate. Untersuchungen an entzun-detem Gewebe und an Gewebskulturen. Arch Exp Zellforsch 4:1

54. McDonald JC et al (1999) Editorial: chrysotile, tremolite and fibrogenicity. Ann Occup Hyg 43(7):439–442

55. McQualter JL et al (2010) Evidence of an epithelial stem/progenitor cell hierarchy in the adult mouse lung. Proc Natl Acad Sci 107(4):1414–1419

56. Merewether ERA (1934) A memorandum on asbestosis. Tubercle 75:69–81, 109–118, 152–159

57. Merewether ERA, Price CW (1930) Report on the effects of asbestos dust on the lungs and dust suppression in the asbestos industry. Her Majesty's Stationery Office, London

58. Mossman BT et al (1986) Alteration of super-oxide dismutase activity in tracheal epithelial cells by asbestos and inhibition of cytotoxicity by antioxidants. Lab Invest 54:204

59. Murphy RLH et al (1972) Low exposure to asbestos. Gas exchange in ship pipe coverers and controls. Arch Environ Health 25:253

60. Newhouse ML, Thompson H (1965) Epidemi-ology of mesothelial tumors in the London area. Ann NY Acad Sci 132:579–588

61. Rees D et al (2001) Asbestos lung fibre concen-trations in South African chrysotile mine work-ers. Ann Occup Hyg 45:473–477

62. Reid A et al (2007) Age and sex differences in malignant mesothelioma after residential exposure to blue asbestos (crocidolite). Chest 131:376–382

63. Riddell RH et al (1981) Peritoneal malignant mesothelioma in a patient with recurrent perito-nitis. Cancer 48:134

64. Risberg B et al (1980) Familial clustering of malignant mesothelioma. Cancer 45:2422

65. Roggli VL et al (1997) Malignant mesothe-lioma in women. Anat Pathol 2:147–163

66. Rovario GC et al (1982) The association of pleural mesothelioma and tuberculosis. Am Rev Respir Dis 126:569

67. Sebastien P, McDonald JC (1997) Mesothelioma in Quebec chrysotile miners and millers: epide-miology and aetiology. Ann Occup Hyg 41(6):707–719

68. Sheers G (1980) Mesothelioma risks in a naval dockyard. Arch Environ Health 35:276–282

69. Sheers G, Templeton AR (1968) Effects of asbestos in dockyard workers. Br Med J 11:574

70. Spirtas R et al (1994) Malignant mesothelioma: attributable risk of asbestos exposure. Occup Environ Med 51:804–811

71. Stanton MF, Wrench C (1978) Mechanisms of mesothelioma induction with asbestos and fibrous glass. J Natl Cancer Inst 48:797

72. Stock RJ et al (1979) Malignant peritoneal mesothelioma following radiotherapy for semi-noma of the testis. Cancer 44:914

73. Stout AP, Murray MR (1942) Localized pleural mesothelioma: investigation of its characteris-tics and histogenesis by the method of tissue culture. Arch Pathol 34:951

74. Stumphius J (1971) Epidemiology of mesothe-lioma on Waicheren Island. Br J Ind Med 28:59

75. Suzuki Y et al (1976) Ultrastructure of human malignant diffuse mesothelioma. Am J Pathol 85:241

76. Tagnon I et al (1980) Mesothelioma associated with the shipbuilding industry in coastal Virginia. Cancer Res 40:3875

77. Timbrell V (1965) The inhalation of fibrous dusts. Ann NY Acad Sci 132:255

78. Tossavainen A (2004) Global use of asbestos and the incidence of mesothelioma. Int J Occup Environ Health 10:22–25

79. Wagner E (1870) Das tuberkelahnliche lymph-adenom (der cytogene oder reticulierte Tuberkel). Arch Heilk 11:497

80. Wagner JC (1991) The discovery of the associ-ation between blue asbestos and mesotheliomas and the aftermath. Br J Ind Med 48:399–403

81. Wagner JC, Sleggs CA, Marchand P (1960) Diffuse pleural mesothelioma and asbestos exposure in the North Western Cape Province. Br J Ind Med 17:260

82. Webster I (1973) Asbestos and malignancy. S Afr Med J 47:165

83. Wedler HW (1943) Asbetsose und lungenkrebs bei asbestoste. Dtsch Arch Klin Med 191:189

84. Wedler HW (1943) Asbetsose und lungenkrebs. Dtsch Med Wochenschr 69:575

85. Whitwell F, Rawcliffe RM (1971) Diffuse malignant pleural mesothelioma and asbestos exposure. Thorax 26:6–22

Abstract Malignant pleural mesothelioma (MPM) is an asbestos-related neoplasm that originates in pleural mesothelial cells and progresses locally along the pleura until it encases the lungs and mediastinum, ultimately causing death. Imaging plays a crucial role in diagnosis and optimal management. Computed tomography (CT) continues to be the primary and initial imaging modality. Magnetic resonance imaging (MRI) complements CT scan and is superior in determining chest wall and diaphragmatic invasion. FDG18-PET/CT provides anatamometabolic information and is superior to both CT and MRI in overall staging and monitoring response to therapy. This chapter will detail the imaging finding of MPM and role of imaging in guiding management.

3.1
Introduction

Malignant pleural mesothelioma (MPM) is an asbestos-related neoplasm that is refractory to current therapies and associated with poor prognosis. The disease originates in pleural mesothelial cells and progresses locally along the pleural reflections until it encases the lungs and mediastinum, ultimately causing death. MPM has been designated as a worldwide epidemic, which is predicted to peak in the next decade (2015–2019) in most Western countries [28]. Patients with mesothelioma have an average survival of 7–12 months [32, 33]; however, trimodality therapy with cytoreductive surgery followed by radiotherapy and chemotherapy can prolong survival [5, 7, 23, 29, 30].

The three distinct histologic subtypes – epithelial, sarcomatoid (sarcomatous), and mixed (biphasic) – cannot be distinguished by imaging. Even though contrast-enhanced CT is the preferred technique for evaluating suspected malignant pleural disease, histological sampling and immunohistocytochemistry can only reliably diagnose MPM. The complex morphology and growth pattern of MPM make it an imaging enigma. This chapter aims to highlight the practical aspects of imaging of MPM with an emphasis on guiding management.

R.R. Gill
Department of Radiology,
Brigham and Women's Hospital,
75 Francis Street, Boston, MA, USA
e-mail: rgill@partners.org

A. Tannapfel (ed.), *Malignant Mesothelioma*, Recent Results in Cancer Research 189,
DOI: 10.1007/978-3-642-10862-4_3, © Springer-Verlag Berlin Heidelberg 2011

3

3.2
Patterns of Presentation and Imaging Features

MPM has varied and nonspecific imaging appearances ranging from pleural effusion, focal pleural thickening, diffuse circumferential pleural thickening, pleural nodularity to pleural masses [13–15, 36]. Calcified and noncalcified bilateral pleural plaques coexist with pleural thickening. Pleural thickening can be focal or circumferential and extends along the mediastinal, diaphragmatic surface of the pleura and along fissures. Nodal involvement and contiguous invasion of adjacent chest wall and direct intra-diaphragmatic extension can be seen in later stages. Contralateral disease can be in the form of pleural effusion or pulmonary nodules. Brain and osseous metastases can be seen in later stages, as well.

The constellation of findings ranges from unilateral pleural effusion, circumferential nodular pleural thickening, pleural masses, and invasion of adjacent structures, to adenopathy, osseous, pulmonary and distant metastases in the later stages [13–15, 36]. Pleural thickening and/or effusions also represent early presentation and are nonspecific without histological confirmation. Rind-like circumferential pleural thickening is seen as the disease progresses, with the disease process often starting from the diaphragmatic surface of the pleura extending upward [27, 34] (Figs. 3.1 and 3.2). Apical involvement is considered a bad prognostic factor and is seen in later stages. Volume loss and mediastinal shift can be seen secondary to encasement of the lung. Sixty percent of the time the disease is seen on the right and is only bilateral in 10% cases [22].

Biphasic and sarcomatoid subtypes have more aggressive behavior and can present with

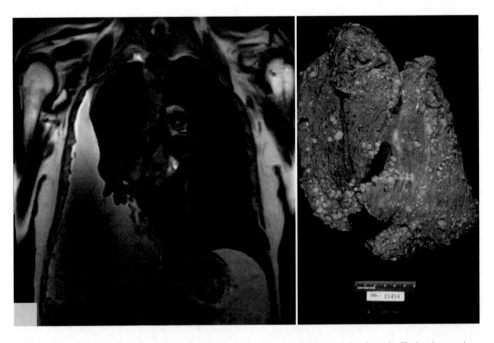

Fig. 3.1 Circumferential nodular pleural thickening and an associated large right pleural effusion in a patient with epithelial MPM

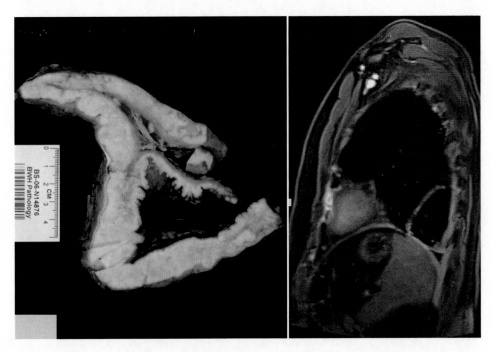

Fig. 3.2 Saggital post-contrast VIBE image showing rind-like circumferential pleural thickening extending along the diaphragm and fissures and reflections of the pleura

distant and osseous metastases in early stages of the disease.

3.3
Preoperative Evaluation of MPM

MPM patients are considered surgical candidates if the disease is confined to the ipsilateral hemithorax and there is no evidence of spread to mediastinal lymph nodes ($N=0$) or distant metastases ($M=0$). Current methods for predicting resectability of patients undergoing extrapleural pneumonectomy for macroscopic complete resection of MPM are limited. Despite improvements in diagnostic imaging over several decades, the proportion of patients who are unable to complete resection after thoracotomy remains high at 25% [27]. Using current methods of preoperative evaluation for patients with malignant pleural mesothelioma, evidence of local invasion of contiguous structures, transdiaphragmatic or transmediastinal invasion, and diffuse chest wall invasion are clear indicators of unresectability (Figs. 3.3–3.6).

Computed tomography (CT) is the mainstay in preoperative evaluation and is complemented by magnetic resonance imaging and ^{18}F-FDG positron tomography [34]. Plain radiography plays a limited role due to varied and nonspecific appearances ranging from pleural effusion to lobulated pleural thickening and pleural masses (Fig. 3.7). Pleural plaques, the hallmark of asbestos exposure, further limit evaluation on radiographs and can potentially obscure contralateral involvement and can obscure pulmonary nodules.

CT continues to be the initial and primary modality for diagnosis, staging, and monitoring

3

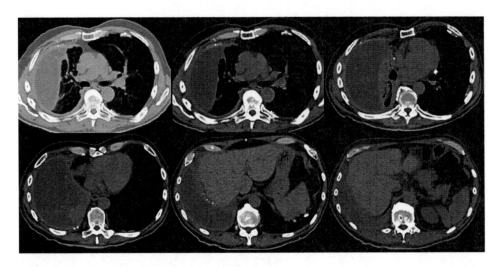

Fig. 3.3 Serial axial CT images showing pleural effusion, thickening, and masses

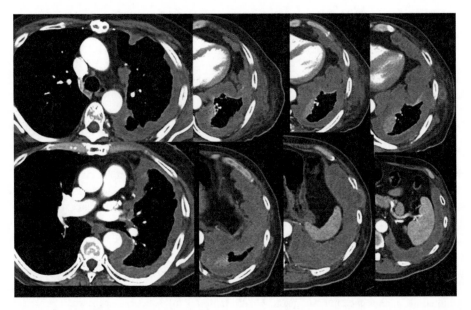

Fig. 3.4 Serial contrast-enhanced axial CT images showing later presentation of epithelial mesothelioma, confined to the left hemithorax, this patient underwent successful extrapleural pneumonectomy

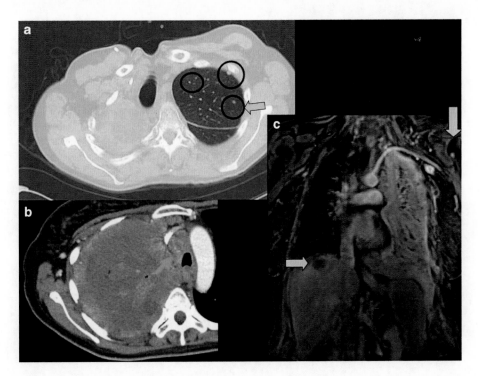

Fig. 3.5 Axial CT images showing (**a**) contralateral pulmonary nodules, (**b**) mediastinal invasion and adenopathy (*arrow*), (**c**) coronal contrast-enhanced MR image showing hepatic metastasis and osseous left humeral head metastasis

of therapeutic response in MPM [25]. Even though CT can easily depict the overall extent of the pleural abnormality, early chest wall invasion, peritoneal involvement, and lymph node metastases can be challenging even on a contrast-enhanced CT scan. Subtle transdiaphragmatic extension can also be difficult to identify on CT.

CT image data can also be effectively reconstructed in three-dimensional planes to yield multi-planar reformats and volume rendered images to simulate the anatomical detail for surgical planning. Three-dimensional (3-D) volume rendered images are increasingly becoming popular to show association with adjacent structures and encasement or encroachment of vascular structures by the tumor [13, 15]. Maximum intensity projections depict the course of vessels

encased by the pleural rind and are helpful during surgery. The 3-D images are intuitive and provide the surgeons an overview of the tumor in vitro, thereby aiding the surgeons during resection. These images also provide patients an overview and extent of their disease during management discussions (Fig. 3.8).

Furthermore, volumetric assessment of MPM can be easily acquired by serially segmenting the tumor using Hounsfield thresholding [6, 24, 27, 31]. Tumor and lung volumes can be generated and have been proven to be prognostically significant (Fig. 3.9).

Ultrasound has a limited role in diagnosis and management of MPM; however, the fluid attenuation of the tumor provides a diagnostic window for the ultrasound, thus enabling ultrasound-guided biopsy and thoracentesis, thereby

3

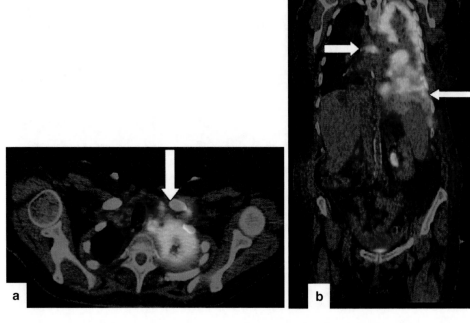

Fig. 3.6 (**a**) and (**b**) Fused ^{18}F-FDG images in a patient with advanced epithelial MPM, with left supraclavicular nodes (*arrow*), mediastinal nodes, and intra-abdominal extension (*arrows*)

improving the diagnostic yield of pleural biopsy [20] (Fig. 3.10).

MRI is superior to CT both in the differentiation of malignant from benign pleural disease due to its superior signal-to-noise ratio and is the modality of choice in the assessment of chest wall and diaphragmatic invasion by MPM [19]. Dynamic contrast-enhanced (DCE) MRI is a promising technique and has the ability to correlate histology and pathology [17, 18] (Giesel 2008).

MRI not only confirms the CT findings such as diffuse pleural thickening and pleural effusion, but is superior in delineating contiguous invasion of adjacent structures. MPM has intermediate to slightly high signal intensity on T1-weighted images (T1-WI) and moderately high signal intensity on T2-weighted images (T2-WI) as compared to adjacent chest wall musculature [13–15, 34] and shows moderate enhancement after administration of gadolinium. MRI has a higher sensitivity and specificity to CT in detecting early chest wall and subdiaphragmatic involvement. Linear enhancing foci in the chest wall depicting sites of previous biopsy, thoracotomy, or chest tube tracts are also relatively more easily seen on MRI than on CT.

Additional techniques such as fat suppression and subtraction images further increase the sensitivity in detecting fissural involvement and invasion of the adjacent structures [14]. Sagittal and coronal reformats are very important in delineating transdiaphragmatic, chest wall, and direct mediastinal involvement, and thus are key sequences in predicting resectability. Patz et al.

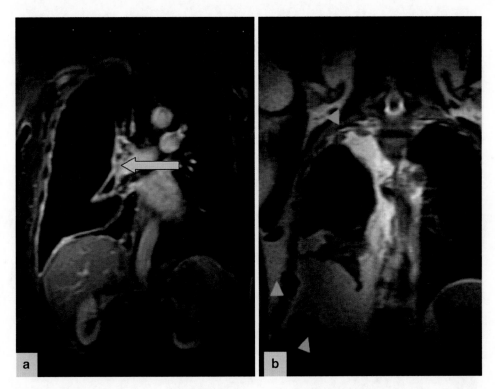

Fig. 3.7 (**a**) Early presentation of MPM, coronal post-contrast VIBE image showing a large right pleural effusion with complete atelectasis of the right lung (*arrow*). (**b**) Combined pleural effusion and pleural-based masses (*arrow heads*) as seen on a coronal T2W MR image

compared the values of the two modalities in predicting resectability and reported high sensitivity for both CT and MRI in evaluating resectability of MPM in relation to the diaphragm and chest wall (94% and 93% sensitivity for CT, and 100% and 100% for MRI); however, MRI was found to be superior [27]. Heelan et al. also found MRI superior to CT in revealing invasion of the diaphragm (55% accuracy for CT vs 82% for MRI) and in showing involvement of endothoracic fascia and solitary resectable foci of chest wall invasion (46% accuracy for CT vs 69% for MRI) [19].

MR imaging of MPM can be severely limited due to artifacts such as susceptibility artifact, aliasing, and motion artifact. However, optimization of imaging sequences with optimal cardiac gating, respiratory compensation, and utilization of fat suppression techniques can help limit artifacts. Additionally, the use of 3-D gradient echo sequences such as FAME (Fast Acquisition with Multiphase Efgre3D), VIBE (Volumetric Interpolated Breath-Hold Examination), and LAVA (Liver Acquisition with Volume Acquisition) are based on a 3-D spoiled gradient echo pulse sequence. The optimized inversion pulse and a new fat suppression technique (called segmented special) provide enhanced image contrast and uniform fat suppression. Array spatial sensitivity encoding technique (ASSET) with partial data filling and shorter TR/TE enables the use of short breath holds for dynamic imaging with multiple phases [14].

3

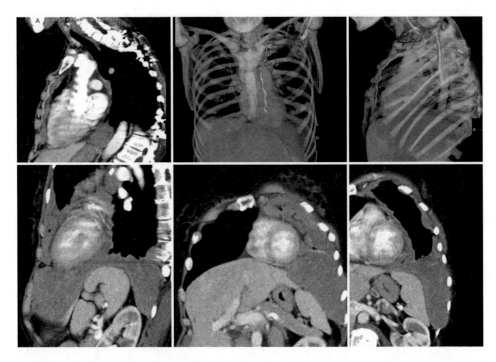

Fig. 3.8 Multi-planar and Volume-rendered CT images showing relationship to mediastinal structures and vessels

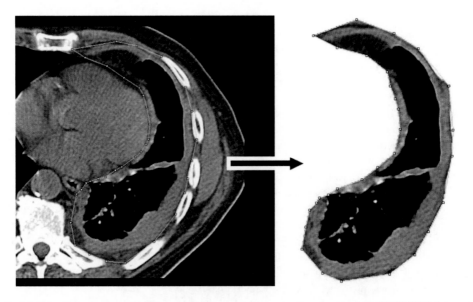

Fig. 3.9 Volumetric assessment of tumor using Image J to segment pleural tumor from CT DICOM data and calculating overall tumor volume from axial images

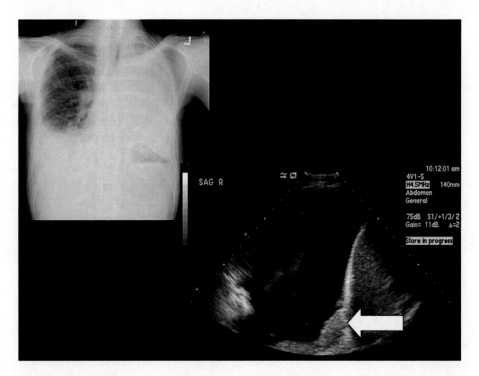

Fig. 3.10 PA and lateral chest x-ray obtained 5 years following left EPP shows interval appearance of a right pleural effusion, rind-like encasement of the right lung and right lung volume loss from MPM. Note the hyperechoic diaphragmatic mass (*white arrow*) seen on a thoracic ultrasound used to guide intraoperative pleural biopsy

Diffusion weighted MRI [16] can give us information on the cellularity of MPM and the ADC values can be correlated with the histological subtypes. Parallel MRI allows for a quantitative assessment of tumor mobility and local lung motion. Parallel MRI acquisition techniques (PAT) such as generalized autocalibrating partially parallel acquisition (GRAPPA), TrueFISP (fast imaging with steady precession), and fast low angle shot (FLASH) can help in delineating subtle invasion of mediastinal structures and the chest wall [17] and are especially useful when direct invasion of mediastinal, vascular structures, and myocardium is suspected.

Functional imaging with PET ^{18}F-Fluorodeoxyglucose (FDG) facilitates noninvasive evaluation of tumor pathophysiology and details anatomo-metabolic extent of MPM, thus enabling preoperative staging. MPM has moderate to high ^{18}F-FDG uptake depending on histological cell type [9, 10]. Gerbaudo et al. have correlated tumor distribution with four different patterns of FDG uptake, namely, focal (type1), linear (type 2), mixed (type 3), and encasing (type 4) [10]. Their study comprised of a semiquantitative analysis of serial dual-phase FDG images, which demonstrated that radiotracer uptake increased over time in both normal tissue and MPM [9]. In the normal lung, the rise in FDG uptake was $6\pm4\%$ in 2 h, between the early and late images; however, the increment of FDG uptake in MPM was higher in stage IV patients ($97\pm25\%$) when compared to stage I ($13\pm1\%$), stage II ($34\pm2\%$), and stage III patients ($57\pm3\%$), thereby predicting that as the stage of MPM increases, the FDG uptake in the tumor also increases. Currently, PET/CT is superior to other imaging modalities in overall staging and selection of patients for surgery due to its ability to detect occult metastases and extensive disease [10] (Fig. 3.7).

3

3.4
Postoperative Evaluation

Curative treatment for MPM is with extrapleural pneumonectomy. Localized disease or minimal disease is treated with local resection or radical pleurectomy or pleural decortication. Radiographs are used to follow patients postoperatively, reserving CT for evaluating complications.

After pneumonectomy, the pneumonectomy space fills up with fluid, generally at the rate of one intercostal space per 7 days, and can be monitored by serial radiographs. Controlled filling of the pneumonectomy space helps control mediastinal shift [35]. Rapid filling of the pneumonectomy space is worrisome and is of concern for hemorrhage within the pneumonectomy space or a Chyle leak. Slow filling of the pneumonectomy space or decreasing fluid level is worrisome for a bronchopleural fistula, or leakage of fluid into the abdomen along the diaphragmatic reconstruction, both these scenarios are secondary to infection (Figs. 3.11 and 3.12).

MDCT with the help of multi-planar reformats and 3-D imaging can help delineate the BPF [13, 15]. The data can also be interpolated to provide measurements for personalized stents [13, 15]. Ventilation scans can help delineate a tiny central BPF. Marsupialization of the pneumonectomy space and Clagette window creation are the treatments of choice for a central BPF. The pneumonectomy space is opened and cleaned and packed with antibiotic soaked packing in an attempt to heal the infection and then the cavity is closed and packed with a muscle flap, generally the latissimus dorsi or the omentum [14].

CT and PET ^{18}F-Fluorodeoxyglucose scans are also used to identify and biopsy possible sites of recurrence (Fig. 3.13).

Another complication seen especially with a left-sided pneumonectomy is herniation of stomach along the medial aspect of the pneumonectomy space. Plain radiographs are the best at depicting the herniation of the gastric bubble above the gortex reconstruction, usually seen on the first postoperative radiograph [14] (Fig. 3.14). Post-pneumonectomy syndrome, another rare complication, can also be assessed by CT. The left main stem bronchus gets stretched over the vertebral body due to severe mediastinal shift to the right post-pneumonectomy [14]. The mediastinal shift can be corrected by putting in a saline-filled implant into the pneumonectomy space, with an aim to displacing the mediastinal structure (Fig. 3.15). MR is a very useful modality when Chyle leak is suspected and helps in identifying the site of leak and the thoracic duct prior to embolization.

Recurrence and/or progressive metastatic disease are generally evaluated by contrast-enhanced CT scan. Multiple patterns of recurrence are seen mostly as enlarging soft tissue masses along the resection margins, ascites, and peritoneal thickening, which is a manifestation of intra-abdominal disease, new pulmonary nodules, and increasing size of mediastinal nodes [21]. FDG/PET is very useful in restaging and also monitoring response to therapy [10, 27, 34].

Post-radical pleurectomy, the granulation tissue along resection margins can be irregular and nodular, thus often raising concern for recurrence; however, serial FDG/PET can help distinguish between the two by semiquantitative evaluation of tracer uptake. Tumor will show progressive increase in uptake of tracer as opposed to granulation tumor, which slowly, over a period of time, will either regress or remain stable [10] (Fig. 3.16).

3.5
Unresectable Disease

Extensive chest wall invasion, direct mediastinal invasion, positive mediastinal nodes, contiguous intra-abdominal disease, and contralateral

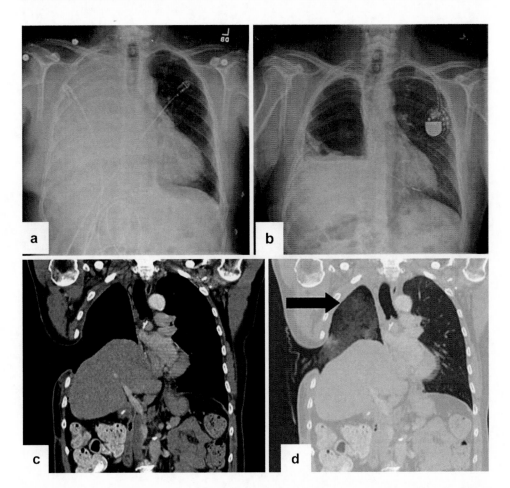

Fig. 3.11 (**a**) Three months post extrapleural pneumonectomy showing complete filling of right pneumonectomy space, (**b**) complete loss of fluid at 4 months signified a bronchopleural fistula, patient underwent exploration and was found to have an infected right pneumonectomy space (**c**) and (**d**) showing a right-sided Clagette window with packing material

involvement are features that are hallmarks of unresectable disease. When patients are deemed unresectable, they are referred for chemotherapy and or palliative debulking surgery. Imaging helps quantify tumor extent, delineate morphology, depict angiogenesis, and identify patients who will potentially respond to chemotherapy [4].

Volumetric analysis is done by using DICOM CT images to generate volume data using Hounsfield thresholding. Volumetric measurements may prove to be more reproducible and accurate than RECIST and modified RECIST criteria in evaluating response to therapy as MPM due to its complex morphology and tendency to grow along pleural reflections. Therefore, it is challenging to acquire reproducible and reliable orthogonal measurements [1–3, 26].

Dynamic contrast-enhanced (DCE) MRI using gadolinium-based contrast material (Gd-CM) can be used for the assessment of perfusion,

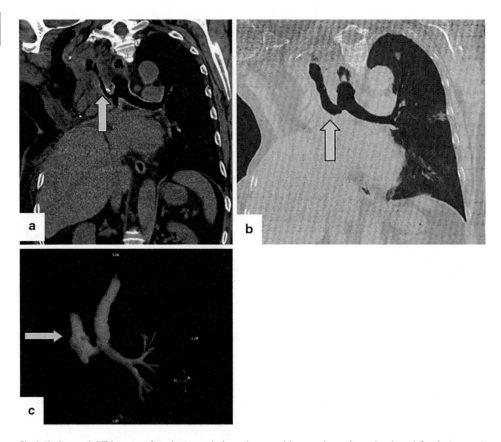

Fig. 3.12 Coronal CT images after clagette window closure with a persistent bronchopleural fistula (*arrows*)

vascularity, and vascular permeability of tumors [17, 18]. The two-compartment model can be applied to the pharmacokinetic analysis of DCE MRI yielding parameters such as redistribution rate contrast (kep) and elimination rate contrast (kel) and amplitude [17, 18]. These parameters can predict the therapeutic efficacy of chemotherapy in MPM. Giesel et al. evaluated the feasibility of DCE MRI in monitoring therapeutic effect of chemotherapy in MPM by comparing pharmacokinetic parameters, including kep and kel, to early clinical response and survival [12]. They found that nonresponders to the therapy showed a higher kep value (3.6 min) than clinical responders(2.6 min), which in turn correlated to shorter survival (460 vs 780 days) [11]. Even though these results are promising, this concept

requires testing in larger cohorts. Direct comparison between perfusion MRI parameters and angiogenesis factors, such as VEGF expression, is also required and correlation with other prognostic indicators needs to be studied.

FDG/PET can also be used to assess treatment response by semiquantitative evaluation of tracer uptake and direct comparison between pretreatment and posttreatment scans [8].

3.6
Future Directions

Dynamic contrast-enhanced MRI can be used to map the heterogeneity of microcirculation in MPM and can be used to predict therapeutic

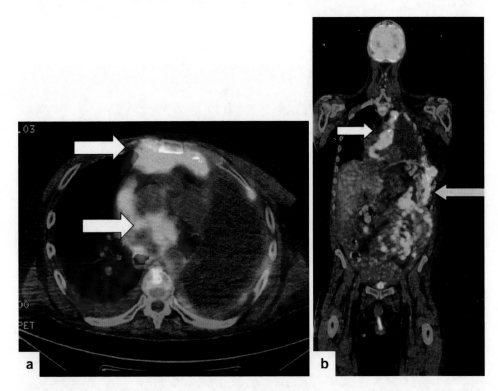

Fig. 3.13 (**a**) and (**b**) axial and Coronal ^{18}F-FDG fused images showing recurrent disease involving the mediastinum, left lateral chest wall and intra-abdominal disease post left extrapleural pneumonectomy (*white arrows*)

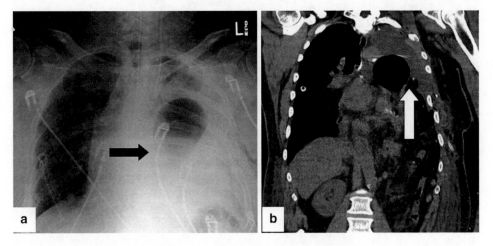

Fig. 3.14 (**a**) Radiograph showing herniation of stomach above the diaphragmatic reconstruction. (**b**) Coronal reformat showing the stomach above the gore-tex reconstruction (*white arrow*)

3

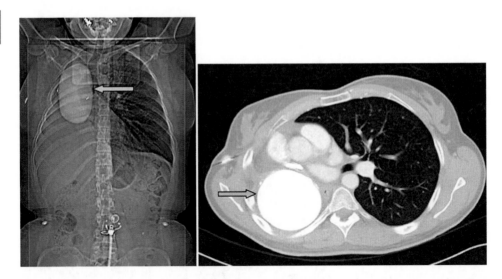

Fig. 3.15 Coronal and axial images showing a (*arrow*) saline implant used to displace the mediastinal structures to the left in order to treat post-pneumonectomy syndrome

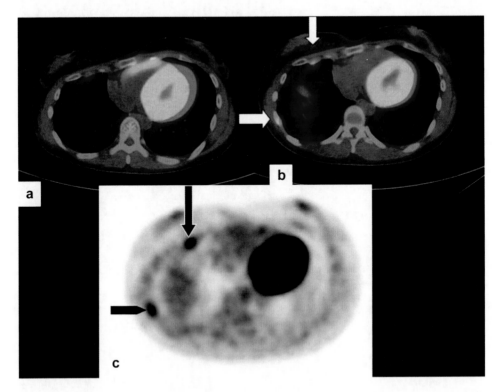

Fig. 3.16 (**a**) Baseline fused ¹⁸F-FDG axial image post right radical pleurectomy (**b**) (*white arrows*) and (**c**) (*black arrows*) 50% increase in SUV; these two areas were subsequently resected

response and stratify survival. The development of such a quantitative technique will bring new measures essential to the diagnosis and management of patients with MPM, and will enable an objective assessment of new pharmacologic agents and serve as a possible tumor biomarker enabling prediction of outcomes. Diffusion MRI, combined with DCE MRI, can be a powerful tool. ADC maps derived by plotting intensity from multiple b values can be used to measure tumor cellularity. However, these techniques need to be validated and studied before they can be adapted into clinical practice.

3.7
Summary

Imaging plays a key role in diagnosis, management, and follow-up of patients with MPM. CT is the primary diagnostic modality in diagnosis, staging, and posttreatment management of MPM. MRI and PET provide additional and complementary information to CT. Optimization of current MR protocols will provide more efficient and valuable MR applications and potentially serve as an imaging biomarker. Larger population studies and correlation of imaging to pathology and genomic profiles can help improve survival.

References

 1. Armato SG III, Ogarek JL, Starkey A et al (2006) Variability in mesothelioma tumor response classification. AJR Am J Roentgenol 186:1000–1006
 2. Armato SG III, Oxnard GR, Kocherginsky M et al (2005) Evaluation of semi-automated measurements of mesothelioma tumor thickness on CT scans. Acad Radiol 12:1301–1309
 3. Armato SG III, Oxnard GR, MacMahon H et al (2004) Measurement of mesothelioma on thoracic CT scans: a comparison of manual and computer-assisted techniques. Med Phys 31: 1105–1115
 4. Drevs J, Schneider V (2006) The use of vascular biomarkers and imaging studies in the early clinical development of anti-tumor agents targeting angiogenesis. J Intern Med 260(6): 517–529
 5. Flores RM (2005) Induction chemotherapy, extrapleural pneumonectomy, and radiotherapy in the treatment of malignant pleural mesothelioma: the Memorial Sloan-Kettering experience. Lung Cancer 49(Suppl 1):S71–74
 6. Flores RM, Akhurst T, Gonen M et al (2003) Positron emission tomography defines metastatic disease but not locoregional disease in patients with malignant pleural mesothelioma. J Thorac Cardiovasc Surg 126(1):11–16
 7. Flores RM, Pass HI, Seshan VE (2008) Extrapleural pneumonectomy versus pleurectomy/decortication in the surgical management of malignant pleural mesothelioma: results in 663 patients. J Thorac Cardiovasc Surg 135: 620–626
 8. Gerbaudo VH, Mamede M, Trotman-Dickinson B (2007) PET/CT patterns of treatment failure of malignant pleural mesothelioma. J Nucl Med 48(Suppl 2):360
 9. Gerbaudo VH, Sugarbaker DJ, Britz-Cunningham S et al (2002) Assessment of malignant pleural mesothelioma with ^{18}F-FDG dual-head gamma-camera coincidence imaging: comparison with histopathology. J Nucl Med 43:1144–1149
10. Gerbaudo VH, Sugarbaker DJ, Britz-Cunningham S et al (2003) Metabolic significance of the pattern, intensity and kinetics of ^{18}F-FDG uptake in malignant pleural mesothelioma. Thorax 58(12):1077–1082
11. Giesel FL, Bischoff H, von Tengg-Kobligk H et al (2006) Dynamic contrast-enhanced MRI of malignant pleural mesothelioma: a feasibility study of noninvasive assessment, therapeutic follow-up, and possible predictor of improved outcome. Chest 129(6):1570–1576
12. Giesel FL, Choyke PL, Mehndiratta A et al (2008) Pharmacokinetic analysis of malignant pleural mesothelioma – initial results of tumor microcirculation and its correlation to microvessel density (CD-34). Acad Radiol 15(5):563–570
13. Gill RR, Gerbaudo VH, Jacobson FL et al (2008) MR imaging of benign and malignant

pleural disease. Magn Reson Imaging Clin N Am 16(2):319–339

14. Gill RR, Gerbaudo VH, Sugarbaker DJ et al (2009) Current trends in radiologic management of malignant pleural mesothelioma. Semin Thorac Cardiovasc Surg 21(2):111–120

15. Gill RR, Poh AC, Camp PC et al (2008) MDCT evaluation of central airway and vascular complications of lung transplantation. AJR Am J Roentgenol 191(4):1046–1056

16. Gill RR, Umeoka S, Mamata H, Tilleman TR, Stanwell P, Woodhams R, Padera RF, Sugarbaker DJ, Hatabu H (2010) Diffusion-weighted MRI of malignant pleural mesothelioma: preliminary assessment of apparent diffusion coefficient in histologic subtypes. AJR Am J Roentgenol. 195(2):W125–130

17. Hatabu H, Gaa J, Kim D et al (1996) Pulmonary perfusion: qualitative assessment with dynamic contrast-enhanced MRI using ultra-short TE and inversion recovery turbo FLASH. Magn Reson Med 36:503–508

18. Hatabu H, Tadamura E, Levin DL et al (1999) Quantitative assessment of pulmonary perfusion with dynamic contrast enhanced MRI. Magn Reson Med 42:1033–1038

19. Heelan RT, Rusch VW, Begg CB et al (1999) Staging of malignant pleural mesothelioma: comparison of CT and MR imaging. AJR Am J Roentgenol 172(4):1039–1047

20. Heilo A, Stenwig AE, Solheim OP (1999) Malignant pleural mesothelioma: US-guided histological core-needle biopsy. Radiology 211: 657–659

21. Jänne PA, Baldini EH (2004) Patterns of failure following surgical resection for malignant pleural mesothelioma. Thorac Surg Clin 14(4): 567–73

22. Kawashima A, Libshitz HI (1990) Malignant pleural mesothelioma: CT manifestations in 50 cases. AJR Am J Roentgenol 155(5):965–969

23. Krug LM, Pass HI, Rusch VW et al (2009) Multicenter phase II trial of neoadjuvant pemetrexed plus cisplatin followed by extrapleural pneumonectomy and radiation for malignant pleural mesothelioma. J Clin Oncol 27(18): 3007–3013

24. Matsuoka S, Tilleman RT, Mueller J et al (2008) Semi-automated tumor volume method: a practical and reproducible volume measurement for malignant pleural mesothelioma from standard CT images. International conference of the international mesothelioma interest group (IMIG), Amsterdam, September 2008

25. Metintas M, Ucgun I, Elbek O et al (2002) Computed tomography features in malignant pleural mesothelioma and other commonly seen pleural diseases. Eur J Radiol 41(1):1–9

26. Pass HI, Temeck BK, Kranda K et al (1998) Preoperative tumor volume is associated with outcome in malignant pleural mesothelioma. J Thorac Cardiovasc Surg 115(2):310–317

27. Patz EF, Shaffer K, Piwnica-Worms DR et al (1992) Malignant pleural mesothelioma: value of CT and MR imaging in predicting resectability. AJR Am J Roentgenol 159(5):961–966

28. Pelucchi C, Malvezzi M, La Vecchia C et al (2004) The mesothelioma epidemic in Western Europe: an update. Br J Cancer 90(5): 1022–1024

29. Sugarbaker DJ, Flores RM, Jaklitsch MT (1999) Resection margins, extrapleural nodal status, and cell type determine postoperative long-term survival in trimodality therapy of malignant pleural mesothelioma: results in 183 patients. J Thorac Cardiovasc Surg 117:54–63; discussion 63–5

30. Tilleman RT, Mujoomdar AA, Richards WG et al (2008) cMED: Mediastinal lymph node dissection and preoperative and postoperative staging of 180 consecutive mesothelioma patients –a single center experience. In: International conference of the international mesothelioma interest group (IMIG), Amsterdam, September 2008

31. Tilleman RT, Richards GW, Zellos L et al (2009) Extrapleural pneumonectomy followed by intracavitary intraoperative hyperthermic cisplatin with pharmacologic cytoprotection for treatment of malignant pleural mesothelioma: a phase II prospective study. J Thorac Cardiovasc Surg 138:405–441

32. Van Meerbeeck JP, Gaafar R, Manegold C et al (2005) Randomized phase III study of cisplatin with or without raltitrexed in patients with malignant pleural mesothelioma: an intergroup study of the European Organisation for Research and Treatment of Cancer Lung Cancer Group and the National Cancer Institute of Canada. J Clin Oncol 23:6881–6889

33. Vogelzang NJ, Rusthoven JJ, Symanowski J et al (2003) Phase III study of pemetrexed in combination with cisplatin versus cisplatin

alone in patients with malignant pleural mesothelioma. J Clin Oncol 21:2636–2644

34. Wang ZJ, Reddy GP, Gotway MB et al (2004)
Malignant pleural mesothelioma: evaluation
with CT, MR imaging, and PET. Radiographics
24(1):105–119

35. Wolf AS, Jacobson FL, Tilleman TR (2010)
Managing the pneumonectomy space after

extrapleural pneumonectomy: postoperative
intrathoracic pressure monitoring. Eur J
Cardiothorac Surg 37(4):770–775, Epub 2010
Jan 6

36. Yamamuro M, Gerbaudo VH, Gill RR (2007)
Morphologic and functional imaging of malignant pleural mesothelioma. Eur J Radiol 64(3):
356–366, Epub 2007 Oct 22

Biopsy Techniques for the Diagnosis of Mesothelioma

4

J. Walters and Nick A. Maskell

Abstract The incidence of mesothelioma continues to increase in the Western world and is likely to do so until 2011–2015. It commonly presents with breathlessness secondary to a pleural effusion, and whilst guidelines still advise thoracocentesis as the first line investigation, the sensitivity of this is low and a tissue diagnosis is usually required. Abrams needle biopsy also has a low diagnostic yield and high complication rate and is not recommended in guidelines on the investigation of mesothelioma. Computed tomography–guided biopsy or thoracoscopy both have a comparable sensitivity and low complication rates. Local anaesthetic thoracoscopy is increasingly used by respiratory physicians and has a comparable diagnostic sensitivity to Video-Assisted Thoracoscopic Surgery (VATS) without the need for a general anaesthetic. The requirement for prophylactic radiotherapy after pleural procedures in cases of mesothelioma is contentious, as the results from early trials suggesting it reduces tract seeding have been disputed by more recent trials.

J. Walters
North Bristol Lung Centre, Southmead Hospital,
Bristol BS10 5NB, UK
e-mail: james@drwalters.co.uk

N.A. Maskell (✉)
Department of Clinical Sciences,
Learning and Research Centre, Southmead Hospital,
University of Bristol, Bristol BS10 5NB, UK
e-mail: nick.maskell@bristol.ac.uk

4.1
Introduction

The incidence of mesothelioma continues to increase; it has a poor prognosis and definitive diagnosis is often difficult to obtain [56]. In Europe, 5,000 people die annually from mesothelioma [47] and in Britain the incidence is projected to peak in 2011–2015 at 1,950–2,450 deaths per year [29]. The prognosis is poor with a study in the USA [52] showing a 1-year survival of 64% from onset of symptoms and median survival of 10 months. A British study [61] found a median survival of 14 months from the onset of symptoms.

A. Tannapfel (ed.), *Malignant Mesothelioma*, Recent Results in Cancer Research 189,
DOI: 10.1007/978-3-642-10862-4_4, © Springer-Verlag Berlin Heidelberg 2011

4

4.2
Clinical Presentation

The most common clinical presentation for patients is progressive dyspnoea and/or chest wall pain [17]. Dyspnoea at presentation is usually caused by a pleural effusion but as the disease progresses this can be caused by pleural restriction. At presentation 90% patients have a pleural effusion with 10% patients having little or no fluid [30]. The effusion is usually unilateral (95%). The chest wall pain is usually caused by significant chest wall invasion. Other symptoms include a dry cough, weight loss, fever, fatigue or night sweats. The patient may also present after abnormalities are found on a routine chest radiograph [2] or present with minimal non-specific symptoms with the diagnosis only becoming apparent with time.

A detailed occupational history is important, although sometimes difficult because of the time that has elapsed since the exposure. Common prior occupational exposures include laggers, pipefitters, plumbers, heavy construction or shipbuilding industry workers and those working aboard ships, especially in the boiler room.

4.3
Investigation of Pleural Effusion

Mesothelioma may be suspected on presentation because of the history, including exposure and symptoms, and abnormalities on the chest radiograph. If a pleural effusion is present then the initial investigations should be a diagnostic/therapeutic pleural aspiration and contrast-enhanced computed tomography (CT) [62]. The contrast allows differentiation between thickened pleura, pleural effusion and underlying collapsed or aerated lung, allowing a detailed look at the pleura including whether the pleural thickening is irregular, circumferential and involves the mediastinal border. It also aids decisions regarding the next, most appropriate, investigation. Pleural aspiration is a simple investigation that can be performed, under ultrasound guidance, in clinic at the initial review and should be sent for cytology with immunocytochemistry if appropriate [2].

4.3.1
Cytology

The diagnostic sensitivity of pleural cytology with malignancy has been reported at about 60% [24, 43]; however, the reported sensitivity for mesothelioma has been reported as much lower than this at 20–32% [32, 51]. This number included those that were suspicious but not diagnostic for mesothelioma. If only the positive results were included and the suspicious results excluded, the sensitivity decreased to 16%. However, it is worth noting that if cytology is positive then the median time to diagnosis is reduced. In one study, this time was reduced from an average of 12 to 4 weeks. It often proves difficult to differentiate between reactive mesothelial cells secondary to an inflammatory response and malignant cells; therefore, pleural tissue is often required to confirm the diagnosis. Immunocytochemistry can help to differentiate between mesothelioma and adenocarcinoma [23]. Sending a second sample if the first was negative has been shown to increase the yield for malignancy by a further 27% [24]; however, in the case of mesothelioma it is unlikely to be this successful and likely to delay diagnosis further. Repeated thoracocentesis has also been shown to increase the number of pleural loculations [16] which could have an impact on later investigations such as thoracoscopy.

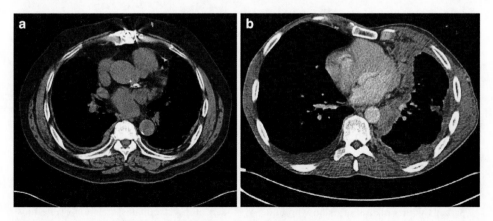

Fig. 4.1 (**a, b**) Benign and malignant pleural thickening on CT scan

The European Respiratory Society (ERS) and European Society of Thoracic Surgeons (ESTS) guidelines on the management of mesothelioma state that it is not recommended to make a diagnosis of mesothelioma based on cytology alone because of the high risk of diagnostic error.

4.4
Investigation of Pleural Thickening with No Effusion

Benign causes of pleural thickening commonly include previous pleural infection or haemothorax and benign asbestos-related pleural thickening. When seen at the lung apices it is generally due to prior infection from tuberculosis or fungi [17]. It is uncommon for asbestos to cause apical pleural thickening.

CT changes suggesting malignancy as opposed to benign pleural thickening are (1) circumferential thickening, (2) nodular pleural thickening, (3) parietal pleural thickening >1 cm and (4) mediastinal pleural involvement [35]. Whilst these changes were specific (100%, 94%, 94% and 88%, respectively), they were not overly sensitive (41%, 51%, 36% and 56%, respectively), and did not allow differentiation of mesothelioma from other cancers. If there is evidence suggesting malignancy, these patients will require a pleural biopsy. The thoracic CT scan is helpful in deciding which method would be most suitable (Fig. 4.1a, b).

4.5
Percutaneous Pleural Biopsy Techniques

4.5.1
Abrams Needle

The use of a blind closed needle biopsy (BCNB) was first described by Abrams in 1958 [3]. It provided an alternative to an open pleural biopsy, which requires a general anaesthetic [7]. Compared to other pleural biopsy techniques it

4

is inexpensive and can be carried out under local anaesthetic. Chakrabarti et al. found no difference in the diagnostic sensitivity between respiratory registrars and their more junior counterparts [13]. Although low yields were reported when diagnosing mesothelioma, it was hoped that this might be improved with the advent of improved histopathological tests [7].

Abrams needle biopsy has been shown to increase the yield in diagnosing malignancy over cytology by 7–27% [43, 48]. There have been two recent reviews of BCNB. In one, of 75 patients with a pleural effusion who underwent BCNB, 46 patients were ultimately diagnosed with malignancy. The initial Abrams biopsy was diagnostic in 20 of the 46 patients diagnosed with malignancy (43%). In those diagnosed with mesothelioma the Abrams biopsy was diagnostic in 4 of 13 cases (31%) [13]. In another review of 119 patients ultimately diagnosed with mesothelioma who underwent BCNB, a definitive diagnosis was made in 44 (46%) whilst the result was suspicious in 20 (21%) [37]. The results in an earlier trial were higher, with five of seven (71%) patients with mesothelioma being diagnosed with an Abrams needle biopsy [7]. A recent trial attempted to increase the sensitivity of an Abrams needle biopsy by determining the entry site with the use of a contemporaneous thoracic CT and measuring the distance between entry and target site two dimensionally on the CT [39]. The sensitivity for diagnosing mesothelioma was 80%. Other attempts have been made to increase the sensitivity by methods such as pleural brushings [6], but diagnostic yields are no greater than 50%. The only randomised controlled trial directly comparing CT-guided cutting needle to blind Abrams biopsy [36] looked at 50 consecutive patients. It showed a significantly increased sensitivity with a CT-guided cutting needle (87%) compared to the Abrams biopsy (47%) in the diagnosis of malignancy and the results were similar when looking at mesothelioma.

Complications of Abrams biopsy include site pain (1–15%), pneumothorax (3–15%), vasovagal reaction (1–5%), haemothorax (<2%), site haematoma (<1%), transient fever (<1%) and very rarely death secondary to haemorrhage.

4.5.2
Radiologically Guided Percutaneous Pleural Biopsy

Pleural thickening, whether benign or malignant, is frequently not uniform, and image-guided biopsy facilitates selection of the most appropriate biopsy site. It also enables safe biopsies in the absence of a pleural effusion. Percutaneous pleural biopsy has been described with both transthoracic ultrasound (US) and CT as image guidance modalities.

US has been used increasingly by respiratory physicians to assess pleural effusions as it has become clear that it increases the success of pleural aspiration and reduces complications [25, 33] and is now recommended in the 2010 BTS pleural disease guidelines for all pleural procedures performed on the ward [62]. US allows real-time images of the biopsy, is readily available and has no radiation risk to the patient. In one review of US-guided cutting needle biopsy versus Abrams needle biopsy, 49 patients underwent pleural biopsy, 25 with an US-guided Tru-Cut needle and 24 with an Abrams needle [14]. In the subgroup diagnosed with mesothelioma, the sensitivity was higher with a US-guided Tru-cut needle with a trend towards statistical significance. Another study looked at the sensitivity and safety of using an US-guided Tru-Cut needle in the diagnosis of pleurally based abnormalities >20 mm in the absence of a pleural effusion (those with effusions underwent aspiration +/− thoracoscopy) [20]. Ninety-one patients underwent biopsies by either a respiratory physician or a registrar under supervision. Of these, 10 had mesothelioma and all were diagnosed on the first biopsy. Helio et al. found similar sensitivities for diagnosing mesothelioma with a US-guided cutting needle [28]. Of 52 patients diagnosed with mesothelioma, 40 (77%) were diagnosed after their first biopsy attempt.

CT-guided biopsy permits access to areas not easily accessible to ultrasound such as pleural lesions near or behind ribs or along the paravertebral surfaces [50]. Higher sensitivities have been reported with CT than with US-guided biopsies although there have been no trials directly comparing them [49]. Metintas et al. looked at 30 patients with mesothelioma who underwent CT-guided closed needle biopsy. This was diagnostic in 25 (83.3%) [41]. Adams et al. reviewed 21 cases of mesothelioma that had received an image-guided biopsy in their work up (6 US and 15 CT) [5]. Their diagnostic sensitivity was 86%. It is also worth noting that of these, four patients had a pleural thickness of less than 5 mm and all of these biopsies were successful.

Cutting needle biopsy has been shown to be more sensitive than fine needle aspiration in the diagnosis of malignancy and the difference is even more marked with mesothelioma [4, 5] with a sensitivity of 93 versus 50% in favour of using a cutting needle. The overall sensitivity can be increased with a combination of both techniques.

Complications occur in less than 5% patients using image-guided pleural biopsy techniques [50] and include pneumothorax, intrapleural bleeding, subcutaneous haematoma and damage to the diaphragm and abdominal viscera.

One study of 85 image-guided biopsies showed their rate of new pneumothoraces was 11% but only 4.7% patients had a new pneumothorax visible on chest radiograph [8]. Of these patients two already had a chest drain in situ and six had had a drain inserted as part of the procedure for drainage of pleural fluid. Therefore, no patient required insertion of a chest drain solely for drainage of a biopsy-induced pneumothorax. 7.5% CT-guided biopsies were associated with

significant bleeding but all remained haemodynamically stable.

4.5.3
Positron Emission Tomography (PET) CT

PET scans are increasingly being used in the evaluation of patients with mesothelioma [58]. F-fluoro-2-deoxy-D-glucose (FDG)–PET has been shown to accurately differentiate benign pleural disease from mesothelioma. In one study of 98 patients with 63 pleural malignancies, FDG-PET had a sensitivity for detecting malignancy of 96.8% and a specificity of 88.5% and appeared to confirm malignant pleural disease that cannot be identified at CT [21]. Neither of the two malignancies that did not show FDG were mesothelioma.

Another study of nine patients with mesothelioma [45] showed that all the primary tumours were FDG positive.

Although no trials have looked at PET-CT being used to increase the diagnostic yield of CT-guided biopsies, there may be a role for this in the future, particularly in those patients who clinically appear to have mesothelioma but have already had negative biopsies and are not suitable for thoracoscopic/surgical biopsies.

4.6
Thoracoscopy

Thoracoscopy was first described in 1910 [31]. It provides a means of diagnosis for effusions of unknown cause and is particularly important in the diagnosis and management of malignant pleural mesothelioma [2]. It is now recommended by the European Respiratory Society and the European Society of Thoracic Surgeons [56] and the British Thoracic Society [63] early in the diagnostic pathway of patients with a symptomatic exudative pleural effusion

4

of unknown cause. Thoracoscopy can be performed by surgeons under general anaesthetic – Video-Assisted Thoracoscopic Surgery (VATS) but increasingly is being performed by physicians under local anaesthetic – Local Anaesthetic Thoracoscopy (LAT). In the UK the number of centres offering LAT has increased from 11 in 1999 to 37 in 2009 [63].

Thoracoscopy allows direct visual assessment of the pleura and subsequent biopsy of the abnormal areas as well the option of a therapeutic talc poudrage at the same time. Success rates for pleurodesis via thoracoscopy are generally very good and can be as high as 86% [38] at 1 month.

4.6.1
Local Anaesthetic Thoracoscopy

This allows direct visualisation of the pleura and the option of a therapeutic procedure without the need for a general anaesthetic. This is an important advantage over VATS as many patients requiring thoracoscopy have comorbidities and a reduced performance status leading to significant risk from a general anaesthetic. It should, however, be noted that across Europe many physicians carrying out thoracoscopy choose to perform this in the presence of an anaesthetist (and often a GA). Boutin et al. reviewed 188 cases of mesothelioma that had undergone thoracoscopy [10]. 185/188 (98.4%) were diagnosed after thoracoscopy with a 100% specificity. These results have been mirrored in a number of recent studies [9, 22, 38, 42, 54, 57, 59] with the sensitivity for the diagnosis of mesothelioma ranging from 88% to 100% with a specificity of 100% (see Table 4.1).

The thoracoscope can be flexible, semirigid or rigid. One study comparing the use of rigid with flexible thoracoscope [18] looked at 30 consecutive patients with pleural effusion of unknown cause. The first 10 underwent rigid thoracoscopy whilst the following 20 underwent thoracoscopy with both rigid and flexible

thoracoscope. Of those with a final diagnosis of mesothelioma 13/15 (87%) were diagnosed at thoracoscopy. Three biopsies were more informative with the flexible thoracoscope whilst eight were more informative with the rigid thoracoscope. Two biopsies from the flexible thoracoscope were upgraded from reactive pleurisy to mesothelioma by the rigid thoracoscope biopsies. Overall, it was felt that the rigid instrument was superior because it was easier to manipulate and obtain larger biopsies. Munavvar et al. [42] trialled the use of a semirigid thoracoscope, hoping to combine the advantages of the flexible and rigid instruments. They correctly diagnosed 15/15 patients with mesothelioma and did not appear to experience the difficulties previously described with the flexible thoracoscope.

Most centres require at least some pleural fluid to be able to perform thoracoscopy. One centre found approximately 10% of pleural effusions too small for a standard thoracoscope and therefore trialed a smaller instrument [59]. They used a minilaparoscope, which was 3.3 mm rather than the standard 7 mm. They were able to they were able to use this on small, loculated effusions inaccessible to the larger instrument, but no figures were given. They felt that the histological samples were comparable although the samples were smaller with the 3.3mm instrument, only 8F drains could be used, the procedure was 20% longer and conversion to conventional thoracoscopy was sometimes used.

Autofluorescence has also been used to try and improve diagnostic yield by correct identification of the abnormal area to biopsy and to aid with staging by helping to delineate the tumour margins [15]. Preliminary results from 24 patients showed that in all 16 cases of pleural malignancy (seven of whom had mesothelioma) the colour of the affected area changed from white/pink to red, giving a sensitivity of 100%. However, in 2/8 cases of chronic pleurits, there was a similar colour change giving a specificity of 75%.

Alternative forceps has also been used to try and increase the yield. Sasada et al. [55] have used an insulated-tip diathermic knife and

Table 4.1 Results from local anaesthetic thoracoscopy reported since 2000

Trial	Number of thoracoscopies for undiagnosed pleural effusion	Number of patients where biopsies possible	Diagnostic yield %[a]	Number diagnosed with malignancy/total with malignancy (sensitivity)	Number with mesothelioma	Number diagnosed with mesothelioma
Tassi et al. [59]	30	30	93.4	12/13 (92.3%)	5	5 (100%)
Medford et al.[b] [38]	125	117	90.4	57/60 (95%)	30	29 (96.6%)
Fletcher et al. [22]	50	47	90	37/42 (88.1%)	35	31 (88.6%)
Munavvar et al.[b] [42]	57	54	86.0	32/37 (86.5%)	15	15 (100%)
Blanc et al. [9]	149	142	93.3	77/85 (90.6%)	48	42 (87.5%)
Simpson et al. [57]	89	89	95.5	69/73 (94.5%)	25	24 (96%)
Sakuraba et al. [54]	138	138	97.1	25/27 (92.6%)	10	10 (100%)

[a]Diagnostic yield includes patients where biopsy attempts were unsuccessful
[b]Data not available on patients where biopsies not taken therefore not included when calculating sensitivity for diagnosing malignancy or mesothelioma

compared this to standard flexible forceps in 20 cases. There overall diagnostic yield was low using the standard forceps at 60% and this was increased to 85% with the use of the diathermic knife. Combined, they achieved a sensitivity of 100%. It is worth noting, however, that the diagnosis of mesothelioma was only reached in 3/6 patients using the diathermic knife and in all 6 with the standard forceps.

The main reason for failure or 'non-diagnosis' with LAT was inability to visualise the presence of all the pleural space or significant adhesions, making further investigation too difficult or unsafe. Major complications following thoracoscopy are rare. The BTS guidelines for thoracoscopy reviewed 47 trials that reported complications [63]. Death occurred in 16/4,736 cases (0.34%) but was reduced to 0/2,421 when only studies involving diagnostic thoracoscopy were included. A major contribution to the mortality (9/16 deaths) occurred in a trial of talc poudrage in the USA where ungraded talc particles were used.

Major complications (empyema, haemorrhage, port site tumour growth, bronchopleural fistula, post-operative pneumothorax or air leak and pneumonia) were reported in 1.8% cases whilst minor complications (subcutaneous emphysema, minor haemorrhage, operative skin site infection, hypotension during procedure, raised temperature and atrial fibrillation) were reported in 7.3% cases.

4.6.2
Video-Assisted Thoracoscopic Surgery

VATS usually requires general anaesthesia and the placement of a dual lumen tube. VATS is therefore more expensive and time consuming than LAT [53]. There have been no trials directly comparing it to LAT; however, the diagnostic efficacy of the two methods appears comparable. Harris et al. performed VATS on 182 patients [27]. Of the 98 patients with malignancy 29

4

(30%) had mesothelioma. Their diagnostic sensitivity for malignancy was 95% with a specificity of 100% though they did not state what malignancies the 5 false negatives were. Grossebner et al. reported on 25 patients referred with suspected mesothelioma [26]. Of these 23 had mesothelioma and all were diagnosed from VATS biopsy.

Comparing complications and length of stay in hospital is difficult because more extensive procedures are often carried out in the VATS groups and there are no recent trials looking purely at diagnosis with or without pleurodesis. Studies looking at complications from VATS often include patients with conditions such as empyema that require the extensive breaking down of adhesions, which is more difficult with LAT. However, complications do seem higher with VATS; de Groot et al. reported that nine (26%) of their patients had a major complication [19] whilst Harris et al. reported one death (due to pulmonary laceration), major complications in 15% (haemorrhage, prolonged air leak, empyema, pneumonia, wound infection, congestive cardiac failure, entering peritoneum, biopsy pneumothorax, myocardial infarction, post operative seizure) and minor complications in 8% (subcutaneous emphysema, fever, hypotension, intercostal neuritis) [27]. However, Viskum et al. reported no deaths in their series of 566 examinations with air embolism and cardiac dysrhythmias occurring in less than 1% [60].

4.7
Open Biopsy

Prior to thoracoscopy, this was the next stage in the diagnostic pathway if closed needle biopsy failed. It is now required only if there is obliteration of the pleural space and CT-guided biopsy is not possible or has failed to reach a diagnosis [46].

Its main complication is intractable chest wall pain [7]. Of all the pleural biopsy techniques,

this technique has the highest rate of tract seeding [34, 40].

4.8
Prophylactic Radiotherapy

Mesothelioma seeding along pleural intervention tracts is well recognised and present as subcutaneous nodules of varying size. O'Rourke et al. recorded the characteristics of 12 patients that had subcutaneous nodules [44]. 75% reported mild pain, 17% slight pain and 8.3% moderate pain with ulceration in 1 patient. A review of the literature on tract seeding of mesothelioma [34] found that this ranged from 0% to 48% with the risks highest after thoracotomy (24%) and thoracoscopy (9–16%) and lower for smaller incisions such as needle biopsy (0–22%). A recent study of 212 patients who did not receive prophylactic radiotherapy showed that there was an overall rate of tract seeding of 13.2% [40]. Seeding was more common after thoracotomy (25.8%) versus thoracoscopy and closed needle biopsy or CT-guided biopsy (11.0%). 157 patients received chemotherapy and 26 received multi-modal therapy which may explain why the recurrence rate was lower than the 40% reported by Boutin et al. [11] in the control arm of their trial of prophylactic radiotherapy. Boutin showed no tumour seedling in the intervention arm (21 Gy in three fractions) and this trial result led to national guidelines promoting the practise of giving prophylactic radiotherapy after pleural interventions in patients with mesothelioma [1, 2]. Recent trials, however, have failed to support its use. Bydder et al. randomised 43 patients (58 sites) to receive a single dose of radiotherapy (10 Gy) or no radiotherapy [12] whilst O'Rourke et al. recruited 61 patients (60 sites) to have three fractions of 7 Gy or no radiotherapy. Both studies showed no difference in tumour seeding between their control and treatment groups

(10% control vs 7% radiotherapy and 10% control vs 13% radiotherapy, respectively). Important differences between the trials were that all of the patients in Boutin's original trial underwent a thoracoscopy (with a large chest wall incision) whilst only 23–39% in the two more recent trials did. There was also a difference in the radiotherapy regime in Bydder trial. All of these trials are underpowered and there is therefore still the need for a definitive trial to inform practise.

References

1. American Thoracic Society (2000) Management of malignant pleural effusions. Am J Respir Crit Care Med 162:1987–2001
2. British Thoracic Society Standards of Care Committee (2007) BTS statement on malignant mesothelioma in the UK, 2007. Thorax 62(Suppl 2):ii1–ii19
3. Abrams LD (1958) A pleural-biopsy punch. Lancet 1:30–31
4. Adams RF, Gleeson FV (2001) Percutaneous image-guided cutting-needle biopsy of the pleura in the presence of a suspected malignant effusion. Radiology 219:510–514
5. Adams RF, Gray W, Davies RJ, Gleeson FV (2001) Percutaneous image-guided cutting needle biopsy of the pleura in the diagnosis of malignant mesothelioma. Chest 120:1798–1802
6. Aksoy E, Atac G, Sevim T, Gungor G, Torun T, Maden E, Tahaoglu K (2005) Diagnostic yield of closed pleural brushing. Tüberk Toraks 53:238–244
7. Beauchamp HD, Kundra NK, Aranson R, Chong F, MacDonnell KF (1992) The role of closed pleural needle biopsy in the diagnosis of malignant mesothelioma of the pleura. Chest 102:1110–1112
8. Benamore RE, Scott K, Richards CJ, Entwisle JJ (2006) Image-guided pleural biopsy: diagnostic yield and complications. Clin Radiol 61:700–705
9. Blanc FX, Atassi K, Bignon J, Housset B (2002) Diagnostic value of medical thoracoscopy in pleural disease: a 6-year retrospective study. Chest 121:1677–1683
10. Boutin C, Rey F (1993) Thoracoscopy in pleural malignant mesothelioma: a prospective study of 188 consecutive patients. Part 1. Diagnosis. Cancer 72:389–393
11. Boutin C, Rey F, Viallat JR (1995) Prevention of malignant seeding after invasive diagnostic procedures in patients with pleural mesothelioma. A randomized trial of local radiotherapy. Chest 108:754–758
12. Bydder S, Phillips M, Joseph DJ, Cameron F, Spry NA, DeMelker Y, Musk AW (2004) A randomised trial of single-dose radiotherapy to prevent procedure tract metastasis by malignant mesothelioma. Br J Cancer 91:9–10
13. Chakrabarti B, Ryland I, Sheard J, Warburton CJ, Earis JE (2006) The role of Abrams percutaneous pleural biopsy in the investigation of exudative pleural effusions. Chest 129:1549–1555
14. Chang DB, Yang PC, Luh KT, Kuo SH, Yu CJ (1991) Ultrasound-guided pleural biopsy with Tru-Cut needle. Chest 100:1328–1333
15. Chrysanthidis MG, Janssen JP (2005) Autofluorescence videothoracoscopy in exudative pleural effusions: preliminary results. Eur Respir J 26:989–992
16. Chung CL, Chen YC, Chang SC (2003) Effect of repeated thoracenteses on fluid characteristics, cytokines, and fibrinolytic activity in malignant pleural effusion. Chest 123:1188–1195
17. Cugell DW, Kamp DW (2004) Asbestos and the pleura: a review. Chest 125:1103–1117
18. Davidson AC, George RJ, Sheldon CD, Sinha G, Corrin B, Geddes DM (1988) Thoracoscopy: assessment of a physician service and comparison of a flexible bronchoscope used as a thoracoscope with a rigid thoracoscope. Thorax 43:327–332
19. de Groot M, Walther G (1998) Thoracoscopy in undiagnosed pleural effusions. S Afr Med J 88:706–711
20. Diacon AH, Schuurmans MM, Theron J, Schubert PT, Wright CA, Bolliger CT (2004) Safety and yield of ultrasound-assisted transthoracic biopsy performed by pulmonologists. Respiration 71:519–522
21. Duysinx B, Nguyen D, Louis R, Cataldo D, Belhocine T, Bartsch P, Bury T (2004) Evaluation of pleural disease with 18-fluorodeoxyglucose positron emission tomography imaging. Chest 125:489–493
22. Fletcher SV, Clark RJ (2007) The Portsmouth thoracoscopy experience, an evaluation of

service by retrospective case note analysis. Respir Med 101:1021–1025

23. Froudarakis ME (2008) Diagnostic work-up of pleural effusions. Respiration 75:4–13

24. Garcia LW, Ducatman BS, Wang HH (1994) The value of multiple fluid specimens in the cytological diagnosis of malignancy. Mod Pathol 7:665–668

25. Grogan DR, Irwin RS, Channick R, Raptopoulos V, Curley FJ, Bartter T, Corwin RW (1990) Complications associated with thoracentesis. A prospective, randomized study comparing three different methods. Arch Intern Med 150: 873–877

26. Grossebner MW, Arifi AA, Goddard M, Ritchie AJ (1999) Mesothelioma–VATS biopsy and lung mobilization improves diagnosis and palliation. Eur J Cardiothorac Surg 16:619–623

27. Harris RJ, Kavuru MS, Mehta AC, Medendorp SV, Wiedemann HP, Kirby TJ, Rice TW (1995) The impact of thoracoscopy on the management of pleural disease. Chest 107:845–852

28. Heilo A, Stenwig AE, Solheim OP (1999) Malignant pleural mesothelioma: US-guided histologic core-needle biopsy. Radiology 211: 657–659

29. Hodgson JT, McElvenny DM, Darnton AJ, Price MJ, Peto J (2005) The expected burden of mesothelioma mortality in Great Britain from 2002 to 2050. Br J Cancer 92:587–593

30. Ismail-Khan R, Robinson LA, Williams CC Jr, Garrett CR, Bepler G, Simon GR (2006) Malignant pleural mesothelioma: a comprehensive review. Cancer Control 13:255–263

31. Jacobeus HC (1910) Uber die Mogllichkeit die Zystoskope bei untersuchung seroser hohlungen anzuwenden. Münch Med Wochenschr 40: 2090–2092

32. Johnston WW (1985) The malignant pleural effusion. A review of cytopathologic diagnoses of 584 specimens from 472 consecutive patients. Cancer 56:905–909

33. Kohan JM, Poe RH, Israel RH, Kennedy JD, Benazzi RB, Kallay MC, Greenblatt DW (1986) Value of chest ultrasonography versus decubitus roentgenography for thoracentesis. Am Rev Respir Dis 133:1124–1126

34. Lee C, Bayman N, Swindell R, Faivre-Finn C (2009) Prophylactic radiotherapy to intervention sites in mesothelioma: a systematic review

and survey of UK practice. Lung Cancer 66: 150–156

35. Leung AN, Muller NL, Miller RR (1990) CT in differential diagnosis of diffuse pleural disease. AJR Am J Roentgenol 154:487–492

36. Maskell NA, Gleeson FV, Davies RJ (2003) Standard pleural biopsy versus CT-guided cutting-needle biopsy for diagnosis of malignant disease in pleural effusions: a randomised controlled trial. Lancet 361:1326–1330

37. McLaughlin KM, Kerr KM, Currie GP (2009) Closed pleural biopsy to diagnose mesothelioma: dead or alive? Lung Cancer 65: 388–389

38. Medford AR, Agrawal S, Free CM, Bennett JA (2009) A local anaesthetic video-assisted thoracoscopy service: prospective performance analysis in a UK tertiary respiratory centre. Lung Cancer 66:355–358

39. Metintas M, Ak G, Dundar E, Yildirim H, Ozkan R, Kurt E, Erginel S, Alatas F, Metintas S (2010) Medical thoracoscopy versus computed tomography guided Abrams Pleural needle biopsy for diagnosis of patients with pleural effusions: a randomized controlled trial. Chest 137(6): 1362–1368

40. Metintas M, Ak G, Parspour S, Yildirim H, Erginel S, Alatas F, Batirel HF, Sivrikoz C, Metintas S, Dundar E (2008) Local recurrence of tumor at sites of intervention in malignant pleural mesothelioma. Lung Cancer 61:255–261

41. Metintas M, Ozdemir N, Isiksoy S, Kaya T, Ekici M, Erginel S, Harmanci E, Erdinc P, Ulgey N, Alatas F (1995) CT-guided pleural needle biopsy in the diagnosis of malignant mesothelioma. J Comput Assist Tomogr 19:370–374

42. Munavvar M, Khan MA, Edwards J, Waqaruddin Z, Mills J (2007) The autoclavable semirigid thoracoscope: the way forward in pleural disease? Eur Respir J 29:571–574

43. Nance KV, Shermer RW, Askin FB (1991) Diagnostic efficacy of pleural biopsy as compared with that of pleural fluid examination. Mod Pathol 4:320–324

44. O'Rourke N, Garcia JC, Paul J, Lawless C, McMenemin R, Hill J (2007) A randomised controlled trial of intervention site radiotherapy in malignant pleural mesothelioma. Radiother Oncol 84:18–22

45. Otsuka H, Terazawa K, Morita N, Otomi Y, Yamashita K, Nishitani H (2009) Is FDG-PET/CT useful for managing malignant pleural mesothelioma? J Med Invest 56:16–20

46. Pass HI (2001) Malignant pleural mesothelioma: surgical roles and novel therapies. Clin Lung Cancer 3:102–117

47. Peto J, Hodgson JT, Matthews FE, Jones JR (1995) Continuing increase in mesothelioma mortality in Britain. Lancet 345:535–539

48. Prakash UB, Reiman HM (1985) Comparison of needle biopsy with cytologic analysis for the evaluation of pleural effusion: analysis of 414 cases. Mayo Clin Proc 60:158–164

49. Qureshi NR, Gleeson FV (2006) Imaging of pleural disease. Clin Chest Med 27:193–213

50. Rahman NM, Gleeson FV (2008) Image-guided pleural biopsy. Curr Opin Pulm Med 14:331–336

51. Renshaw AA, Dean BR, Antman KH, Sugarbaker DJ, Cibas ES (1997) The role of cytologic evaluation of pleural fluid in the diagnosis of malignant mesothelioma. Chest 111:106–109

52. Ribak J, Selikoff IJ (1992) Survival of asbestos insulation workers with mesothelioma. Br J Ind Med 49:732–735

53. Rodriguez-Panadero F, Janssen JP, Astoul P (2006) Thoracoscopy: general overview and place in the diagnosis and management of pleural effusion. Eur Respir J 28:409–422

54. Sakuraba M, Masuda K, Hebisawa A, Sagara Y, Komatsu H (2006) Diagnostic value of thoracoscopic pleural biopsy for pleurisy under local anaesthesia. ANZ J Surg 76:722–724

55. Sasada S, Kawahara K, Kusunoki Y, Okamoto N, Iwasaki T, Suzuki H, Kobayashi M, Hirashima T, Matsui K, Ohta M, Miyazawa T (2009) A new electrocautery pleural biopsy technique using an insulated-tip diathermic knife during semirigid pleuroscopy. Surg Endosc 23:1901–1907

56. Scherpereel A, Astoul P, Baas P, Berghmans T, Clayson H, de Vuyst P, Dienemann H, Galateau-Salle F, Hennequin C, Hillerdal G, Le Pechoux C, Mutti L, Pairon JC, Stahel R, van Houtte P, van Meerbeeck J, Waller D, Weder W (2010) Guidelines of the European Respiratory Society and the European Society of Thoracic Surgeons for the management of malignant pleural mesothelioma. Eur Respir J 35:479–495

57. Simpson G (2007) Medical thoracoscopy in an Australian regional hospital. Intern Med J 37: 267–269

58. Subramaniam RM, Wilcox B, Aubry MC, Jett J, Peller PJ (2009) 18F-fluoro-2-deoxy-D-glucose positron emission tomography and positron emission tomography/computed tomography imaging of malignant pleural mesothelioma. J Med Imaging Radiat Oncol 53:160–169, quiz 170

59. Tassi G, Marchetti G (2003) Minithoracoscopy: a less invasive approach to thoracoscopy. Chest 124:1975–1977

60. Viskum K, Enk B (1981) Complications of thoracoscopy. Poumon Coeur 37:25–28

61. Yates DH, Corrin B, Stidolph PN, Browne K (1997) Malignant mesothelioma in south east England: clinicopathological experience of 272 cases. Thorax 52:507–512

62. Hooper C, Lee YC, Maskell NA (2010) Investigation of a unilateral pleural effusion in adults: British Thoracic Society pleural disease guideline 2010. Thorax 65(suppl 2):ii4–ii17

63. Rahman NM, Ali NJ, Brown G, Chapman SJ, Davies RJO, Downer NJ, Gleeson FV, Howes TQ, Treasure T, Singh S, Phillips GD (2010) Local anaesthetic thoracoscopy: British Thoracic Society pleural disease guideline 2010. Thorax 65(suppl 2):ii54–ii60

Pathohistological Diagnosis and Differential Diagnosis

5

Iris Tischoff, Matthias Neid, Volker Neumann, and Andrea Tannapfel

Abstract Malignant mesothelioma is a rare aggressive tumour arising from mesothelial cells of the pleural and peritoneal cavity including pericardium and tunica vaginalis testis. Malignant mesothelioma occurs predominantly in men (>90%). Asbestos exposure is the best known and evaluated risk factor with a long latency period between exposure and onset of malignant mesothelioma ranging from 15 to 60 years. Exposure to erionite leads to higher incidences of mesothelioma and play an important role in environmental exposure (Turkey). Other possible risk factors are radiation, recurrent pleuritis/peritonitis and simian virus 40 (SV 40).

Malignant pleural mesothelioma is most common, whereas malignant peritoneal mesothelioma accounts only for 6–10%. Infrequent sites of origin are the pericardium and tunica vaginalis in 1–2%.

Malignant mesothelioma shows either diffuse growth pattern or occurs as a localised tumour mass. Diffuse type represents an aggressive tumour with poor prognosis and is incurable in most cases.

According to the WHO classification, three histological subtypes are distinguished: epithelioid, sarcomatoid and biphasic malignant mesothelioma.

Rare variants are desmoplastic type, a subtype of sarcomatoid mesothelioma, undifferentiated type and deciduoid type. Epithelioid type is the most frequent one, but biphasic malignant mesothelioma occurs in 30%. Pure sarcomatoid or biphasic type is seen less frequently in malignant peritoneal mesothelioma than in its pleural counterpart.

Well-differentiated papillary mesothelioma is a generally non-invasive mesothelioma with low malignant potential that arises mostly in females in the peritoneal cavity. Histological type is an important prognostic marker. Longest survival is seen in patients with epithelioid malignant mesothelioma. Sarcomatoid subtype has the worst prognosis.

Malignant mesothelioma shows macroscopical and microscopical similarities to benign lesions and other malignancies. Therefore, reactive mesothelial proliferations on the one hand and secondary tumours resembling mesothelial cells as well as benign or rare mesothelial tumours on the other hand have to be

I. Tischoff, M. Neid, V. Neumann, and A. Tannapfel (✉)
Institut für Pathologie, Ruhr-Universität Bochum, BG Kliniken Bergmannsheil, Bürke-de-la-Camp Platz 1, 44789 Bochum, Germany
e-mail: andrea.tannapfel@ruhr-uni-bochum.de

5

distinguished. Additional immunohistochemistry is essential in histopathological assessment using a marker panel of antibodies.

5.1
Introduction

Malignant mesothelioma is a malignant tumour originating from mesothelial cells. Most frequently, it arises in the pleura (70–95%). Primary peritoneal mesothelioma is less frequent (6–10%) [22, 33, 53]. Rarely, the primary site of malignant mesothelioma is the pericardium or the tunica vaginalis of the testis [34]. The most frequent pleural and peritoneal tumour is metastatic carcinoma [32]; therefore morphological diagnosis by the surgical pathologist has to take into account clinical history and radiology [76].

Asbestos exposure is the highest risk factor of pleural and peritoneal malignant mesothelioma and reported in approximately 54–90% of the patients [53, 70]. The mean latency period between exposure and tumour diagnosis ranges from 35 to 40 years [53]. In peritoneal mesothelioma, an increased pulmonal asbestos exposure of the lung can be observed in 85% of the patients. Further, patients with peritoneal mesotheliomas have a higher pulmonal asbestos exposure than those with pleural mesotheliomas [54].

The incidence of malignant pleural mesothelioma shows marked variation in different countries. The highest incidence rates are reported from Great Britain, Belgium and Australia with annual incidences from about 30 cases per million [14, 72].

In women, occupational asbestos exposure plays a minor role than in men. It has been found in approximately 23%. No occupational asbestos exposure has been found in young patients with malignant peritoneal mesothelioma. In women, malignant peritoneal mesothelioma occurs in younger age and is associated with better prognosis [15]. Two percent to 5% arise in the first 2 decades of life.

Other possible risk factors for malignant mesothelioma are radiation, recurrent peritonitis and simian virus 40 (SV 40). The association between Simian virus 40 (SV 40) and risk of mesothelioma development remains a controversial discussion [5, 6, 62]. Exposure to erionite (zeolith mineral fibre similar in appearance with amphibole asbestos) leads to higher incidences of mesothelioma and plays an important role in environmental exposure (Turkey).

Prognosis is dependent on histological type. Longest survival can be seen in patients with epithelioid malignant mesothelioma. Patients with sarcomatoid malignant mesothelioma have the worst prognosis and prognosis of biphasic malignant mesothelioma lies in between [53, 76]. Grading has not been proven to correlate with prognosis [23].

For differential diagnosis between metastasis, primary malignant mesothelioma or reactive mesothelial proliferation, not only histology but also a panel of immunohistological markers is essential.

5.2
Malignant Mesothelioma of the Pleura

The most common primary tumour of the pleura is diffuse malignant mesothelioma (WHO nomenclature), but often this tumour is designated as malignant mesothelioma or simply as mesothelioma [23].

5.2.1
Morphology

5.2.1.1
Macroscopy and Tumour Spread

Early malignant mesothelioma begins as multiple nodules, usually in the parietal pleura and less frequently in the visceral pleura. Later, nodules become confluent and diffuse tumour growth leads to pleural mass, pleural thickening (more than 1 cm to several cm) and effusion. Parietal and visceral pleura are both involved and cannot be separated. The tumour has a firm, sometimes gelatinous consistency, and spreads throughout the pleura, grows along interlobular spaces and encloses the lung. Hyaline pleural plaques are often present – up to 40% [54].

In advanced stage, diffuse malignant mesothelioma infiltrates the underlying lung tissue, and primarily the chest wall and diaphragm as well as the mediastinal pleura, pericardium and the contralateral pleura. This results in lung compression and consecutive dyspnoea with susceptibility to pneumonia. Tumour infiltration can be seen along needle channels or surgical sites after diagnostic biopsy. Penetration of the diaphragm and involvement of the intraabdominal cavity is associated with ascites. Invasion into lymph vessels is frequent and intrapulmonal metastasis may occur. Metastasis to hilar and mediastinal lymph nodes emerge in late stage disease as do distant metastasis to the liver, adrenal gland, brain, bone and kidney [23].

5.2.1.2
Histological Patterns

Malignant mesothelioma has the capability to reveal either epithelial or mesenchymal differentiation or both. Depending on the histological growth pattern, epithelioid, sarcomatoid, biphasic and desmoplastic malignant mesothelioma are distinguished according to the WHO-classification [23].

Epithelioid Mesothelioma

The most frequent one is epithelioid malignant mesothelioma. It shows different growth patterns, mostly tubular or tubulopapillar. Tubules are small and papillary structures have

vasculated stroma cores [4, 10, 19]. Papillary areas may show psammoma bodies. Sheet-like or microglandular (also revered to as adenomatoid) growth pattern can also be seen and are admixed with tubulopapillar areas [4, 10, 19]. Sometimes pseudo-signet ring cells are demonstrable (negative for mucine) or clear cell differentiation [4, 19].

Uniform histological appearance may occur, particularly in small biopsies, but in most cases, several growth patterns exist, tubulopapillar is the most frequent one [4, 19, 23]. Most mesotheliomas show a monotonous growth with bland cells and little mitosis (Fig. 5.1). Cytology of tumour cells is uniform, showing cuboidal or flat medium size cells with eosinophilic cytoplasm and round nuclei [10, 19]. Pleomorphism, giant cells and increased mitotic count might be encountered but are less numerous. Partial deciduoid differentiation with large, eosinophilic tumour cells, distinct cell borders and round, vesicular nuclei resembling decidua is often found, but usually occurs focally and does not predominate throughout the whole tumour tissue [4, 10, 19]. Very rarely, small cell differentiation of epithelioid malignant mesothelioma occurs [4, 10]. Circumscribed myxoid changes reveal floating tumour cell nests within Alzianblue positive hyaluronate. Tumour stroma is

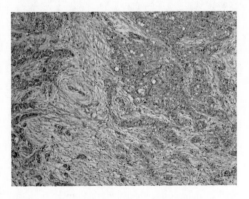

Fig. 5.1 Epithelioid mesothelioma. Epithelioid tumour cell nests within a bland fibrous stroma

diverse and ranges from paucicellular with sclerotic, hyalinised collagen deposits to hypercellular, difficult to distinguish from biphasic tumour differentiation [10, 23].

Sarcomatoid Mesothelioma

Sarcomatoid malignant mesothelioma shows spindle cells, which are arranged in a haphazard pattern, or giant cells with anaplasia. Tumour growth resembles fibrosarcoma or malignant fibrous histiocytoma (Fig. 5.2). Focal areas of osteosarcomatous or chondrosarcomatous differentiation can be found. In sarcomatoid malignant mesothelioma, greater atypia, mitotic activity and more necrosis can be found compared to epithelial mesothelioma [4].

Biphasic Mesothelioma

Biphasic malignant mesothelioma comprises both the aforementioned components, showing an epithelioid and sarcomatoid differentiation (Fig. 5.3). At least 10% of the tumour should be represented by one of the components to be called biphasic. About 30% of all mesotheliomas are biphasic [23, 53], but the more tumour tissue

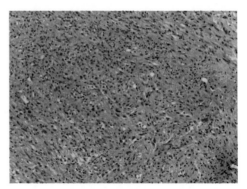

Fig. 5.3 Sarcomatoid malignant mesothelioma. Malignant spindle cells without epithelioid component

sampled, the higher percentage of biphasic differentiation can be detected. Spindle cell differentiation of tumour cells must not be confused with pronounced stroma reaction in epithelioid mesothelioma. Focal osseous differentiation is possible [26].

Rare Forms of Mesothelioma

In desmoplastic malignant mesothelioma, dense eosinophilic stroma of desmoplastic type predominates throughout at least 50% of the tumour (Figs. 5.4 and 5.5). Atypical spindle cells are distributed in a patternless manner [23, 45]. Particularly in small biopsies, desmoplastic malignant mesothelioma may be confused with reactive sclerosing pleuritis (Fig. 5.6) as there might not be overt infiltration of fat or muscle tissue or sarcomatoid differentiation to prove malignancy. Desmoplastic mesothelioma can be regarded as a subtype of sarcomatoid malignant mesothelioma.

Rare forms of tumour differentiation comprise lymphohistiocytoid, small cell and pleomorphic pattern [4]. Lymphohistiocytoid pattern is characterised by discohesive cell growth within a dense lymphocytic inflammatory infiltrate. Small cell differentiation resembles small

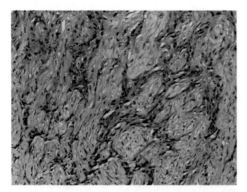

Fig. 5.2 Biphasic malignant mesothelioma. Neoplastic epithelioid cells surrounded by neoplastic spindle cells

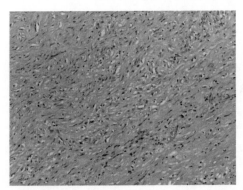

Fig. 5.4 Desmoplastic malignant mesothelioma. Uniform small spindle cells within a hyalinised desmoplastic stroma

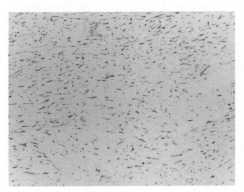

Fig. 5.5 CK5/6 highlights mesothelial origin of spindle cells in desmoplastic malignant mesothelioma

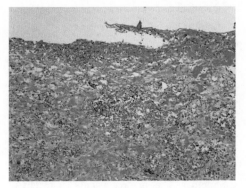

Fig. 5.6 Chronic pleuritis. Dense stroma with fibroblast proliferation and inflammatory cells

cell lung carcinoma and in pleomorphic malignant mesothelioma, multiple giant cells can be detected [4].

Very rarely, a localised subtype of malignant epithelioid mesothelioma occurs without diffuse growth. Histologically, it is identical to epithelioid malignant mesothelioma described above [23].

5.3
Differential Diagnosis of Malignant Mesothelioma and Pleural Metastases

Although diffuse malignant mesothelioma is the most common primary neoplasm arising in the pleura, metastatic carcinoma by far is the most frequent pleural tumour overall [4, 32]. In daily routine pleural biopsy diagnostic, one has to deal with the question, if mesothelial proliferation is reactive or neoplastic, primary mesothelioma or metastatic. Histology is the gold standard of diagnostic, but morphology alone cannot solve the problem and needs to be accomplished by additional immunohistochemical analyses [45].

5.3.1
Morphological Differences

Epithelioid malignant mesothelioma needs to be distinguished from metastatic carcinoma, particularly of the lung, breast, gastrointestinal tract and prostate. To separate malignant mesothelioma from metastases, immunohistochemistry is essential, but some morphological characteristics narrow the possible differential diagnosis [46, 50].

Clear cell differentiation of mesothelioma can be misdiagnosed for metastatic renal cell carcinoma, clear cell adenocarcinoma of the lung or malignant melanoma [2, 4]. Sarcomatoid malignant mesothelioma raises the possible differential diagnosis of spindle cell carcinoma, different types of sarcoma (leiomysarcoma, synovial sarcoma, angiosarcoma, pleomorphic sarcoma and others) and again sarcomatoid renal cell carcinoma or malignant melanoma. Macroscopic appearance of the tumour is important, since malignant mesothelioma usually shows diffuse growth and metastases of the above-mentioned tumours are mainly circumscribed [38].

Thymoma and solitary fibrous tumour, respectively, has to be taken into consideration as well [61]. Reactive changes like sclerosing pleuritis (Fig. 5.6) or papillary mesothelial hyperplasia need to be ruled out.

Nuclei in malignant mesothelioma usually are bland and round and cells are cuboidal or flat. Columnar tumour cells or elongated, eccentric nuclei could be suspected of causing metastatic adenocarcinoma [17]. PAS-positive material can be identified in malignant mesothelioma. But after digestion with diastase PAS (Diastase Periodic-Schiff) mesothelioma shows negative reaction whereas mucine in adenocarcinoma remains positive after this treatment.

Pleomorphic malignant mesothelioma can mimic pleural metastasis of pleomorphic carcinoma, mostly of the lung, or pleomorphic sarcoma (malignant fibrous histiocytoma) [4, 17]. Psammoma bodies can be seen in metastasis of serous ovarian cancer, primary peritoneal carcinoma, papillary lung or renal carcinoma as well as in papillary or tubulo-papillary malignant mesothelioma [17]. They do not prove the metastatic origin of the tumour.

Rarely, malignant mesothelioma reveals small cell differentiation. The most important differential diagnoses of course are small cell lung cancer and malignant lymphoma. But any other tumours with small, round and blue cell morphology comes into question, for instance desmoplastic small round cell tumour of the pleura, metastasis of Ewing sarcoma/PNET or alveolar rhabdomyosarcoma [4]. Noteworthy,

small cell malignant mesothelioma usually does not show typical karyorhexis and crush artefacts like small cell lung cancer or malignant lymphoma do [4].

All the above-mentioned differential diagnoses cannot be accomplished without additional immunohistochemistry.

5.3.2
Immunohistochemistry

Immunohistochemistry is essential for diagnosis of epithelioid malignant mesothelioma, for delineating reactive from neoplastic mesothelial proliferation and for excluding or ascertaining pleural metastases, mainly adenocarcinoma. With the exception of TTF-1, there is no other single immunohistochemical marker which is able to prove or exclude malignant mesothelioma, yet. A panel of different immunohistochemical markers has to be applied [38, 44, 47, 55, 56, 79].

5.3.2.1
Important Markers for Differential Diagnosis

Pancytokeratin

Epithelioid mesothelioma is strongly positive for pancytokeratin. More than 70% of sarcomatoid mesotheliomas are positive with the broad spectrum cytokeratin in the cytoplasm [7].

CK 5/6

64–100% of epithelioid malignant mesotheliomas express CK5/6 [55, 56] and it also helps to highlight tumour cells in desmoplastic malignant mesothelioma (Fig. 5.5). The marker serves to distinguish mesothelioma from lung adenocarcinomas. This marker usually characterises squamous cell differentiation but can also be found in adenocarcinoma of the lung in 2–19% [38, 55, 56].

Calretinin

Calretinin is one of the best known and most specific positive mesothelioma markers. It is positive in almost all epithelioid mesotheliomas with a nuclear and cytoplasmatic staining pattern (Fig. 5.7). Nevertheless, specificity is not 100%, because focal cytoplasmatic expression can be found 0–38% of lung carcinomas [47, 55, 56], whereas positive nuclear staining is only found in mesothelioma [17, 55, 56].

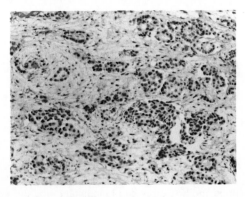

Fig. 5.8 Nuclear expression of WT1 in epithelioid tumour cells

lung [55]. Serous adenocarcinoma of the ovary also shows positive WT-1 reaction.

WT-1

WT-1 is negative in adenocarcinoma of the lung, and cells of malignant mesothelioma show positive reaction in 75–90% [30, 38, 55, 56] (Fig. 5.8). In recent studies none of the lung adenocarcinomas were found to express WT-1 [38, 55, 56]. It is one of the best markers to distinguish malignant mesothelioma from adenocarcinoma of the

D2-40

Malignant mesothelioma shows membrane positivity of D2-40 (podoplanin) in more than 96% (Fig. 5.9), adenocarcinoma of the lung focally in up to 7% [38]. D2-40 is a marker that stains a protein which is expressed in lymphatic endothelial cells [9, 40]. It can be a very useful marker in histological specimens to diagnose

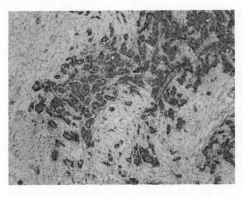

Fig. 5.7 Calretinin expression of epithelioid tumour cells

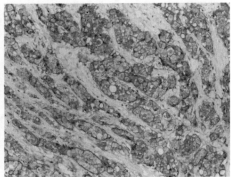

Fig. 5.9 Membrane staining of D2-40 in epithelioid tumour cells

malignant mesothelioma [55, 56] but not in serous effusion cytological smears, because it does not distinguish mesothelioma cells from metastatic cells of serous adenocarcinoma, seminoma or malignant peripheral nerve sheath tumour, which are also positive [9, 40].

TTF-1

To our knowledge, TTF-1 has never been proven to be expressed in malignant mesothelioma [55, 56] but is positive in about 85% of lung adenocarcinoma (nuclear expression), but not in squamous cell carcinoma. Reversely, it does not prove the pulmonary origin of pleural metastases because thyroid carcinoma is also positive and some other primary tumours rarely show TTF-1 expression, one among them being adenocarcinoma of the colon in 10% [25, 58].

BerEP4

Adenocarcinoma of the lung is positive for BerEP4 (also known as HEA) in more than 95%. Malignant mesothelioma focally expresses BerEP4 in up to 20% [38, 55, 56]. Fifty-five percent to 90% of pulmonary adenocarcinomas are positive for CEA and malignant mesothelioma expresses this marker in less than 5% [38, 55, 56].

MOC-31

MOC-31 is another useful immunohistochemical marker to separate malignant mesothelioma from pulmonary adenocarcinoma [55, 56, 79]. This antibody reacts with most carcinomas and only patchily with epithelioid mesothelioma. It is positive in more than 95% of adenocarcinoma and in up to 10% of malignant mesothelioma [38, 55, 56].

BG8

Analogous expression is achieved with BG8 [38, 55, 56], which shows diffuse strong positivity in 98–100% of adenocarcinoma. Only weak and focally staining in 3–7% of malignant mesothelioma have been described [38, 55, 56, 79]. BG 8 could be useful in differentiating epithelioid mesothelioma from lung adenocarcinoma and serous carcinomas.

Claudin

Claudin 4 is a marker, which is expressed in pleural metastasis of adenocarcinoma of the lung, breast, gastrointestinal tract and ovary in 100% [29]. The majority of epithelioid and sarcomatoid malignant mesotheliomas are negative, but positivity may be found in a minority of cases [69].

5.3.2.2
Conclusions Immunohistochemistry

At least two positive mesothelioma markers, two positive carcinoma markers (Table 5.1), and one pancytokeratin are requested according to

Table 5.1 Immunohistochemical markers expressed in malignant epithelioid mesothelioma or in metastasis of adenocarcinoma (modified according to the International Consensus Statement of Pathologic Diagnosis of Malignant Mesothelioma [38]. Sensitivity of the markers is 80% or more. At least two mesothelioma/carcinoma markers should be applied

Positive in malignant epithelioid mesothelioma	Positive in metastasis of adenocarinoma
Calretinin	BerEP4
WT-1	MOC-31
D2-40/Podoplanin	CEA
CK5/6	BG8
	TTF-1 (lung)
	Claudin 4

the International Consensus Statement of Pathologic Diagnosis of Malignant Mesothelioma [38]. Sensitivity of each marker should be at least 80%. When there are discordant findings, additional markers should be performed.

Positivity of calretinin, especially nuclear expression, and/or another of the mesothelioma markers in combination with expression of CK5/6 is very suggestive of malignant mesothelioma. Expression of CK5/6 together with negative mesothelioma markers and positive carcinoma markers is found in metastasis of squamous cell carcinoma and in a minority of adenocarcinoma or adenosquamous carcinoma of the lung [38].

Additional markers like CK7, CK20, CDX-2, TTF-1, PSA or hormone receptors help to precise primary tumour origin of pleural metastases in the breast, lung prostate or gastrointestinal tract [8, 11, 55, 56, 79]. CK7 is useful for proving adenocarcinoma but rarely can be found focally in malignant mesothelioma, also. Positive or negative reaction of mesothelioma/carcinoma markers in the panel usually helps to confirm the right diagnosis. TTF-1 expression in the nucleus in most of the cases is very suggestive of metastasis of lung cancer (primary thyroid carcinoma has to be excluded), adenocarcinoma of the lung is positive in 85% [11].

Nevertheless, immunohistochemical results need to be handled with care, since carcinomas may show unusual expression patterns [11, 55, 56] or malignant epithelioid mesothelioma can show expression pattern like renal cell carcinoma with positive reaction for CD10, erythropoietin or renal cell carcinoma marker [17, 19].

In biphasic mesothelioma, mainly the epithelioid component shows immunohistochemical expression of mesothelioma markers. Sarcomatoid malignant mesothelioma can raise difficulties in differential diagnosis between pleomorphic carcinoma of the lung or metastasis, [23], because expression of mesothelioma markers in sarcomatoid malignant mesothelioma is not reliable, even calretinin can be negative [11, 55, 56]. To differentiate renal cell carcinoma from sarcomatoid

mesothelioma can be particularly difficult when D2-40 is used because both can express it [40]. Clinical history and gross appearance have to be considered in these cases.

5.4
Reactive Versus Neoplastic Mesothelial Proliferation

In small, superficial pleural biopsies, differentiation between reactive or neoplastic mesothelial proliferations can be difficult. Macroscopic appearance in important and need to includes into the diagnosis [20] and has to take into account if the lesion is diffuse or circumscribed, inflammation, pneumonia of the lung, bilateralism, involvement of parietal or visceral pleura.

Papillary mesothelial proliferation occurs in reactive hyperplasia and malignant epithelioid mesothelioma. Cytological atypia can be more pronounced in reactive hyperplasia, whereas malignant mesothelioma cells usually are uniform and bland [17, 20, 63]. Proliferation, for example, Ki67, in malignant mesothelioma is higher than in reactive changes [43]. Fibrovascular cores in papillary lesions are a clue for malignancy; papillary proliferations in reactive changes mainly consist of epithelial cells [2].

Although mesothelial proliferation in pleuritis can be pronounced, the lesion is more superficial and shows zonation with fewer cells in deeper regions. Malignant mesothelioma usually comprises the whole thickness of the pleura with greater cellularity. Tubular structures can be found in the connective tissue underneath the surface in perpendicular arrangement and growth is disorganised [20]. Infiltration favours malignant epithelioid mesothelioma but can be difficult to detect in heavy inflammation and must be separated from artificially entrapped mesothelial cells in prolonged pleuritis [2]. Infiltration of the underlying fat tissue usually allows the diagnosis of malignant mesothelioma [20]. Differential

Table 5.2 Expression pattern of reactive versus neoplastic mesothelial proliferation. EMA-clone E29 should be used. Clone Mc5 is specific to discriminate reactive from neoplastic mesothelial proliferation

	Reactive	Neoplastic
EMA	–	+
Desmin	+	–
Ki67	Low	High

diagnosis of sclerosing pleuritis on the one hand and desmoplastic or sarcomatoid malignant mesothelioma as well as other spindle cell tumours on the other hand can sometimes be very difficult even after immunohistochemistry.

Reactive mesothelial proliferations tend to express desmin and are negative for EMA whereas neoplastic mesothelial cells show a contrarious pattern [2, 7] (Table 5.2). It is very important, which EMA-clone is applied for immunohistochemistry: clone E29 should be used and is positive in 75% of malignant mesothelioma and negative in reactive mesothelial proliferation. Clone Mc5 is not specific and positive in 70% of malignant mesothelioma and 60% of reactive changes [63].

If the existence of malignant mesothelioma remains unclear because infiltration cannot be detected due to superficial biopsy, but papillary growth of atypical mesothelial cells is seen, the diagnosis of atypical mesothelial proliferation should be made. At present, there are no reliable morphological features for mesothelioma in situ in the absence of overt infiltration, hence this term should not be used in this case [2, 20].

5.5
Primary Pleural Tumours Other than Malignant Mesothelioma

Several other tumours arise in the pleura, benign and malignant. Adenomatoid tumour is a benign mesothelial tumour mostly seen in the tunica vaginalis of the genital tract but it can develop in the pleura also. It is a circumscribed, solitary tumour with epithelioid morphology, tubular structures and fibrous stroma. Pseudo-signet ring cells can be found and may be mistaken for metastasis of signet ring cell carcinoma. Cytology usually is uniform [2, 23].

Well-differentiated papillary mesothelioma rarely develops in the pleura. It is mainly seen in the peritoneum and is described below.

Synovial sarcoma is a biphasic tumour and is very rarely seen in the pleura. Differential diagnosis is biphasic malignant mesothelioma [52]. Most synovial sarcomas are pleural metastases and only a minority is primary to the pleura. Patients usually are younger than patients with malignant mesothelioma; the average age is 33 years [2]. They are localised compared to the diffuse growth of malignant mesothelioma. Epithelioid component can be difficult to detect, tumour growth is more compact with long spindle cell fascicles compared to malignant mesothelioma, which tends to have smaller, less cellular fascicles with greater pleomorphism [2]. It is important to know that synovial sarcoma can be positive for calretinin and malignant mesothelioma for CD99 [2]. Demonstration of Syt-translocation t(X;18) provides the diagnosis [52].

Solitary fibrous tumour presents itself as a mesenchymal tumour of fibroblastic origin and was first described in the pleura, but can evolve in other sites as well. Size can be up to 10 cm [33]. It arises in the visceral pleura, lung or mediastinum as a solitary, sometimes pedunculated tumour. Histologically, it shows a haemangiopericytoma-like growth pattern of spindle cells with hypercellular and wirelike fibrous areas [11, 74]. Myxoid areas can be found. Immunohistochemistry is helpful and these tumours express CD34 and bcl-2. They may express D2-40 [51] which is important to know if this marker is used for differential diagnosis of malignant mesothelioma, but are negative von cytokeratin. Most solitary fibrous tumours are benign but malignant forms do occur and reveal higher mitotic activity (>4 per 10 HPF).

Calcifying fibrous tumour is a circumscribed mass ranging from 1.5 to 12.5 cm in diameter. It is rare and evolves in the extremities, trunk, scrotum, axilla and visceral pleura [32]. Typical psammomatous calcifications lie within a hyalinised, nearly acellular stroma [74].

Malignant vascular tumours primary to the pleura are angiosarcoma and epithelioid haemangioendothelioma [2]. These tumours can mimic malignant mesothelioma due to diffuse growth. Tumour cells may weakly express cytokeratin, whereas malignant mesothelioma is strongly positive. Blood vessels in epithelioid haemangioendothelioma can be very small and intraluminal erythrocytes sparse. Detection of vascular markers (CD34, CD31, factor VIII) confirms the diagnosis [74].

Malignant lymphoma can be secondary or evolve primary to the pleura. Primary effusion lymphoma develops in the absence of a mass within the effusion. It is mainly seen in patients with acquired immunodeficiency syndrome and is associated with EBV and HHV-8 infection. Cells are large and most of the lymphomas are of B-cell origin but T-cell lymphomas also do occur. Prognosis is poor, median survival is 6 months [32].

Pyothorax-associated lymphoma in contrast to primary effusion lymphoma presents as a pleural mass and is also associated with EBV infection. It is a B-cell lymphoma with immunoblastic morphology within a longstanding pyothorax and in patients without immunodeficiency [23].

Further, very rare primary malignancies of the pleura are desmoplastic small round cell tumour, pleural lipsarcoma and pleuropulmonal blastoma. Desmoplastic small round cell tumour shows multiple nodular lesions and evolves very rarely in the pleura and more often in the abdomen. Histologically, they consist of small round blue cells within a desmoplastic stroma [74]. Cells express cytokeratin, EMA, NSE and focally desmin (dotlike pattern). Diagnosis is made by demonstrating t(11;22)(p13;q12) translocation [32].

Morphology of liposarcoma is identical to soft tissue liposarcoma and may present as well-differentiated lipomatous tumour/lipoma-like liposarcoma, myxoid or round cell liposarcoma [32]. Very rarely, pleural infiltration of thymous tumours or Askin tumour has to be considered.

5.5.1
Peritoneal Mesothelioma

5.5.1.1
Pathohistological Diagnosis

Malignant peritoneal mesothelioma is characterised by a peritoneal tumour mass with unspecific clinical symptoms like abdominal pain, abdominal swelling, anorexia, weight loss, and/or ascites. Radiological features are non-specific [72]. Therefore, the histological examination is essential to yield correct diagnosis. Examination of ascites or fine-needle aspiration can be useful but is of low diagnostic potential because of the small numbers of malignant cells in the fluid and their cytological resemblance to normal mesothelial cells. The use of immunocytology can be useful in some cases. But in general, sampling of tumour biopsy has a higher diagnostic significance whereas immunohistochemical examination is indispensable in distinguishing MPM from other lesions and neoplasias.

Macroscopy

Malignant peritoneal mesothelioma consists of multiple or innumerable nodules approximately 1.5 cm in diameter. The tumour mass is undistinguishable from peritoneal metastases or primary peritoneal carcinoma. The cut surface is frequently heterogeneous with solid regions and embedded cystic or mucoid areas into the tumour mass.

The localised subtype forms a typically circumscribed mass invading adjacent organs without a diffuse growth through the abdominal cavity. In contrast, the diffuse type shows a widespread expansion and involvement of the abdominal organs along parietal and visceral peritoneum [41, 42]. Infiltrating per continuitatem into the stomach from serosa to the mucosa is seen in every fourth case [41]. Involvement of liver, abdominal wall, pancreas, bladder, retroperitoneum or diaphragm with invasion into the pleural cavity are less common [48].

In 7% of the cases, abdominal, thoracic or inguinal lymph node metastases are found. Haematogenous metastases are seen in the liver, lung, pleura, pericard, kidney, pancreas or in bones [41].

Microscopy

Analogue to pleural mesotheliomas, malignant peritoneal mesothelioma is divided into three different major histological types: epithelioid mesothelioma, sarcomatoid mesothelioma and the mixed or biphasic type. There are further rare subtypes like the undifferentiated type (poor differentiated) or lymphohistiocytoid and desmoplastic mesothelioma (that belongs to the sarcomatoid subtype). The most common type of malignant peritoneal mesothelioma is the epithelioid subtype in more than 50%. In approximately 25% of MPM, a sarcomatoid component can be found, but pure sarcomatoid mesothelioma is very infrequent in the peritoneum and more commonly seen in the pleura [8, 53, 55].

In women, a deciduoid subtype has been described, that can be mistaken for an extensive ectopic decidual reaction. This subtype can be found in women during pregnancy as well as in women of advanced age. Patients with this subtype have a worse prognosis with a median survival rate of 7 months. Asbestos exposure can be found in 35–80% [35, 49, 68, 71].

75% of malignant peritoneal mesotheliomas are epithelioid mesotheliomas resembling normal mesothelial cells. They are composed of trabecular, papillary or tubulo-papillary formed tumour nests (Figs. 5.10 and 5.11). Microglandular or signet-ring cell patterns are also found. The tumour cells invade submesothelial connective tissue, fatty tissue and muscle which help to distinguish malignant mesothelioma from reactive mesothelial hyperplasia.

The sarcomatoid mesothelioma shows typically closely packed polymorphic spindle cells with sparse cytoplasm and mitotic figures. Malignant osteoid, chondroid or muscle elements within the tumour mass may be found. In biphasic type, histomorphological features of epithelioid and sarcomatoid are found.

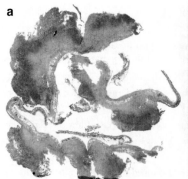 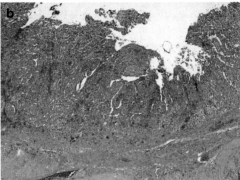

Fig. 5.10 (**a, b**) Epithelioid subtype of malignant peritoneal mesothelioma (HE)

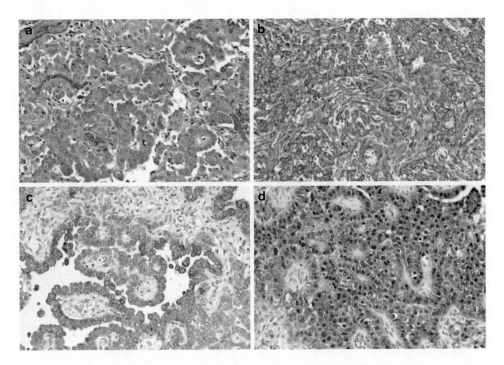

Fig. 5.11 (a) Papillary tumour nest in malignant peritoneal mesothelioma (HE), (b) MNF expression, (c) CK5/6 expression, (d) nuclear positivity for Calretinin

5.5.2
Malignant Mesothelioma of Tunica Vaginalis Testis

Malignant mesothelioma of tunica vaginalis testis is a rare tumour that belongs to malignant peritoneal mesothelioma because during embryonal period, tunica vaginalis testis evolves from invagination of the abdominal peritoneal membrane and is covered by mesothelial cells [59]. Less than 5% of malignant peritoneal mesotheliomas are localised primarily in the tunica vaginalis testis [39, 54]. Several studies evaluated that mesotheliomas of tunica vaginalis testis are asbestos related in case of significant asbestos burden [45, 59, 65].

5.5.3
Well-Differentiated Papillary Mesothelioma

Well-differentiated papillary mesothelioma is a rare subtype of epithelioid mesothelioma with low malignant potential in contrast to malignant peritoneal mesothelioma. It occurs more frequently in the peritoneum than in the pleura and it is typically most common in young woman without asbestos exposure, but its relation to asbestos exposure remains still unclear. One study group reported an occupationally asbestos exposure in 42% of all examined patients [31].

Macroscopically, the tumour size ranges from 1 cm to more than 3 cm, but more than half of the cases of well-differentiated papillary mesotheliomas are smaller than 1 cm [36, 57]. Furthermore, it can occur as solitary type or multifocal type. The latter shows more aggressive behaviour. In some cases, patients with initial well-differentiated papillary mesothelioma die from diffuse malignant mesothelioma during the course of disease [16, 18].

Histologically, well-differentiated papillary mesothelioma is characterised by a generally

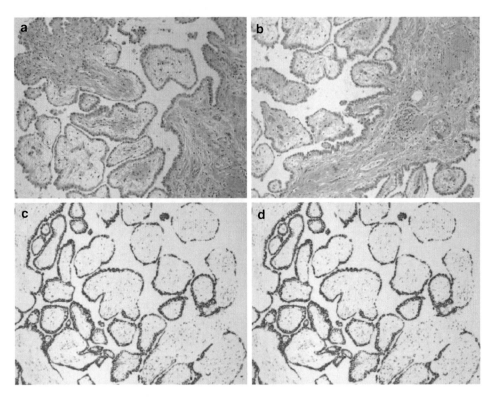

Fig. 5.12 (**a**, **b**) Well-differentiated papillary mesothelioma (HE), (**c**) Immunohistochemical staining of MNF116, (**d**) Immunohistochemical staining of Calretinin

non-invasive papillary or tubulo-papillary tumour formation. The papillae and tubules are lined by a single layer of uniform, cuboidal and flattened neoplastic mesothelial cells with bland nuclear features (Fig. 5.12). Psammon bodies are seen in some cases. The tumour stroma can show extensive fibrosis that causes glandular irregularity and confusing invasive foci of malignant mesotheliomas or metastases of adenocarcinoma.

5.5.4
Prognosis and Predictive Factors

The diffuse type of malignant mesothelioma is a highly aggressive tumour, whereas no characteristic features were found to distinguish favourable or less favourable groups. Women have a better outcome but the reason still remains unclear [78]. Well-differentiated papillary mesothelioma is associated with better prognosis. Distinction between histological subtypes is an important predictive value because epithelioid mesothelioma has a better prognosis than the sarcomatoid or biphasic subtype.

Several studies investigated on the value of potential prognostic factors. Male gender, age <53 years, loss of weight, tumour volume, sarcomatoid or biphasic histological subtype, mitotic count and nuclear size were identified as negative prognostic factors, but further studies are needed to evaluate these features [3, 6, 21, 27, 28, 78].

5.5.5
Differential Diagnosis

Several neoplastic and non-neoplastic processes have to be excluded due to the infrequent incidence of malignant peritoneal mesothelioma and certain histomorphological similarities to other benign lesions and malignancies whereas malignant peritoneal mesotheliomas remains still a differential diagnosis.

Non-neoplastic lesions include inflammatory processes like reactive mesothelial proliferations related to peritonitis, tuberculosis, sarcoidosis or foreign body reaction and adhesions that develop after surgical intervention. In women, endometriosis and endosalpingiosis or decidual knots formed during pregnancy caused by decidual transformation of the serosal membrane can impress as tumourous process.

Neoplastic lesions have to be distinguished from peritoneal metastases, primary peritoneal

carcinoma, lymphoma, sarcoma and benign lesions/tumours like benign multicystic mesothelioma, adenomatoid tumour, leiomyomatosis peritonealis disseminata and gliomatosis peritonei (see Table 5.3).

5.5.6
Benign Lesions

5.5.6.1
Benign Multicystic Peritoneal Mesothelioma

Benign multicystic peritoneal mesothelioma arises in pelvic serosa and forms a mulitcystic tumour mass occurring predominantly in young and middle-aged women. In less than 20%, benign multicystic peritoneal mesothelioma can be found in males [35]. In contrast to malignant peritoneal mesothelioma, asbestos exposure is not found. The tumour comprises a multicystic tumour mass that is either solitary or in most cases diffuse or multilocated. The tumour cysts are translucent, filled with serous fluid and confluent and delimited by a fibrous band. The cysts measures less than 1 cm up to 20 cm in diameter [77]. The multicystic mesothelioma has a benign or indolent course and is inclined to recur in one-half of the cases between 1 and 27 years. In rare cases, multiple recurrence and malignant transformation to malignant mesotheliomas have been observed [31, 77].

5.5.6.2
Adenomatoid Tumour

Adenomatoid tumour – also designated as benign mesothelioma – is a very rare benign mesothelial tumour that forms gland-like tumour nests with adenoid, angiomatous or cystic structures with smooth muscle proliferations embedded in a fibromatous stroma. It occurs most frequently in the tunica vaginalis testis. Macroscopically, the

Table 5.3 Summary of peritoneal tumours [73]

Primary tumours	Secondary tumours (metastases)
Malignant peritoneal mesothelioma	Ovarian carcinoma
Primary peritoneal carcinoma	Colorectal carcinoma
Extragonadal germ cell tumours	Gastric carcinoma
GIST	Pancreatic carcinoma
Lymphoma	Gallbladder carcinoma
Sarcoma	Uterus carcinoma
Benign multicystic mesothelioma	Lung carcinoma
Adenomatoid tumour	Lymphoma
Leimyomatosis disseminata peritonealis	GIST
Gliomatosis peritonei	Germ cell tumours
	Seminoma
	Sarcoma

tumour is solitary and less than 2 cm in diameter with a white-grey cut surface. After resection, recurrence is very rare [2, 35].

5.5.7
Malignant Lesions

5.5.7.1
Peritoneal Metastases

Peitoneal metastases are secondary tumours of the peritoneum and the most common tumours of the peritoneum. Ovarian carcinoma, colorectal cancer and gastric cancer just as carcinomas of the pancreas, gallbladder, uterus and lung are the most frequent tumours that show peritoneal involvement. Peritoneal metastases represent advanced tumour stage and are associated with a poor prognosis.

In patients with colorectal carcinoma, peritoneal metastases occur in 10–15%. Primary ovarian carcinomas show peritoneal metastases in 65–70%, pancreatic carcinomas in 35% and gastric cancer in 25–30%. Peritoneal metastases caused by separation of individual tumor cells from the primary tumour. The invasion of these dissociated tumour cells depends on the location of the primary tumour. Invasion in blood and lymphatic vessel is characteristic for carcinomas of the gastrointestinal tract. Tumours that are adherent to the peritoneum, like ovarian carcinomas, show direct peritoneal involvement [10, 73].

Frequently, peritoneal metastases show similar histological pattern like their primary tumour; most of peritoneal metastases are adenocarcinomas. Tumour heterogeneity, like differences of tumour grading, causes diagnostic problems. Peritoneal metastases of a primary low-grade adenocarcinoma can show a high-grade pattern, for example. Loss of original histological pattern can occur in tumours after

chemotherapy. In such cases, clinical informations about pretreatment or knowledge of primary tumour site is helpful to confirm the correct diagnosis. Particularly, in case of mixed carcinomas like adenocarcinoma with partial endocrine type or adenosquamous carcinoma, peritoneal metastases can consist of only one of the histological pattern. A correct diagnosis on the basis of conventional histology is difficult in most cases and additional immunohistochemistry is required.

5.5.7.2
Carcinoma of Unknown Primary (CUP)

Carcinoma of unknown primary (CUP) is seen in 3–5% of all tumour diseases. In 5–10% the peritoneum is involved (Muir 1995). On the other hand, 2–4% of primary peritoneal tumours represent the origin of CUP [1]. Histologically, most peritoneal metastases are adenocarcinomas in 40–60%, undifferentiated carcinomas in 15–30%, squamous carcinomas in 15–20% and in 3–5% small cell carcinomas or endocrine tumours are observed. Therefore, immunohistochemistry is necessary to classify tumour infiltration but in some cases the assignment to the localisation of the primary tumour site is not possible [73].

5.5.7.3
Primary Peritoneal Carcinoma

Primary peritoneal carcinoma (PPC) is an extraovarian neoplasia that resembles surface epithelial tumours of ovarian origin. It occurs exclusively in middle-aged women between 53 and 62 years. Fifteen percent of 'typical ovarian cancers' are primary peritoneal carcinomas [66, 67]. It consists of confluent tumour masses transforming omentum and mesenteriums to tumour bulks and involving the surface of the liver, anterior abdominal wall and the peritoneal side of the diaphragm. The most common histological subtype is serous adenocarcinoma whereas, like in surface carcinoma of the ovary, transitional cell, clear cell, mucinous or squamous cell carcinomas have been reported. Histologically and immunohistologically, PPC is undistinguishable from ovarian carcinoma. To separate these two tumour entities, certain criteria have been developed [60, 75].

Distinction between malignant peritoneal mesothelioma, especially the epithelioid subtype, and primary peritoneal carcinoma/peritoneal metastases of primary ovarian carcinoma is very difficult because of overlapping histomorphological similarities. Only use of immunohistochemistry based on the combination of different markers makes it possible to distinguish these tumour entities (discussed below, and see Table 5.5 that shows a panel of antibodies).

5.5.7.4
Primary Peritoneal Borderline Tumour

Primary peritoneal borderline tumour is a rare neoplasia of the peritoneum that only arises in women mostly between 16 and 67 years of age. Median age is 32 years [13]. Characteristically, this tumour shows morphological similarities to serous borderline tumour of the ovary but arises from the peritoneum without or with minimal involvement of the ovarian surface [12].

Macroscopically, the tumour nodules appear like non-invasive implants of ovarian borderline tumour with smaller knots or adhesions. Only in rare cases, tumour mass is found [12]. Like ovarian borderline tumour, most tumours are of serous types with psammoma bodies [13].

5.5.8
Immunohistochemistry

Malignant peritoneal mesothelioma shows the same immunohistochemical staining pattern like the pleural counterpart expressing calretinin, WT1 (Wilm's tumour antigen 1), EMA, Cytokeratin 5/6, D2-40. Characteristically, they are negative for CEA, TTF-1, BerEp-4 (HEA), B72.3, MOC-31, BG8 and Claudin-4 [29, 38]. A marker panel including antibodies that are frequently positive in mesotheliomas should be used.

EMA and desmin help to distinguish benign mesothelial lesions from MPM in most cases. Up to 80% of malignant mesotheliomas show positive immunostaining of EMA and up to 85% of benign mesothelial lesions express desmin. But both, EMA and desmin, have a low sensitivity and specificity of 70–75% differentiating benign from malignant mesothelial lesions, because weak membrane positivity of EMA can be found in reactive mesothelial proliferation. On the other hand, some cases of malignant mesothelioma are EMA negative [37, 43, 64].

To separate mesotheliomas from sarcomas, lymphomas or melanomas, the use of cytokeratin is helpful.

Discrimination between malignant peritoneal mesothelioma and peritoneal metastases, especially in case of CUP, is difficult and requires further immunohistochemical staining. Peritoneal metastases show frequently the same histological typing and grading with similar immunohistochemical pattern like their primary tumour. The most common histological type that is seen in peritoneal metastases are adenocarcinomas. Peritoneal metastases, as mentioned, are mostly seen in ovarian, gastric, pancreatic, colon, gallbladder, uterus and breast cancer. But to confirm correct diagnosis, targeted antibody markers should be applied in dependence of clinical questions (see Table 5.4).

5

Table 5.4 Immunohistochemical marker panel to distinguish between malignant peritoneal mesothelioma (MPM) and primary adenocarcinoma of digestive tract [38]

Marker	MPM	PC	CRC	GC
Calretinin	+	(+)	−	−
WT1	+	−		−/(+)
D2-40 (Podoplanin)	+	−		−
CK5/6	+	+/−	−	−
MOC-31	−/(+)	+	+	+
BG8	−/(+)	+	+	+
Ber-EP4 (HEA)	−/(+)	+	+	+
B72.3	−(+)	+	+	
CEA	−	+	+	+
CDX2	−	−/(+)	+	+/−

MPM malignant peritoneal mesothelioma, *PC* pancreatic ductal adenocarcinoma, *CRC* Colorectal carcinoma, *GC* gastric carcinoma
+ positive; − negative; +/− both positive and negative; −/(+) mostly negative, rarely positive

5.6
Primary Peritoneal Carcinoma/Metastases of Serous Ovarian Cancer Versus Malignant Peritoneal Mesothelioma

Epithelioid type of malignant peritoneal mesothelioma shows close overlapping histomorphological similarities to primary peritoneal carcinoma/metastases of serous ovarian cancer; therefore, distinction of these tumour entities is very important for further therapy, because MPM is a radio- and chemotherapy-resistant malignancy with poor prognosis. Several studies evaluated expression of immunohistochemical markers to differentiate malignant mesotheliomas from primary peritoneal carcinoma/metastases of serous ovarian carcinoma. A high sensitivity of h-Caldesmon, Calretinin and D2-40 as well as a high specificity of calretinin and D2-40 (95%) has been reported in mesotheliomas. In primary peritoneal carcinomas/metastases of serous ovarian carcinoma, estrogen receptor and BerEp4 show a

high sensitivity, and non-mesothelioma markers (like estrogen receptor, progesterone receptor, B72.3, CA19-9, CD15 and to a lesser extent BerEp-4) are characterised by a high specificity [8, 24]. In case of D2-40, some studies reported a limited use because D2-40 is expressed in 13–65% of primary peritoneal carcinomas/metastases of serous ovarian carcinoma [9, 38]. Estrogen receptor, BerEp-4, MOC-31 and BG8 are expressed in primary peritoneal carcinomas/metastases of serous ovarian carcinoma to a high extent but are negative or infrequently detectable in malignant mesotheliomas [38].

In general, to differentiate malignant peritoneal mesothelioma from primary peritoneal carcinomas/metastases of serous ovarian carcinoma, a panel including antibodies that are frequently positive in mesotheliomas (like Calretinin and WT-1) on the one hand and non-mesothelial markers (like estrogene receptor, BerEP-4, MOC-1 and BG8) on the other hand should be used (see Table 5.5).

Table 5.5 Immunohistochemical marker panel to distinguish between malignant peritoneal mesothelioma (MPM) and primary peritoneal carcinoma/peritoneal metastasis of serous ovarian carcinoma (PCC/MPOC) [38, 73]

Marker	MPM	PPC/PMOC
Calretinin	+	−
WT1	+	+
D2-40 (Podoplanin)	+	−/(+)
CK5/6	+	−/(+)
Estrogen receptor	−	+/−
Progesterone receptor	−	+/−
Thrombomodulin	+	−/(+)
MOC-31	−/(+)	+
BG8	−/(+)	+
Ber-EP4 (HEA)	−/(+)	+
B72.3	−(+)	+

MPM malignant peritoneal mesothelioma, *PPC* primary peritoneal carcinoma, *PMOC* peritoneal metastases of serous ovarian carcinoma
+ positive; − negative; +/− both positive and negative; −/(+) mostly negative, rarely positive

References

1. Abbruzzese JL, Abbruzzese MC, Hess KR, Raber MN, Lenzi R, Frost P (1994) Unknown primary carcinoma: natural history and prognostic factors in 657 consecutive patients. J Clin Oncol 12:1272–1280
2. Addis B, Roche H (2009) Problems in mesothelioma diagnosis. Histopathology 54:55–68
3. Achermann YIZ, Welch LS, Bromley CM et al (2003) Clinical presentation of peritoneal mesothelioma. Tumori 89:255–258
4. Allen TC (2005) Recognition of histopathologic patterns of diffuse malignant mesothelioma in differential diagnosis of pleural biopsies. Arch Pathol Lab Med 129:1415–1420
5. Antman KH, Corson JM, Li FP, Greenberger J, Sytkowski A, Henson DE, Weinstein L (1983) Malignant mesothelioma following radiation exposure. J Clin Oncol 1:693–700
6. Antman K, Hassan R, Eisner M et al (2005) Update on malignant mesotheliomas. Oncology 19:1301–1309
7. Attanoos RL, Griffin A, Gibbs AR (2003) The use of immunohistochemistry in distinguishing reactive from neoplastic mesothelium. A novel use for desmin and comparative evaluation with epithelial membrane antigen, p53, platelet-derived growth factor-receptor, P-glycoprotein and Bcl-2. Histopathology 43:231–238
8. Barnetson RJ, Burnett RA, Downie I et al (2006) Immunhistochemical analysis of peritoneal mesothelioma and primary and secondary serous carcinoma of the peritoneum: antibodies to estrogen and progesterone receptors are useful. Am J Clin Pathol 125:67–76
9. Bassarova AV, Nesland JM, Davidson B (2006) D2-40 is not a specific marker for cells of mesothelial origin in serous effusions. Am J Surg Pathol 30:878–882
10. Battifora H, McCaughey WTE (1995) Tumours of the serosal membranes. In: Atlas of tumour pathology. Third series. Fascicle 15. Armed Forces Institute of Pathology, Washington, DC
11. Beasley MB (2008) Immunohistochemistry of pulmonary and pleural neoplasia. Arch Pathol Lab Med 132:1062–1072
12. Bell DA, Scully RE (1990) Serous borderline tumours of the peritoneum. Am J Surg Pathol 14:230–239
13. Biscotti CV, Hart WR (1992) Peritoneal serous micropapillomatosis of low malignant potential (serous borderline tumours of the peritoneum). Am J Surg Pathol 16:467–475
14. Bofetta P (2007) Epidemiology of peritoneal mesothelioma: a review. Ann Oncol 18:985–990
15. Bridda A, Padoan I, Mencarelli R et al (2007) Peritoneal mesothelioma: a review. MedGenMed 9:32–41
16. Bürrig K, Pfitzer P, Hort W (1990) Well differentiated papillary mesothelioma of the peritoneum: a borderline mesothelioma: report of two cases and review of literature. Virchows Arch 417:443–447
17. Butnor KJ (2005) My approach to the diagnosis of mesothelial lesions. J Clin Pathol 59:564–574
18. Butnor KJ, Sporn T, Hammar S et al (2001) Well differentiated papillary mesothelioma. Am Surg 25:1304–1309
19. Butnor KJ, Nicholson AG, Allred DC, Zander DS, Henderson DW, Barrios RB, Haque AK, Allen TC, Killen DE, Cagle PT (2006) Expression of renal cell carcinoma-associated markers erythropoietin, CD10, and renal cell carcinoma marker in diffuse malignant mesothelioma and metastatic renal cell carcinoma. Arch Pathol Lab Med 130:823–827
20. Cagle P, Churg A (2005) Differential diagnosis of benign and malignant mesothelial proliferation on pleural biopsies. Arch Pathol Lab Med 129:1421–1427
21. Cerruto CA, Brun EA, Chung D et al (2006) Prognostic significance of histomorphologic parameters in diffuse malignant peritoneal mesothelioma. Arch Pathol Lab Med 130:1654–1661
22. Chua TC, Yan TD, Morris DL (2009) Surgical biology for the clinician: peritoneal mesothelioma: current understanding and management. Can J Surg 52:59–64
23. Churg A, Roggli V, Galateau-Salle F, Cagle PT, Gibbs AR, Hasleton PS, Henderson DW, Vignaud JM, Inai K, Praet M, Ordonez NG, Hammar SP, Testa JR, Gazdar AF, Saracci R, Pugatch R (2004) Mesothelioma. In: Travis WD, Brambilla E, Müller-Hermelink HK, Harris CC (eds) World Health Organization classification of tumours. Pathology and genetics of tumours of the lung, pleura, tymus and heart. IARC Press, Lyon

24. Comin CE, Calogero S, Messerini L (2007) h-Caldesmon, calretinin, estrogen receptor, and BerEP-4: a useful combination of immunohistochemical markers for differentiating epithelioid peritoneal mesothelioma from serous papillary carcinoma of ovary. Am J Surg Pathol 31:1139–1148

25. Comperat E, Zhang F, Perrotin C, Molina T, Magdeleinat P, Marmey B, Régnard JF, Audouin J, Camilleri-Broët S (2005) Variable sensitivity and specificity of TTF-1 antibodies in lung metastatic adenocarcinoma of colorectal origin. Mod Pathol 18:1371–1376

26. Demirag F, Unsal E, Tastepe I (2007) Biphasic malignant mesothelioma cases with osseous differentiation and long survival: a review of the literature. Lung Cancer 57:233–236

27. De Pangher MV, Recchia L, Cafferata M et al (2010) Malignant peritoneal mesothelioma: a multicenter study on 81 cases. Ann Oncol 21(2):348–353, Epub 2009 Jul 27

28. Deraco M, Nonaka D, Baratti D et al (2006) Prognostic analysis of clinicopathological factors in 49 patients with diffuse malignant peritoneal mesothelioma treated with cytoreductive surgery and intraperitoneal hyperthermic perfusion. Ann Surg Oncol 13:229–237

29. Facchetti F, Lonardi S, Gentili F, Bercich L, Falchetti M, Tardanico R, Baronchelli C, Lucini L, Santin A, Murer B (2007) Claudin 4 identifies a wide spectrum of epithelial neoplasms and represents a very useful marker for carcinoma versus mesothelioma diagnosis in pleural and peritoneal biopsies and effusions. Virchows Arch 451:669–680

30. Foster MR, Johnson JE, Olson SJ, Allred DC (2001) Immunohistochemical analysis of nuclear versus cyoplasmatic staining of WT1 in malignant mesotheliomas and primary pulmonary adenocarcinomas. Arch Pathol Lab Med 125:1316–1320

31. Gonzales-Moreno S, Yan H, Alcorn K et al (2002) Malignant transformation of benign cystic mesothelioma of the peritoneum. J Surg Oncol 79:234–251

32. Guinee DG, Allen TC (2007) Primary pleural neoplasia. Arch Pathol Lab Med 132:1149–1157

33. Guinee DG, Allen TC (2008) Primary pleural neoplasia: entities other than diffuse malignant mesothelioma. Arch Pathol Lab Med 132:1149–1170

34. Hammar Sp (2006) Macroscopic, histologic, histochemical, immunohistochemical, and ultrastructural features of mesothelioma. Ultrastruct Pathol 30:3–17

35. Hassan R, Alexander R (2005) Nonpleural mesothelioma: mesothelioma of the peritoneum, tunica vaginalis and pericardium. Hemtol Oncol Clin North Am 19:1067–1087

36. Hoekstra AV, Riben MW, Frumovitz M et al (2005) Well differentiated papillary mesothelioma of the peritoneum: a pathohistological analysis and review of the literature. Gynecol Oncol 98:161–167

37. Hurllimann J (1994) Desmin and neural marker expression in mesothelial cells and mesotheliomas. Hum Pathol 25:753–757

38. Husain AN, Colby TV, Ordonez NG, Krausz T, Borczuk A, Cagle PT, Chiriac LR, Churg A, Galateau-Salle F, Gibbs AR, Gown AM, Hammar SP, Litzky LA, Roggli VL, Travis WD, Wick MR (2009) Guidelines for pathologic diagnosis of malignant mesothelioma. Arch Pathol Lab Med 133:1317–1331

39. Ikegami Y, Kawai N, Tozawa K et al (2008) Malignant mesothelioma of the tunica vaginalis testis related to asbestos. Int J Urol 15:560–561

40. Kalof AN, Cooper K (2008) D2-40 immunohistochemistry – so far! Adv Anat Pathol 16:62–64

41. Kannerstein M, Churg M (1977) Peritoneal mesothelioma. Hum Pathol 8:83–94

42. Kerrigan SA, Turnnir RT, Clement PB, Young RH, Churg A (2002) Diffuse malignant epithelial mesotheliomas of the peritoneum in woman: a clinicpathologic study of patients. Cancer 94:378–385

43. King J, Thatcher N, Pickering C, Hasleton P (2006) Sensitivity and specificity of immunohistochemical antibodies used to distinguish between benign and malignant pleural disease: a systematic review of published reports. Histopathology 49:561–568

44. Klebe S, Nurminen M, Leigh J, Henderson DW (2009) Diagnosis of epithelial mesothelioma using a tree-based regression analysis and a minimal panel of antibodies. Pathology 41:140–148

45. Krismann M, Müller K (2000) Malignes mesotheliom der pleura, des perikards und des peritoneums. Chirurg 71:877–886

46. Krismann M, Müller KM, Jaworska M, Johnen G (2004) Pathological anatomy and molecular pathology. Lung Cancer 45:29–33

47. Kushitani K, Takeshima Y, Amatya VJ, Furonaka O, Sakatani A, Inai K (2007) Immunihistochemical marker panels for distinguishing between epitheliod mesothelioma and lung adenocarcinoma. Pathol Int 57:190–199

48. Mayhall FG, Gibbs AR (1991) Malignant peritoneal giving rise to multiple intestinal polyps. Histopathology 20:47–50

49. Mourra N, Chaisemartin C, Vesini I et al (2005) Malignant deciduoid mesothelioma. Arch Pathol Lab Med 129:403–406

50. Muir C (1995) Cancer of unknown primary site. Cancer 75(1 Suppl):353–356

51. Naito Y, Ishii G, Kawai O, Hasebe T, Nishiwaki Y, Nagai K, Ochiai A (2007) D2-40-positive solitary fibrous tumors of the pleural: diagnostic pitfall of biopsy specimen. Pathol Int 57:618–621

52. Ng SB, Ahmed Q, Tien SL, Sivaswaren C, Lau LC (2003) Primary pleural synovial sarcoma. Arch Pathol Lab Med 127:85–90

53. Neumann V, Gunther S, Muller KM et al (2001) Malignant mesothelioma – German mesothelioma register 1987-1999. Int Arch Occup Environ Health 74:383–395

54. Neumann V, Löseke S, Tannapfel A (2009) Medical insurance aspects of peritoneal tumors with particular attention to peritoneal mesotheliomas. Med Klin (Munch) 104:765–771

55. Ordonez NG (2005) Immunohistochemical diagnosis of epithelial mesothelioma: an update. Arch Pathol Lab Med 129:1407–1414

56. Ordonez NG (2006) The diagnostic utility of immunhistochemistry and electron microscopy in distinguishing between peritoneal mesotheliomas and serous carcinomas: a comparative study. Pathology 19:34–48

57. Park JY, Kim KW, Kwon HJ et al (2008) Peritoneal mesotheliomas: clinicopathological features, CT findings, and differential diagnosis. AJR 191:814–825

58. Penman D, Downie I, Roberts F (2006) Positive immunostaining for thyroid-transcription factor-1 in primary and metastatic colonic adenocarcinoma: a note of caution. J Clin Pathol 59:663–664

59. Plas E, Riedl C, Plueger H (1998) Malignant mesothelioma of the tunica vaginalis testis.

Review of the literature and assessment of prognostic parameters. Cancer 83:2437–2446

60. Ransom DT, Patel SR, Keeney CL, Malkasian GD, Edmondson JH (1990) Papillary serous carcinoma of the peritoneum. A review of 33 cases treated with platin-based chemotherapy. Cancer 66:1091–1094

61. Rdzanek M, Fresco R, Pass HI, Carbone M (2006) Spindle cell tumors of the pleura: differential diagnosis. Semin Diagn Pathol 23: 44–55

62. Riddell RH, Goodman MJ, Moossa AR (1981) Peritoneal malignant mesothelioma in a patient with recurrent peritonitis. Cancer 48: 134–139

63. Saad R, Cho P, Liu Y, Silverman JF (2004) The value of epithelial membrane antigen expression in separating benign mesothelial proliferation from malignant mesothelioma: a comparative study. Diagn Cytopathol 32:156–159

64. Salman WD, Eyden B, Shelton D et al (2009) An EMA negative, desmin positive malignant mesothelioma: limitations of immunohistochemistry? J Clin Pathol 62:651–652

65. Schneider J, Woitowitz H (2001) Fallbericht: absestverursachtes malignes mesotheliom der tunica vaginalis testis. Zentralbl Chir 126: 229–232

66. Schorge JO, Muto MG, Lee SJ, Huang LW, Welch WR, Bell DA, Keung EZ, Berkowitz RS, Mok SC (2000) BRCA-1 related papillary serous carcinoma of the peritoneum has a unique molecular pathogenesis. Cancer Res 60: 1361–1364

67. Schorge JO, Muto MG, Welch WR, Bandera CA, Rubin SC, Bell DA, Berkowitz RS, Mok SC (1998) Molecular evidence for multifocal papillary serous carcinoma of the peritoneum in patients with germline BRCA-1 mutations. J Natl Cancer Inst 90:841–845

68. Shia J, Erlandson R, Klimstra D (2002) Deciduoid mesothelioma: a report of 5 cases and literature review. Ultra Pathol 26:355–363

69. Soini Y, Kinnula V, Kahlos Km Päkkö P (2005) Claudins in differential diagnosis between mesothelioma and metastatic adenocarcinoma of the pleura. J Clin Pathol 59:250–254

70. Steffen HM, Wamnbach G, Hoffmann A, Jaursch-Hancke C, Kaufmann W (1989) Diagnostik und therapie des malignen peritonealen mesothelioms. Med Klin 84:469–473

71. Sugarbaker P, Achermann Y, Brun E (2002) Deciduoid peritoneal mesothelioma. Contemp Surg 58:341–346

72. Tannapfel A, Brücher B, Schlag PM (2009) Peritoneal mesothelioma – rare abdominal tumors. Der Onkologe 15:250–260

73. Tischoff I, Tannapfel A (2007) Pathologic and anatomic evidence of peritoneal metastases. Chirurg 78:1088–1090

74. Travis WD, Churg A, Aubry MC, Ordonez NG, Tazelaar H, Pugatch R, Manabe T, Miettinen M (2004) Mesenchymal tumours. In: Travis WD, Brambilla E, Müller-Hermelink HK, Harris CC (eds) World Health Organization classification of tumours. Pathology and genetics of tumours of the lung, Pleura, thymus and heart. IARC Press, Lyon

75. Truong LD, Maccato ML, Awalt H, Cagle PT, Schwartz MR, Kaplan AL (1990) Serous surface carcinoma of the peritoneum: a clinicopathologic study of 22 cases. Hum Pathol 21:91–110

76. Tsao AS, Wistuba I, Roth JA, Kindler HL (2009) Malignant pleural mesothelioma. J Clin Oncol 27:2081–2090

77. Van Ruth S, Achermann YIZ, Van de Vijver MJ, Hart AAM, Verwaal VJ, Zoetmulder FAN (2003) Pseudomyxoma peritonei: a review of 62 cases. Eur J Surg Oncol 29:682–688

78. Yan TD, Popa E, Brun EA et al (2006) Sex difference in diffuse malignant mesothelima. Br J Surg 93:1536–1542

79. Yazij H, Battifora H, Barry TS, Hwang HC, Bacchi CE, McIntosh MW, Kussick SJ, Gown AM (2006) Evaluation of 12 antibodies for distinguishing epithelial mesothelioma from adenocarcinoma: identification of a three-antibody immunohistochemical panel with maximal sensitivity and specificity. Mod Pathol 19:514–523

Abstract The strong relationship between mesothelioma and asbestos exposure is well established. The analysis of lung asbestos burden by light and electron microscopy assisted to understand the increased incidence of mesothelioma in asbestos mining and consuming nations.

The data on the occupational exposure to asbestos are important information for the purpose of compensation of occupational disease No. 4105 (asbestos-associated mesothelioma) in Germany.

However, in many cases the patients have forgotten conditions of asbestos exposure or had no knowledge about the used materials with components of asbestos. Mineral fiber analysis can provide valuable information for the research of asbestos-associated diseases and

for the assessment of exposure. Because of the variability of asbestos exposure and long latency periods, the analysis of asbestos lung content is a relevant method for identification of asbestos-associated diseases. Also, sources of secondary exposure, so called "bystander exposition" or environmental exposure can be examined by mineral fiber analysis.

Household contacts to asbestos are known for ten patients (1987–2009) in the German mesothelioma register; these patients lived together with family members working in the asbestos manufacturing industry.

Analysis of lung tissue for asbestos burden offers information on the past exposure. The predominant fiber-type identified by electron microscopy in patients with mesothelioma is amphibole asbestos (crocidolite or amosite). Latency times (mean 42.5 years) and mean age at the time of diagnose in patients with mesothelioma are increasing (65.5 years). The decrease of median asbestos burden of the lung in mesothelioma patients results in disease manifestation at a higher age.

Lung dust analyses are a relevant method for the determination of causation in mesothelioma. Analysis of asbestos burden of the lung and of fiber type provides insights into the pathogenesis of malignant mesothelioma. The most important causal factor for the development of mesothelioma is still asbestos exposure.

V. Neumann (✉) and S. Löseke
German Mesothelioma Register,
University Hospital Bergmannsheil,
Bochum, Germany
e-mail: volker.neumann@ruhr-uni-bochum.de

A. Tannapfel
German Mesothelioma Register,
University Hospital Bergmannsheil, Bochum,
Germany and
Institut für Pathologie, Ruhr-Universität Bochum,
BG Kliniken Bergmannsheil, Bürke-de-la-Camp
Platz 1, 44789 Bochum, Germany
e-mail: andrea.tannapfel@ruhr-uni-bochum.de

A. Tannapfel (ed.), *Malignant Mesothelioma*, Recent Results in Cancer Research 189,
DOI: 10.1007/978-3-642-10862-4_6, © Springer-Verlag Berlin Heidelberg 2011

6

6.1
Introduction

Occupational exposure to asbestos dust has been widespread in all industrial nations and exposure still exists in Canada, Russia, China, and Africa. Asbestos is a group of minerals with particular properties but only six asbestiform minerals are of commercial importance. There are two large groups of asbestos fibers, first amphibole asbestos including five asbestiform members (crocidolith, amosite, tremolite, actinolite, anthophyllite) and secondly serpentine asbestos of which chrysotile is the only asbestiform member. Crocidolith, amosite, and chrysotile are the most common commercially used asbestiform minerals. The other amphiboles have only limited commercial importance but are relevant as contaminants of other mineral species. Asbestos minerals have been used in over 3,000 commercial applications [2, 39].

The strong relationship between mesothelioma and asbestos exposure is well established [35, 36, 61, 63, 65, 122, 132]. There is a direct relationship between the national asbestos consumption (kg per head per year) in industrial nations and the number of deaths per million people per year by mesothelioma and asbestosis [75]. Historical asbestos consumption is a significant predictor for death by mesothelioma. Whereas in the so-called normal population mesothelioma have an incidence of 1–2 cases per 1 million inhabitants [83], the number of mesothelioma after asbestos exposure is much higher [32, 96]. The highest incidence rates – about 30 cases per 1 million- were estimated in Australia [72], Belgium [15], and Great Britain [87].

Although the usage of asbestos containing products was forbidden in most industrialized countries long time ago the number of mesothelioma is still growing due to long and variable latency periods (20 up to over 40 years) between exposure and diagnosis [20, 93, 104, 121]. Therefore, the incidence of mesothelioma is expected to peak between the years 2010 and 2020 [9, 64, 103, 106].

The commercial use of asbestos peaked in Germany at more than 200,000 t/year between 1968 and 1977 (Fig. 6.1). At present, as well as

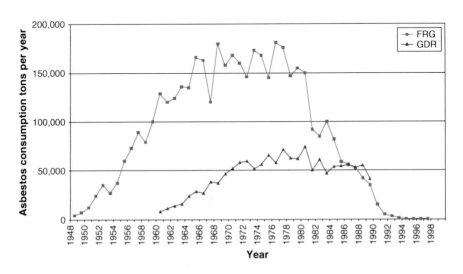

Fig. 6.1 Consumption of asbestos in Germany (GDR/FRG) (German democratic republic/FRG Federal Republik of Germany)

in the near future asbestos-related diseases are considered to be a public health problem in Germany [99].

In 2008, 905 new cases (Fig. 6.2) were recognized as asbestos-related mesothelioma in Germany [38].

Mesothelioma often develop in patients with long-term occupational asbestos exposure, but can also occur in patients with low level or minor exposure to asbestos [59, 93]. Mesothelioma cases have been reported in wives and children of asbestos workers who were exposed to asbestos dust by cleaning and storing workers' clothes [44, 93, 129].

Such household contacts are known for ten patients (1989–2009) in the German mesothelioma register; these patients had lived together with family members working in the asbestos manufacturing industry.

The analysis of asbestos content of lung tissue provides important information concerning the understanding of the relationship between asbestos exposure and causation of asbestos-associated diseases [113].

So mineral fiber analysis is an essential tool to obtain valuable information for the research of asbestos-associated diseases and for the assessment of asbestos exposure [93]. The exact determination of asbestos exposure may often be problematic because of the variability of asbestos exposure in patient's histories, long latency times, and subsequent frequently forgotten episodes of asbestos exposure. So the analysis of asbestos lung content is a relevant method for identification of an asbestos-associated disease. The sole measurement of airborne asbestos fibers by using air samplers has some disadvantages and cannot solve the previously mentioned problems in the evaluation of a patient's individual history of asbestos exposure. The disadvantage of airborne measurements of asbestos fibers is caused by:

- Different sampling techniques over the time.
- Measurement of fibers $\geq$ 5 µm does not differentiate between respirable and nonrespirable.
- No fiber size distributions are given.
- Concentrations based on counts using the phase contrast microscopy.

Only measuring the asbestos content in lung tissue will give the relevant fiber burden retained in the lung at the time of analysis. Thus, this method is able to subsume the deposition and clearance of asbestos fibers in the

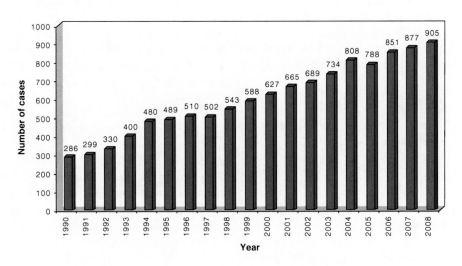

Fig. 6.2 New recognized occupational disease no. 4105 – malignant mesothelioma

6

human lung. An optimal lung dust analysis is based on representative samples, accurate preparation techniques, and a trained and experienced analyst [37]. Other important variables that determine the quality of the information gained from lung tissue analysis include tissue quantity and the method of analysis.

6.2
Techniques for Analysis of Pulmonary Mineral-Fiber Content

There are several established analytical methods for asbestos fiber analysis that differ in their specificity and sensitivity. This diversity is the reason for the poor direct comparability of the results from one laboratory to another. Asbestos fibers are ubiquitous in the air and present in the lung of subjects without any occupational asbestos exposure. So a reliable determination of an elevated pulmonary asbestos fiber content caused by occupational asbestos exposure must be based on the comparison with the so-called normal population. Due to the high variability between different techniques and laboratories, each laboratory has to establish its own reference values for normal lungs in relation to lungs with elevated asbestos burden.

The different analysis techniques can be subdivided into three common operation steps [111]:

1. Dissolving and removal of the organic lung matrix
2. Recovery and concentration of asbestos bodies and mineral fibers
3. Quantification of the asbestos lung tissue burden

6.2.1
Lung Tissue Digests

The sampling of the lung tissue for fiber burden analysis is the first relevant step. If possible, for lung dust analysis, tissue from [55] the upper lobe (right and left side) and the lower lobe (right and left side) should be taken. The used lung tissue should be well inflated and without secondary lung alterations (nontumorous sample, no autolysis and without pneumonia) [14, 55, 93, 94]. There exists a variety of techniques for the extraction of asbestos bodies from lung tissue. Some methods employ chemical digestion, others use low temperature ashing techniques. The tissue digestion must be carefully performed to avoid loss of asbestos bodies, asbestos fibers, or fiber fractions [113]. Any process that may damage fibers by shortening or splitting should be avoided [7, 89]. Drying tissue before digestion leads to fracture of longer asbestos fibers, causing artificial higher results. Introduction of a sonification or hot ashing step of the lung tissue can lead to extended fragmentation of chrysotile fibers and artifactual increase in asbestos fiber numbers [58, 70]. In the German mesothelioma register, we use a direct isolation method without ultrasonification, centrifugation, or drying of the tissue samples.

First step in lung dust analysis procedure is the weighing of the wet lung tissue, followed by a sodium hypochloride-based wet chemical digestion step of the organic lung tissue matrix. Afterward, increasing amounts of the dissolved lung tissue are filtrated through a porous membrane and are concentrated on the filter matrix. These filters are mounted on glass slides and made transparent for light microscopy by acetone vaporization.

The asbestos burden can be given in terms of fibers (or asbestos bodies) per gram of wet tissue, fibers per cm^3 of lung tissue, or fibers per gram of dry lung tissue. These values (units) are not precisely comparable and can vary from case to case, but in general one fiber in wet tissue is approximately equivalent to one fiber in cm^3, corresponding to a concentration of nearly ten fibers per gram of dry tissue [113].

The concentration of asbestos fibers and asbestos bodies depends partly on the density of lung tissue [7]. Increasing density of lung tissue – due to fibrosis or pneumonia – will lead to a decrease of fibers or asbestos bodies per unit weight (wet or dry). Decreasing density of lung tissue – due to emphysema – will lead to an increasing number of fibers or asbestos bodies per unit weight (wet or dry). Thus, the use of surface unit in cm^3 instead of wet or dry weight is the best method to minimize the influence of tissue density on the results of asbestos burden counts [47].

6.3
Methods for Mineral Fiber Analysis

6.3.1
Light Microscopy (LM)

Light microscopy analysis of lung tissue burden is characterized by the following pros and cons:

- Allows the detection of low concentrations (1 asbestos body per cm^3 or gram of wet or dry lung tissue)
- It is a quick and inexpensive method to confirm asbestos burden.
- Limited resolution (0.2 μm) and magnification (400×).
- Consequently only large fibers with a diameter of >0.2 μm can be detected.
- Asbestos bodies formed primarily on asbestos fibers longer than 8–10 μm, thus asbestos bodies present a selected population of long asbestos fibers.

The first description of asbestos bodies goes back to the work of a German pathologist [77] who called them "pigmented crystals." The term "asbestos bodies" was used for the first time in the 1930s. [31, 80].

The majority of asbestos bodies from human lungs have amphibole asbestos cores. Of these asbestos bodies, only 2–7% [23, 60, 92] consist of a chrysotile core and 98% to 93% enclose an amphibole asbestos core. Chrysotile asbestos

fibers cannot be identified by light microscopy due to their very thin diameters. By light microscopy, all structures with a characteristic proteinous envelope containing straight fiber cores that appear colorless, transparent, slight birefringence (under polarized light), and with plan parallel edges [18, 23] are identifiable as asbestos bodies. Most non-asbestos ferruginous bodies or pseudoasbestos bodies can be distinguished from true asbestos bodies at the light microscopic level [18, 26–28, 33, 39, 42]. Therefore, a trained dust analyst can clearly identify asbestos bodies and pseudoasbestos bodies based on the morphological definition of asbestos bodies [39].

The characteristic light microscopical appearance and the identification in histologic sections is an important component of the pathologic diagnosis of asbestosis (I–IV) [94].

So, light microscopy of chemically digested lung tissue at magnifications between 200 and 400× and in combination with polarization techniques is an ideal routine method for the quantification of asbestos bodies and asbestos burden of the lung. [112]. In cases where asbestos bodies cannot be identified by light microscopy and with obvious secondary lung alterations, additional electron microscopic mineral-fiber analysis of digested lung tissue should follow.

6.3.2
Electron Microscopy

Electron microscopical methods with high resolutions (Analytical scanning electron microscope (SEM), Analytical Transmission electron microscope (TEM)) were able to detect thin (diameter 0.05–0.01 μm) and small (down to 0.3 μm in length) fibers. The SEM method allows the detection of asbestos bodies and uncoated fibers in parallel, and this technique has the advantage of a relatively simple preparation of the lung tissue. The option to perform EDX-analysis of each single fiber makes it possible to differentiate between non-asbestos and asbestos fibers and also to discriminate and

6

subtype between different asbestos species. In comparison to TEM-analysis, the SEM method allows the examination of larger proportions of the filter surface and consequently more of the lung tissue. So, the extrapolation of fiber concentration in relation to the total sample volume is more reliable and less prone to over- or underestimation. Due to the more complex preparation techniques and the very small percentage of the sample that can be examined on a single TEM grid, the TEM method is time consuming and only ideal and useful for specialized investigations and where other approaches like light microscopy and SEM techniques have failed.

6.3.3
Comparability of Results Generated by Light or Electron Microscopy

There is a good correlation (correlation coefficient = 0.091, $p < 0.0001$) between asbestos bodies concentrations determined by SEM and LM [113]. Also the asbestos bodies concentration of the lung counted light microscopically correlates well (correlation coefficient 0.79, $p < 0.00019$) with the pulmonary burden of uncoated fibers (≥ 5 μm) measured by SEM [36, 67, 90, 91, 114]. The comparative evaluation of EM and LM lung dust countings has shown, that the ratio of asbestos bodies and asbestos amphibole fibers may range between 1:10 and >1:200 in dependency on tissue preparation and analytical method (SEM/TEM) [28, 30, 49, 97, 101, 108, 110, 113, 126].

6.3.4
Reference Population and Background Lung Asbestos Burden

The evaluation of a maximum standard value for a normal or background fiber burden of the lung is a relevant task and an essential assumption to quantitatively define elevated fiber concentrations. The reference population for the "general population" includes subjects without occupational asbestos exposure living in areas without asbestos deposits or asbestos manufacturing industries. Such a "general population" is only exposed to asbestos up to the general and ubiquitous level of environmental contamination with asbestos fibers [37, 41, 43]. The evaluated content of lung asbestos burden of such a reference population can be used to determine an elevated asbestos concentration in disease cases with an occupational asbestos exposure history.

For light microscopical asbestos burden analysis, there are several studies [19, 39, 40, 45, 114, 115] concluding a burden of 0 up to <22 asbestos bodies per gram wet tissue as representative for the general population. On the electron microscopical level, there is no generally applicable and universal asbestos fiber concentration that might be used by every laboratory to distinguish between fiber burden of the normal population and occupationally exposed individuals [49]. Each laboratory has to establish its own reference values. In the German Mesothelioma Register, our reference values for the general population ($n = 50$) were evaluated for the FE-REM method [14]. Based on these values, "normal" asbestos burdens can extent up to 1.0×10^4 amphibol and 1.8×10^4 chrysotile asbestos fibers (>5 μm in length) per gram wet tissue.

6.3.5
Asbestos Bodies and Fiber Counting

Tissue samples were selected, if possible, from four different locations of both lungs, for the quantification of asbestos body concentrations (asbestos bodies/cm³ lung tissue or g wet tissue). The filter analyses [19, 45] were examined by light microscopy at 200–400 × magnification (differential interference contrast / polarization microscopy). Only characteristic bodies with typical morphology and thin, colorless, and translucent cores were counted as asbestos bodies [18, 113].

Fiber identification and quantification [113, 116, 117] were performed by SEM microscopy 1,000–20,000 magnification. Fibers were defined as particles with a ratio (length / width) of at least 3:1.

6.4
Asbestos Lung Tissue Content in Patients with Mesothelioma

6.4.1
Light Microscopy

The asbestos burdens of the cases recorded in the German mesothelioma register were determined mainly by light microscopy. The pathologic and demographic data are presented in Table 6.1. In most of the mesothelioma patients (84%), we were able to detect an increased asbestos burden (more than 22 asbestos bodies/cm³ = maximum standard value) of the lung. About 30% of these patients had distinctly elevated concentrations (more than 1,000 asbestos bodies / cm³) in lung tissue and 54% of the examined tissue samples contained a slightly to moderately elevated asbestos burden (>22–1,000 asbestos bodies).

Table 6.1 Mesothelioma cases: pathologic and demographic data

		%
Sex		94 (men)
		6 (women)
Pleura mesothelioma		96
Peritoneal mesothelioma		3.0
Pericardial mesothelioma		< 1
Epithelioid subtype		36
Biphasic subtype		52
Sarcomatoid		12
Pleural plaques	Yes	42
	No	15
	Unknown	43
Asbestosis		27

At least 16% of the mesothelioma patients showed no detectable elevated asbestos burden in light microscopy analysis. In about 10% of this patient group, significant secondary alterations such as pneumonia, autolysis, or tumorous infiltrations were seen. These alterations may cause destruction of the asbestos body coats which subsequently become undetectable by light microscopy. This leads to substantial underestimation of the measured concentration values. After excluding these "false negative" cases, a collective of ca. 6% patients with definitively no measurable elevated asbestos burden on the light microscopical level remained. These cases needed further investigation concerning the background of the etiology of their malignant mesotheliomas.

The total group of mesothelioma patients was divided into two parts {(Group I (1989–1999) and Group II (2000–2009)} in order to assess possible changes of asbestos burden in mesothelioma patients during the respective decades.

In comparison to the older cases in study group I (Table 6.2) there is a significant trend toward lower median asbestos burden (320 to 290 asbestos bodies per cm³) in group II.

Also latency times become significantly longer in group II (38–43 years) and patients in group II are significantly older (mean age 65 years) than the patients of group I (mean age 60 years) at the time of diagnosis.

Our data are in line with results of a recent study by Roggli (2008, Table 6.3). He also showed a time-related significant trend toward lower median asbestos burden and older ages with a median of 480 asbestos bodies and a mean age of 62 years in the period from 1980 to 1992 down to a median of 350 asbestos bodies and a mean age of 65 years for the years 1992–2005.

The median asbestos burden of the lung is significantly ($p < 0.05$) higher for patients with peritoneal mesothelioma than for patients with pleural mesothelioma [Neumann 2001].

Table 6.2 Mesothelioma and asbestos burden (light microscopy) and latency period

Light microscopy			
	1989–2009 Asbestos burden (asbestos bodies/cm³ wet tissue)	1989–1999 Asbestos burden (asbestos bodies/cm³ wet tissue)	2000–2009 Asbestos burden (asbestos bodies/cm³ wet tissue)
Median	310	320	290
Minimum	1	1	0
Maximum	990,000	990,000	410,000
Probability		<0.05	
Latency period (in years)	40	38	43
Mean age at diagnosis	–	60	65
Probability		<0.05	

Table 6.3 Mesothelioma and asbestos burden (light microscopy) [117]

Light microscopy			
	Total Group 1980–2005 Asbestos burden (asbestos bodies/g wet tissue)	Subgroup I 1980–1992 Asbestos burden (asbestos bodies/g wet tissue)	Subgroup II 1992–2005 Asbestos burden (asbestos bodies/g wet tissue)
Median	–	480	350
Minimum	1	1	3.3
Maximum	1,600,000	1,600,000	207,000
Probability		$p < 0.05$	

6.4.2
Electron Microscopy

The predominant fiber type identified by electron microscopy in patients with mesothelioma is amphibole asbestos (crocidolite or amosite) [112]. In a study of 94 cases, about 60% of the analyzed fibers were amosite [111]. Patients with mesothelioma show elevated levels of amphibole but not of chrysotile fibers compared to control groups [56, 57, 111, 116]. The lung SEM dust study [18] based on 409 patients with malignant mesothelioma and the measured (SEM) asbestos contents of patients with malignant mesothelioma are summarized in Table 6.4. As seen in data obtained by light microscopy, SEM analysis of this collective also reflects a significant trend

toward lower asbestos bodies and asbestos fiber burden during the decades [18].

The percentage of cases with elevated amphibole fiber burden (over the reference range) in this collective was about 80% [18]. There was a trend for decreasing asbestos fiber burden from group 1 to group 2.

6.4.3
Asbestos Content and Fiber Dimensions in Pleural Samples

The vast majority of studies analyses asbestos fiber burden only in lung parenchyma. Only few studies [17, 41, 43, 57] found long amphibole fibers in different samples of the pleura (pleural

Table 6.4 Mesothelioma and asbestos burden measured by electron microscopy modified from Roggli 2008

	Total Group 1980–2005 Asbestos burden (asbestos bodies/g wet tissue)	Subgroup I 1980–1992 Asbestos burden (asbestos bodies/g wet tissue)	Subgroup II 1992–2005 Asbestos burden (asbestos bodies/g wet tissue)
SEM-Analysis Amosite			
Median	–	17,500	6,330
Minimum	120	120	390
Maximum	11,900,000	11,900,000	2,610,000
Probability		<0.05	
SEM-Analysis Chrysotile			
Median	–	1,800	1,370
Minimum	580	580	590
Maximum	124,000	124,000	4,180
Probability		<0.05	

plaque, diffuse visceral pleural fibrosis) from asbestos workers. One study [17] found especially long commercial amphibole fibers in black spots of the parietal pleura [17]. Another study [127] reported short chrysotile fibers in pleural and mesothelial tissue. The examination of individuals exposed to mixed amphibole and white asbestos [120] showed that short chrysotile fibers (<5 μm) accumulate primarily in the pleura whereas longer amphibole fibers accumulate primarily in lung tissue. In contrast, several other studies [17, 42, 54, 57, 120, 127] provided evidence that short (<5 μm) and long chrysotile and amphibole asbestos fibers are able to reach the pleural tissue. So, it is especially those fiber types and sizes with the highest carcinogenic potential that can be transported to the pleura [113, 128].

6.5
Discussion

The pathogenic response of the lung to inhaled dust depends on the mineral fiber type, exposure conditions (short-time overload or prolonged moderate exposure) and fraction of respirable fibers. The mineral fiber content in the lung reflects the pathogenic fraction of inhaled dust which represents only a minor amount of the total fiber dust exposure prevailing at many workstations [102]. The quantity of mineral fiber asbestos consumption in Europe and other industrial states has changed over the last decades [126]. Therefore, individual asbestos exposure normally changes during lifetime and especially during working life.

6.5.1
Asbestos Bodies and Fiber Burden of the Lung

In lung tissue of most mesothelioma patients (85%) [93], elevated levels of asbestos could be detected by light microscopy. Negative results in lung dust analyses (16%) have to be assessed with caution. After excluding such cases with unsuitable lung tissues only 6% of patients revealed definitely no elevated asbestos burden of the lung. The frequency distribution of light microscopically evaluated asbestos body concentrations does not correlate with a special tumor subtype. All asbestos-related tumor entities were seen within the whole range of asbestos lung concentrations [93, 95]. Other investigators

[1991], too, found no differences in asbestos body concentrations in relation to different tumor subtypes.

Considering only amphibole fibers, there is a known significant relation of asbestos fiber-concentration and the number of asbestos bodies in lung tissue [1, 51, 67, 110]. The results of most studies, however, show that patients with mesotheliomas and occupational asbestos exposure show increased concentrations of amphibole asbestos, but not of chrysotile [89, 130].

6.5.2
Latency Period and Mean Age at Diagnosis of Mesothelioma

As shown in other studies [78, 117], we also observed in our patient group a trend toward longer latency times and an increased average age for the initial diagnosis of mesothelioma. Mesothelioma patients showed an inverse relationship between latency period and pulmonary asbestos burden [117]. So, patients with very high asbestos burdens show significantly shorter latency periods [93]. The observed decrease of the median asbestos burden of the lung from one decade to the other may explain the tendency toward elongated latency periods and higher age of mesothelioma patients.

6.5.3
Clearance and Biopersistence of Asbestos Fibers

The geometry of the tracheobronchial tree and the different clearing mechanisms of the respiratory systems are important factors influencing the deposition of particles and fibers. The clearing mechanisms include fine hairs in the nasal cavity, the mucociliary escalator of the tracheobronchial tree and the alveolar macrophages. Long-term inhalation studies demonstrated that the relative retention of amphibole fibers in the lungs is considerably higher than that for chrysotile [24, 25, 34, 131] and that amphibole fibers accumulate within the lungs to a much greater extent than chrysotile fibers.

The average length of fibers – observed for chrysotile and amphibole – retained within the lung increased in parallel with time after exposure. This observation may be explained by a more effective clearance of shorter fibers [81, 82, 84, 85, 89]. As yet, there is no definite reason for the preferential retention of amphibole fibers in the lung; however, various aspects are in discussion. Important factors could be the tendency of chrysotile to split longitudinally into very small individual fibrils [11, 12] or a different biopersistence of chrysotile in comparison to amphibole asbestos. New experimental animal studies provide very different results for the biopersistence of chrysotile asbestos. One study [12] using a rat model showed that one year after asbestos exposure no chrysotile fibers longer than 20 µm remain in the lungs. Another study with monkeys [125] describes the detection of white asbestos fibers and asbestos bodies containing chrysotile fibers 11.5 years after inhalation of chrysotile asbestos. In some cases [49, 50], elevated levels of chrysotile asbestos in the lung were found as late as 60 years after asbestos exposure.

However, chrysotile is less biopersistent than amphibole asbestos fibers [12, 13A, 29, 30]. Only in patients with massive pulmonary asbestos burdens overload, the amounts of both chrysotile and amphibole fibers are increased [23, 29, 107]. After intermediate time of decades elevated chrysotile burden overload of the lung are rare [49, 51]. So, there is no clear correlation between asbestos bodies and chrysotile concentrations [1, 40, 51, 114], and asbestos bodies with chrysotile as a central core are rare [41, 69]. The results of most studies show that patients with mesothelioma after occupational asbestos exposure possess increased concentrations of amphibole asbestos but no elevated levels of chrysotile [46, 52, 82, 86, 115, 130, 133].

6.5.4
Carcinogenic Potency of Asbestos Fibers

According to results of a cohort study including 3,072 workers from an asbestos textile plant [124], the carcinogenic potential of the fibers is strongly associated with the exposure to long (>10 μm) and thin fibers (<0.25 μm). The detection of short (<5 μm) white asbestos fibers is of questionable relevance, because a convincing pathogenic potency is not attributable to this subclass of chrysotile fibers [113].

The carcinogenic potency of chrysotile asbestos for mesothelioma is discussed controversially [11–13A, 24, 48, 74, 81, 88, 100, 119, 123]. Some cohort studies stated significant positive relations between estimated chrysotile exposure and lung cancer and asbestosis mortality [62].The tendency of chrysotile asbestos [12, 100] to fragment into shorter fibers and its reduced biopersistence are possibly the reasons for the lower carcinogenic potency in comparison to amphibole asbestos [12]. One meta-analysis [64] comes to the conclusion that the relative specific risks to develop mesothelioma after exposure to the three commercially used asbestos types chrysotile, amosite, and crocidolite, can be described by the ratio of 1:100:500, respectively. Whereas some cohort studies demonstrate significant positive relations between estimated chrysotile exposure and lung cancer or asbestosis mortality [62], the majority of studies stated that amphibole asbestos fibers were the primary reason for an elevated risk to develop mesothelioma [29, 30, 82, 86]. Chrysotile asbestos is often contaminated with low doses of tremolite asbestos, one hypothesis is that the tremolite contaminant is the exclusive substance inducing cancer in chrysotile mine workers [53, 54, 62, 84, 101]. Some suggested that workers exposed to "pure" chrysotile have no increased cancer risk. This speculation has been referred to as the amphibole hypothesis [11–13A, 62, 71, 84, 85].

There is new scientific evidence for the missing fibrogenic potency of chrysotile (exception overload situation) [13A]. Futher chrysotile fibers do not migrate to the pleura cavity, the site of mesothelioma origin [13B].

6.5.5
Peritoneal Mesothelioma

Some studies clearly demonstrate a significant relation between the degree of asbestos lung burden and the primary tumor site [8, 73, 93]. Elevated asbestos-concentrations in lung tissue (>5,000 asbestos bodies/cm^3) are significantly higher in patients with peritoneal than those with pleural mesotheliomas. Especially, a high number of asbestos bodies can be found in the group of patients with peritoneal mesotheliomas of the most frequent epithelioid subtype. In contrast to one study [68], our data suggest that the amount of asbestos bodies in lung tissue has no prognostic value and does not correlate with the survival time.

6.5.6
Asbestos-Associated Mesothelioma and Other Possible Causes of Malignant Mesothelioma

According to other studies [134], the percentage of asbestos-associated mesotheliomas is about 90%. Only 5–10% of the patients have no elevated pulmonary asbestos burden.

Exposure to erionite [10, 98], too, leads to higher incidences of mesothelioma and plays an important role in environmental exposure. For example, in some regions of Central Turkey the development of malignant mesothelioma is associated with a ubiquitous presence of erionite. This mineral is a hydrated aluminum silicate of the zeolith mineral family and shows similar characteristics and cancerogenic potencies as amphibole asbestos.

Apart from this, other mesothelioma-inducing factors are in discussion: Infection with SV-40

6

virus [5, 21], Wilms tumor [3, 4], recurring inflammations [105], thorotrast [79, 93], ionized radiation [22], Mediterranean fever [76], and genetic factors [118] are suggested to play a role in the development of malignant mesothelioma.

6.5.7
Threshold or Cut-off Level

There is an ongoing discussion about the definition of a cut-off level of asbestos exposure beyond which the exposure to asbestos does not lead to the development of malignant mesothelioma [63, 66, 82, 107, 109, 121, 128]. However, such a specific threshold based on measurements or assumed levels of asbestos exposure has not yet been determined scientifically [16, 63, 82, 93, 108, 117]. In spite of this, every action taken over the last decades resulting in the reduction and prevention of occupational exposure to asbestos fibers was an important and decisive improvement. With the implementation of these exposure prevention measures, a decrease of average concentrations from about 500 fibers/cm^3 in the early 1950s to less than 1 fiber/cm^3 until the asbestos ban in Germany was achieved [6, 38, 99]. So, the reduction of asbestos doses on different workplaces by effective prevention measures leads to lower asbestos burdens of the lung, resulting in longer latency times, a higher average age of mesothelioma patients, and a shifted peak of mesothelioma development.

6.6
Conclusion

The most important causal factor for the development of mesothelioma is still asbestos exposure. In this context, lung dust analyses are a relevant method for the determination of causation in mesothelioma. Quantitative analysis of asbestos burden of the lung and qualitative differentiation of fiber types provide helpful insights into the pathogenesis of malignant mesothelioma.

It is also possible that patients with asbestos bodies or asbestos fibers counts comparable to the "normal population" develop asbestos-associated mesothelioma. But other possible causes of malignant mesothelioma have to be taken into consideration. Patients with no history of occupational asbestos exposure and without elevated asbestos burden of the lung may develop a so-called background or spontaneous mesothelioma. Are these cases a result of other etiological factors than asbestos or the erionite exposure?

References

1. Albin M, Johansson L, Poley F, Jakobsson K, Attewell R, Mitha R (1990) Mineral fibres, fibrosis and asbestos bodies in lung tissue from deceased asbestos cement workers. Br J Ind Med 47:767–74
2. Albracht G, Schwerdtfeger O (1991) Herausforderung Asbest. Universum Verlag GmbH KG, Wiesbaden
3. Amin KM, Litzky LA, Smythe WR (1995) Wilms tumor 1 susceptibility (WT1) gene products are selectively expressed in malignant mesothelioma. Am J Pathol 246:344–56
4. Antman KH, Ruxer RL, Aisner J, Vawter G (1984) Mesothelioma following Wilms' tumor in childhood. Cancer 54:367–69
5. Aoe K, Hiraki A, Murakami T, Toyooka S, Shivapurkar N, Gazdar A, Sueoka N, Taguchi K, Kamei T, Takeyama H, Sugi K, Kishimoto T (2006) Infrequent existence of simian virus 40 large T antigen DNA in malignant mesothelioma in Japan. Cancer Sci 97:292–295
6. Arendt M, Bauer H, Blome H (2007) BK-Report 1/2007 – FaserjahreBerufsgenossenschaftliche Hinweise zur Ermittlung der kumulativen Asbestfaserstaub-Dosis am Arbeitsplatz (Faserjahre) und Bearbeitungshinweise zur Berufskrankheit Nr. 4104 "Lungenkrebs oder Kehlkopfkrebs". In: Deutsche Gesetzliche Unfallversicherung (DGUV), ed. Sankt Augustin, Germany 2007
7. Ashcroft T, Heppleston A (1973) The optical and electron microscopy determination of pulmonary asbestos fibre concentration and its relation to the human pathological reaction. J Clin Pathol 26:224–234

8. Attanoos R, Gibbs AR (1998) Peritoneal Mesothelioma: clinicopathological analysis of 227 cases from the U.K. mesothelioma register. Arch Anat Cyt Path Clin Exp Path 46:376

9. Bang K, Mazurek J, Storey E, Attfiel M, Schleiff P, Wood J (2009) Malignant mesothelioma mortality – United states 1999–2005. MMWR Morb Wkly Rep 58:393–396

10. Baris YI, Simonato L, Artvinli M (1987) Epidemiological and environmental evidence of the health effects of exposure to erionite fibers: a four study in the Cappadocian region of Turkey. Int J Cancer 39:10–17

11. Berman D, Crump K (2008) A meta analysis of asbestos related cancer risk that addressed fiber size and mineral type. Crit Rev Toxicol 38:49–73

12. Bernstein D, Donaldson K, Decker U, Gaering S, Kunzendorf P, Chevallier J, Holm S (2005) A biopersistence study following exposure to chrysotile asbestos alone or in combination with fine particles. Inhal Toxicol 20:1009–1028

13A. Bernstein D, Hoskins J (2006) The health effects of chrysile: current perspective based upon recent data. Regul Toxicol Pharmacol 45:252–264

13B. Bernstein D, Rogers R, Sepulveda R, Donaldson K, Schuler D, Gaering S, Kunzendorf P, Chevalier J, Holm S. (2010) The pathological response and fate in the lung and pleura of chrysotile in combination with fine particles compared to amosite asbestos following short term inhalation exposure. interim results. Inhal. Toxicol 22:937–962

14. BIA-Arbeitsmappe (2000–2001) Bestimmung von anorganischen Fasern im menschlichen Lungengewebe 26. Lfg 26. III/01 und 24. Lfg. III/00 TEM und REM Methode

15. Bianchi C, Brollo A, Ramani L, Bianchi T (2000) Malignant mesothelioma in Europe. Int J Med Biol Environ 28:103–107

16. Bianchi C, Girelli L, Grandi G, Brillo A, Ramani L, Zuch C (1997) Latency periods in asbestos related mesothelioma of the pleura. Eur J Cancer Prev 6:162–6

17. Boutin C, Dumortiers R, Rey F, Viallat J, DeVuyst P (1996) Black spots concentrate oncogenic asbestos fibers in the parietal pleura. Am J Respir Crit Care Med 153:444–449

18. Brockmann M (1991) Asbestassoziierte Lungen- und Pleuraerkrankungen – pathologische Anatomie. Pneumologie 45:422–428

19. Brockmann M, Fischer M, Müller K (1989) Lungenstaubanalyse bei Bronchialkarzinomen und Mesotheliomen. Atemw Lungenkrankh 6:263–65

20. Browne K, Smither W (1983) Asbestos related mesothelioma factors discriminating between pleural and peritoneal sites. Br J Ind Med 40:145–152

21. Carbone M (1999) New molecular and epidemiological issues in mesothelioma Role of SV40. J Cell Physiol 180:167–72, Review

22. Cavazza A, Travis LB, Travis WD, Wolfe JT, Foo ML, Gillespie DJ, Weidner N, Colby TV (1996) Post irradiation malignant mesothelioma. Cancer 77:1379–1385

23. Churg A (1982) Fiber counting and analysis in the diagnosis of asbestos related diseases. Hum Pathol 13:381–392

24. Churg A (1988) Chrysotile, tremolite and malignant mesothelioma in man. Chest 93:621–28

25. Churg A (1994) Deposition and clearance of chrysotile asbestos. Ann Occup Hyg 38: 625–633

26. Churg A, Warnock M (1981) Asbestos and other ferruginous bodies. Am J Pathol 102:447–456

27. Churg A, Warnock M, Green N (1977) Analysis of the cores ferruginous (asbestos) bodies from the general population. I. Patients with and without lung cancer. Lab Invest 37:280–286

28. Churg A, Warnock M, Green N (1979) Analysis of the core of ferruginous bodies from the general population. II. True asbestos bodies and pseudoasbestos bodies. Lab Invest 40:31–38

29. Churg A, Wiggs H (1984) Fiber size and number of amphibole asbestos induced mesothelioma. Am J Pathol 115:437–442

30. Churg A, Wiggs B, DePaoli L, Kampe B, Stevens B (1984) Lung asbestos content in chrysotile workers with mesothelioma. Am Rev Respir Dis 130:1042–45

31. Cooke W, Hill C (1927) Pulmonary asbestosis. J R Microsc Soc 47:232

32. Craighead J (1987) Current pathogenetic concepts of diffuse malignant mesothelioma. Hum Pathol 18:544–557

33. Crouch E, Churg A (1984) Ferruginous bodies and the histologic evaluation of dust exposure. Am J Surg Pathol 8:109–116

34. Davis J, Beckett S, Bolton R, Collings P, Middleton A (1978) Mass and number of fibers in the pathogenesis of asbestos related lung disease in rats. Br J Cancer 37:673–688

35. Dawson A, Gibbs A, Pooley F, Griffiths D, Hoy J (1993) Malignant mesothelioma in women. Thorax 48:269–74

36. DeKlerk N, Musk A, Williams V, Filion P, Whitaker D, Shilkin K (1996) Comparison of measures of exposure to asbestos in former crocidolite workers from Wittenoom Gorge, W. Australia. Am J Ind Med 30:579–587

37. DeVuyst P, Karjalainen A, Dumortier P, Pairon J, Monso E, Brochard P, Teschler H, Tossavainen A, Gibbs A (1998) Guidelines for mineral fibre analysis in biological samples: report of the ERS Working group. Eur Resp J 11:1416–1426

38. DGUV (2008) Occupational cancer statistics www:///dguv.de/inhalt/zahlen/bk/index.jsp

39. Dodson F, Aktinson M (2006) Measurements of asbestos burden in tissues. Ann NY Acad Sci 1076:281–291

40. Dodson R, O'Sullivan F, Corn C (1996) Relationships between ferruginous bodies and uncoated asbestos fibers in lung tissue. Arch Environ Health 51:462–6

41. Dodson R, O'Sullivan M, Corn M, McLarty J, Hammar S (1997) Analysis of asbestos fiber burden in lung tissue from mesothelioma patients. Ultrastruct Pathol 21:321–36

42. Dodson R, Williams M, Corn C, Brollo A, Bianchi C (1990) Asbestos content of lung tissue, lymph nodes and pleural plaques from former shipyard workers. Am Rev Respir Dis 142:843–847

43. Dodson R, Williams M, Huang J, Bruce J (1999) Tissue burden of asbestos in non-occupationally exposed individuals from east Texas. Am J Ind Med 35:281–286

44. Edge J, Choudhury S (1978) Malignant mesothelioma of the pleura in Barrow in Furness. Thorax 33:26–30

45. Eitner F, Otto H (1984) Zur Dignität von Asbestkörperzählungen im Lungengewebe. Arbeitsmed Sozialmed Präventivmed 19:1–5

46. Elmes P (1994) Mesothelioma and chrysotile. Ann Occup Hyg 38:547–553

47. Ewers U, Fischer M, Müller K, Seemann J, Theile A, Welge P, Wittig P, Wittsiepe J (1999) Multiple inhalative exposure of the human lung to carcinogens, metalloids and asbestos fibers. BAMAS FP 1947–1469

48. Frank A, Dodson R, Williams M (1998) Carcinogenic implications of the lack of tremolite in UICC reference chrysotile. Am J Ind Med 34:314–17

49. Friedrichs K, Brockmann M, Fischer M, Wick G (1992) Electron microscopy analysis of mineral fibers in human lung tissue. Am J Ind Med 22(49):49–58

50. Friedrichs K, Dykers A, Otto H (1995) Material stability of asbestos fibers in human lung tissue [Materialstabilität von Asbestfasern im Lungengewebe]. Arbeits Sozial Umweltm 30: 18–20

51. Friedrichs KH, Otto H, Fischer M (1992) Gesichtspunkte zur Faseranalyse in Lungenstäuben. Arbeits Soz Prävent 27:228–32

52. Gaudichet A, Janson X, Monchaux G (1988) Assessment by analytical microscopy of the total lung fibre burden in mesothelioma patients matched with four other pathological series. Ann Occup Hyg 32(Suppl):213–23

53. Gibbs G (1970) Qualitative aspects of dust exposure in the Quebec asbestos mining and milling industry. In: Walton WH (ed) Inhalated particles 3, Proceeding of the British occupational hygiene society symposium, London, 1970, pp 783–799

54. Gibbs A (1990) Role of asbestos and other fibres in the development of diffuse malignant mesothelioma. Thorax 45:649–54

55. Gibbs A, Attanonous R (2000) Examination of lung specimens. J Clin Pathol 53:507–12

56. Gibbs A, Pooley F (1996) Analysis and interpretation of inorganic mineral fibers in lung tissue. Thorax 51:327–34

57. Gibbs A, Stephens M, Griffiths D, Blight B, Pooley F (1991) Fibre distribution in the lungs and pleura of subjects with asbestos related diffuse pleural fibrosis. Am Rev Respir Dis 142:843–847

58. Glyseth B, Baumann R, Overaae L (1982) Analysis of fibers in human lung tissue. Br J Ind Med 39:191–195

59. Gold C (1971) Asbestos in tumours. J Clin Pathol 24:481

60. Gross P, Treville R, Haller M (1969) Pulmonary ferruginous bodies (asbestos) bodies in city dwellers a study of their central fiber. Arch Environ Health 19:186–191

61. Hammar S, Roggli V, Ovry T, Moffat E (1998) Malignant mesothelioma in women. Lung Cancer 18:38

62. Hein M, Stayner L, Lehmann E, Dement J (2007) Follow up of chrysotile textile workers: cohort mortality and exposure response. Occup Environ Med 64:616–625

63. Hodgson J, Darnton A (2000) The quantitative risk of mesothelioma and lung cancer in relation

to asbestos exposure. Ann Occup Hyg 44: 565–601

64. Hoggson J, McElvenny D, Darnton A, Price M, Peto J (2005) The expected burden of mesothelioma mortality in Great Britain from 2002 to 2050. Br J Cancer 92:587–593

65. Howel D, Gibbs A, Arblaster L, Swinburne L, Schweiger M, Renvoize E, Hatton P, Pooley F (1999) Mineral fibre analysis and routes of exposure to asbestos in the development of mesothelioma in an English region. Occup Environ Med 56:51–58

66. Illgren E, Browne K (1991) Asbestos related mesothelioma: evidence for a threshold in animals and human. Regul Toxicol Pharmacol 13:116–32

67. Karyalainen A, Nurminen M, Vanhala E, Vainio H, Antilla S (1996) Pulmonary asbestos bodies and asbestos fibres as indicators of exposure. Scand J Work Environ Health 22:34–38

68. Kayser K, Becker C, Seeberg N, Gabius HJ (1999) Quantitation of asbestos and asbestos like fibres in human lung tissue by hot and wet ashing and the significance of their presence for survival of lung carcinoma and mesothelioma patients. Lung Cancer 24:89–98

69. Kohyama N, Hiroko K, Kunihiko Y, Yoshizumi S (1992) Evaluation of low level asbestos exposure by transbronchial lung biopsy with analytical electron microscopy. J Electron Microsc 42: 315–327

70. Kohyama N, Suzuki Y (1991) Analysis of asbestos fibres in lung parenchyma, pleural plaques and mesothelioma tissues of north American insulation workers. Ann NY Acad Sci 643:27–52

71. Landrigan P, Nicholson W, Suzuki Y, Ladou J (1999) The hazard of chrysotile asbestos: a critical review. Ind Health 37:271–280

72. Leigh J, Davidson P, Hendrie L, Berry D (2002) Malignant mesothelioma in Australia, 1945–2000. Am J Ind Med 41:188–201

73. Leigh J, Rogers A, Ferguson D, Mulder H, Ackad M, Thompson R (1991) Lung asbestos fiber content and mesothelioma cell type site and survival. Cancer 68:135–141

74. Lidell D (1994) Cancer mortality in chrysotile mining and milling: exposure-response. Ann Occup Hyg 38:519–523

75. Lin R, Takabashi K, Karjalainen A, Hoshuyama T, Wilson D, Kameda T, Chan C, Wen C, Furuya S, Higashi T, Chien L, Ohtaki M (2007) Ecological association between asbestos related diseases and historical asbestos consumption: an international analysis. Lancet 369:844–849

76. Livneh A, Langevitz P, Pras M (1999) Pulmonary associations in familial Mediterranean fever. Curr Opin Pulm Med 5:326–31

77. Marchand F (1906) Über eigentümliche Pigmentkristalle in den Lungen. Verhand Deutsch Pathos Gesell 10:223–228

78. Marinaccio A, Binazzi A, Cauzillo G, Cavone D, DeZottti R, Ferrante P, Gennaro V, Gorini G, Menegozzo M, Mensi C, Merler E, Mirabelli D, Montanaro F, Musti M, Pannelli F, Romanelli A, Scarselli A, Tumino R (2007) Analysis of latency time and its determinants in asbestos related malignant mesothelioma cases of the Italian register. Eur J Cancer 43(18):2722–2728

79. Maurer R, Egloff B (1975) Malignant peritoneal mesothelioma after cholangiography with thorotrast. Cancer 36:1381–85

80. McDonald S (1927) Histology of pulmonary asbestosis. Br Med J 3(2):1025

81. McDonald J (1998) Mineral fibre persistence and carcinogenicity. Ind Health 36:372–5

82. McDonald J, Amstrong B, Case B (1989) Mesothelioma and asbestos fiber type: evidence from lung tissue analyses. Cancer 63:154–1547

83. McDonald J, McDonald A (1996) The epidemiology of mesothelioma in historical context. Eur Respir J 9:1932–42

84. McDonald J, McDonald A (1997) Chrysotile, tremolite and carcinogenicity. Ann Occup Hyg 6:699–705

85. McDonald J, McDonald A, Hughes JM (1999) Chrysotile, tremolite and fibrogenicity. Ann Occup Hyg 43:439–442

86. McDonald AD, McDonald JC, Pooley FC (1982) Mineral fiber content of lung in mesothelioma tumors in North America. Ann Occup Hyg 26:417–422

87. McElvenny D, Darnton A, Price M, Hodgson J (2005) Mesothelioma mortality in Great Britain from 1968 to 2001. Occup Med 55:79–87

88. Mirabelli D, Calisti R, Barone-Adesi F, Foriero E, Merletti F, Magnani C (2008) Excess of mesothelioma after exposure to chrysotile in Balangero, Italy. Occup Environ Med 65:815–819

89. Morgan A, Holmes A (1979) Concentrations and dimensions of coated and uncoated asbestos fibers in the human lung. Br J Ind Med 37:25–32

90. Morgan A, Holmes A (1983) Distribution and characteristics of amphibole asbestos fibres, measured with the light microscope, in the left lung of an insulations worker. Br J Ind Med 40:45–50

6

91. Morgan A, Holmes A (1984) The distribution and characteristics of asbestos fibers in the lungs Finnish anthophyllite mine workers. Environ Res 33:62–75
92. Moulin E, Yourassowsky N, Dumortier P, DeVuyst J, Yernault J (1988) Electron microscopy analysis of asbestos body cores from the Belgian urban population. Eur Respir J 1:818–822
93. Neumann V, Günther S, Müller K, Fischer M (2001) Malignant mesothelioma – German mesothelioma register 1987 to 1999. Int Arch Occup Environ Health 74:383–395
94. Neumann V, Kraus T, Fischer M, Löseke S, Tannapfel A (2009) Relevance of Pathological Examinations and Lung Dust Analyses in the Context of Asbestos-Associated Lung Cancer-No. 4104 of the List of occupational diseases in Germany. Pneumologie 63: 588–593
95. Neumann V, Müller K, Fischer M (1999) Peritoneal mesothelioma – Frequencies and aetiology [Peritoneale Mesotheliome – Häufigkeiten und Ätiologie]. Pathologe 20:169–176
96. Newhouse M, Berry G, Wagner J (1985) Mortality of workers in east London 1933-80. Br J Ind Med 42:4–11
97. Ophus E, Mowe G, Osen K, Glyseth B (1980) Scanning electron microscopy and x-ray microanalysis of mineral deposits in lungs of a patient with pleural mesothelioma. Br J Ind Med 37:375–381
98. Osman E, Hasan B, Meral U, Ercan A, Mehmet T, Nazan B, Ayhan Ö, Erhan E, Öner D (2007) Recent discovery of an old diseases. Malignant pleural mesothelioma in a village in south east turkey. Respirology 12:448–451
99. Pesch B, Taeger D, Johnen G, Gross I, Weber D, Gube M, Müller-Lux A, Heinze E, Wiethege T, Neumann V, Tannapfel A, Raithel H, Brünning T, Kraus T (2010) Cancer mortality in a surveillance cohort of German males formerly exposed to asbestos. Int J Hyg Environ Health 213:44–51
100. Pierce J, McKinley M, Pausenbach D, Finley B (2008) An evaluation of reported no effect chrysotile asbestos exposure for lung cancer and mesothelioma. Crit Rev Toxicol 38: 191–214
101. Pooley F (1976) An examination of the fibrous mineral content of asbestos lung tissue from the Canadian chrysotile mining industry. Environ Res 12:281–298
102. Pooley F, Ranson D (1986) Comparison of the results of asbestos fibers dust counts in lung tissue by analytical electron microscopy and light microscopy. J Clin Pathol 39:313–317
103. Price B, Ware A (2004) Mesothelioma trends in the United states: an update based on surveillance, epidemiology and end results program data for 1973 through 2003. Am J Epidemiol 159:107–12
104. Rees D, Myers J, Goodmann K, Fourie E, Blignaut C, Chapman R, Bachmann M (1999) Case control study of mesothelioma in south Africa. Am Ind Med 35:213–22
105. Ridell RH, Goodman MJ, Moossa AR (1981) Peritoneal malignant mesothelioma in a patient with recurrent peritonitis. Cancer 48:134–139
106. Robinson B, Lake R (2005) Advances in malignant mesothelioma. N Engl J Med 253:1591–603
107. Rödelsperger K, Woitowitz H, Brückel B, Arhelger R, Pohlabeln H, Jöckel K (1999) Dose-response relationship between amphibole fibre lung burden and mesothelioma. Cancer Detect Prev 23:183–93
108. Rogers A (1984) Determination of mineral fiber in human lung tissue by light microscopy and transmission electron microscopy. Ann Occup Hyg 1:1–12
109. Rogers A, Leigh J, Berry G, Fergusond A, Mulder H, Ackad M (1991) Relationship between lung asbestos fiber type and concentration and relative risk of mesothelioma. Cancer 67:1912–20
110. Roggli V (1982) Pulmonary asbestos body counts and electron probe analysis of asbestos body cores in patients with mesothelioma. A study of 25 cases. Cancer 50:2423–2432
111. Roggli V (1992) Quantitative and analytical studies in the diagnosis of mesothelioma. Semin Diagn Pathol 9:162–168
112. Roggli V (2006) The role of analytical SEM in the determination of causation in malignant mesothelioma. Ultrastruct Pathol 30:31–35
113. Roggli V, Oury T, Sporn T (2004) Pathology of asbestos associated diseases, 2nd edn. Springer, New York

114. Roggli V, Pratt P, Brody A (1986) Asbestos content in lung tissue with asbestos associated diseases: a study of 110 cases. Br J Ind Med 43:18–19

115. Roggli V, Pratt P, Brody A (1993) Asbestos fiber type in malignant mesothelioma: an analytical electron microscopy study of 94 cases. Ultrastruct Pathol Am J Ind Med 23:605–614

116. Roggli V, Sanders L (2000) Asbestos content of the lung tissue and carcinoma of the lung: a clinicopathologic correlation and mineral fiber analysis of 234 cases. Ann Occup Hyg 44:109–117

117. Roggli V, Vollmer R (2008) Twenty five years of fiber analysis: what have we learned? Hum Pathol 39:307–15

118. Roushdy-Hammady I, Siegel J, Emri S, Testa J, Carbone M (2001) Genetic-susceptibility factor and malignant mesothelioma in the Cappadocian region of Turkey. Lancet 357:444–455

119. Sakai K, Hisanagna N, Huang J, Chibata E, Ono Y, Aoki T, Tarando T, Yokoi T, Takeuchi Y (1994) Asbestos and non asbestos fiber content in lung tissue of Japanese patients with malignant mesothelioma. Cancer 73:1825–1835

120. Sebastien P, Fondimare A, Bignon J, Monchaux G, Desbordes J, Bonnaud G (1977) Topographic distribution of asbestos fibers in human lung in relation to an nonoccupational exposure. In: Walton W, McGovern E (eds) Inhaled particles IV. Pergamon Press, Oxford, pp 435–444

121. Selikoff I (1986) Asbestos associated diseases. In: Rosenau M (ed) Public Health and preventive medicine, 11th edn. Appleton, Century Crofts, New York, pp 568–598

122. Selikoff I, Lee D (1978) Asbestos and disease. Academic, New York

123. Smith A, Wright C (1996) Chrysotile asbestos is the main cause of pleural mesothelioma. Am J Ind Med 30:252–66

124. Stayner L, Kuempel E, Gilbert S, Hein M, Dement J (2008) An epidemiological study of asbestos fibre dimension in determining respiratory disease risk in exposed workers. Occup Environ Med 65:613–19

125. Stettler L, Sharpnack D, Krieg E (2008) Chronic Inhalation of short asbestos: lung fiber burdens and histopathological for monkeys maintained for 11, 5 years after exposure. Inhal Toxicol 20:63–73

126. Survana K, Layton C (2006) What is a significant lung asbestos fibre result? Histopathology 48:200–19

127. Suzuki Y, Yuen S (2001) Asbestos tissue burden study in human malignant mesothelioma. Ind Health 39:150–160

128. Tomatis L, Susanna C, Francessco C, Merler E, Mollo F, Ricci P, Silvestri S, Vineis P, Teracini B (2007) The role of asbestos fiber dimensions in the prevention of mesothelioma. Int J Occup Environ Health 13:64–69

129. Vianna NJ (1978) Non occupational exposure to asbestos and malignant mesothelioma in females. Lancet 1(8073):1061–1063

130. Wagner J, Berry G, Pooley F (1982) Mesothelioma and asbestos type in asbestos textile workers: a study of lung content. Br Med J 285:603–6

131. Wagner J, Berry G, Skidmore J, Timbrell V (1974) The effects of the inhalation of asbestos in rats. Br J Cancer 29:252–269

132. Wagner JC, Sleggs CA, Marchand P (1960) Diffuse pleural mesothelioma and asbestos exposure in the north western cape province. Br J Ind Med 17:260–71

133. Woitowitz HJ, Hillerdal G, Calazos A (1994) Risiko und Einflussfaktoren des diffusen malignen Mesothelioms (DMM). Research Report series "Arbeit und Technik", Fb 698. Wirtschaftsverlag NW. Federal Institute for occupational Safety and Health, Bremerhaven

134. Yates D, Corrin B, Stidolph P, Browne K (1997) Malignant mesothelioma in south east England: clinicopathological experience of 272 cases. Thorax 52:507–512

Surgical Therapy of Mesothelioma

7

David Rice

Abstract The treatment of malignant pleural mesothelioma is controversial, particularly regarding the role of surgery. Though well accepted as a diagnostic modality, surgery is also frequently used to establish stage, provide palliation, and perhaps most controversially, to offer cytoreduction with the putative goal of delaying tumor progression and prolonging survival. Pleurectomy/decortication (PD) can achieve macroscopic complete resection; however, the ability to deliver effective postoperative radiation treatment is limited because of the risk of lung toxicity. Accordingly, it has been associated with higher rates of local recurrence compared to extrapleural pneumonectomy (EPP). Extrapleural pneumonectomy generally offers a more complete cytoreduction compared to PD but at the cost of increased morbidity and mortality. Adjuvant hemithoracic radiation is feasible following EPP and in most series local recurrence rates are lower after EPP than PD. There are no convincing data, however, to show that one procedure is superior to the other in terms of survival. Furthermore, no randomized data currently exist that demonstrate a survival benefit to any form of surgical cytoreduction over systemic treatment and supportive care. If cytoreductive surgery does have a beneficial effect on long-term survival, it will most likely be realized in patients with epithelioid tumors without nodal metastases.

7.1 Introduction

With the exception of the use of thoracoscopy for diagnosis, indications for surgery in mesothelioma are controversial. Due to the rarity of disease there are no randomized surgical studies on which to base objective treatment decisions, and most of what constitutes current guidelines has been based on single center retrospective studies or phase I/II trials with limited numbers of patients. This chapter will examine the role of surgery for diagnosis, staging, palliation, and therapy for MPM. In understanding the current surgical literature for this disease, the reader is reminded that comparisons between reported series are difficult. Factors that highly influence the outcome such as tumor stage and histology

D. Rice
Department of Thoracic and Cardiovascular Surgery, Unit #445, The University of Texas, M.D. Anderson Cancer Center, 1515 Holcombe Blvd, Houston, TX 77030, USA
e-mail: drice@mdanderson.org

A. Tannapfel (ed.), *Malignant Mesothelioma*, Recent Results in Cancer Research 189,
DOI: 10.1007/978-3-642-10862-4_7, © Springer-Verlag Berlin Heidelberg 2011

7

are not only often difficult to accurately define in an individual patient but are often variably documented in published reports. Furthermore, indications for selection of patients to undergo a given procedure are often poorly explained (if at all) and this inevitably leads to bias when comparisons are performed between different series.

7.2
Natural History

The natural history of mesothelioma is for the tumor to progress locally causing dyspnea, by either lung entrapment or compression from effusion leading to atelectasis and shunting, and pain from chest wall invasion. Death usually occurs within 6–12 months from initial diagnosis. Though autopsy studies reveal that metastases occur in 50–75% of cases, most are clinically occult and are not the cause of death. The majority of patients with MPM are diagnosed when the tumor is at an advanced stage. Many untreated patients with early stage disease (American Joint Commission on Cancer (AJCC) Stage I) will probably survive significantly longer than 12 months. Ruffie et al reported median survival of 6.8 months from date of diagnosis until death in 176 untreated patients from 9 Canadian centers from 1969 to 1984 [55]. Two more recent trials, however, serve as useful contemporary benchmarks for outcome in untreated patients. Merritt et al. reported a median survival of 7.1 months in 101 consecutive patients with MPM treated at two tertiary referral centers in Ontario [40]. Symptom management alone was performed. Patients were not clinically staged, and a relatively large proportion (57%) had non-epithelioid tumors, which are known to have worse outcome. Another trial performed by the Medical Research Council of Great Britain randomized 409 patients to chemotherapy or active symptom control which included use of steroids, appetite stimulants,

bronchodilators, or palliative radiotherapy [44]. Epithelioid tumors occurred in 74% of patients and 79% were AJCC stage III or IV, proportions that are consistent with most clinical series. Median survival calculated from the date of randomization (median 60 days from date of diagnosis) was 7.6 months, and 1-year survival was 29%. Chemotherapy did not have a survival benefit over active symptom control; however, pemetrexed, the current standard chemotherapeutic agent was not included in the drug regimen. Two recent prospective randomized trials using modern platinum/antifolate doublet regimens showed median survival of 11.4 months and 12.1 months, respectively, in non-resectable patients [75, 78]. The median survival for untreated patients is therefore probably between 7 and 10 months from the date of diagnosis and with chemotherapy may extend to 12–13 months, but will be influenced by initial stage and tumor histology. Though these studies provide a rough benchmark on which to base survival comparisons with surgical series. One must remember that subjects in most surgical series are usually a highly select group of good performance status patients. The natural history of MPM in such patients is still poorly defined.

7.3
Diagnosis

7.3.1
Video-Assisted Thoracoscopy

The benefit of video-assisted thoracoscopic surgery (VATS) for the diagnosis of MPM is that it is a safe, simple, widely available, and highly accurate diagnostic procedure. VATS allows large tissue samples to be obtained from multiple areas of the thoracic cavity, an important consideration since there is considerable tumor heterogeneity within individual mesothelioma tumors. In fact it has been shown that sarcomatoid elements within a mesothelioma are not uniformly distributed within the tumor and that the greater the number of separate biopsies that are taken, the higher the likelihood of diagnosing biphasic (or mixed) histologic subtype [5]. As patients with non-epithelioid tumors have significantly worse outcome after cytoreductive surgery than those with epithelioid tumors do, prior knowledge of cell type can greatly influence subsequent therapy. VATS is generally best performed through a single 1–1.5 cm incision placed on the lateral chest wall in line of a potential future thoracotomy. The rationale for this is that MPM can occasionally track along thoracostomy incisions, thus limiting the number of incisions that is beneficial and placement in a region that can be completely excised at the time of future cytoreductive surgery facilitates complete resection without having to perform additional excision of multiple thoracostomy sites. A single 1.5 cm incision will usually allow for placement of a 5 mm angled thoracoscope and an endoscopic biopsy forceps through a soft thoracostomy port. Alternatively, a thoracoscope with a working channel can be used. A single chest drain can subsequently be placed through the same incision, though it is useful to close the fascia and subcutaneous tissue around the chest drain to limit postoperative leakage of pleural fluid. VATS can identify whether tumor involves the visceral pleura as well as the parietal pleura (IMIG/AJCC stage IB) but is otherwise fairly limited as a staging modality. VATS lymphadenectomy is to be avoided as a staging procedure as the interruption of tissue planes may hamper subsequent cytoreductive surgery and it is prone to false positivity due to contamination of specimens from the surrounding tumor. VATS is most easily performed in patients where a large effusive component exists. In this setting, port placement can be easily determined by correlation with axial imaging. In cases where there is significant parietal tumor bulk, it is often best to locate an underlying pocket of fluid first with an 18 gauge spinal needle. Occasionally, tumor burden is such that VATS is impossible and in these instances a small 2 cm incision (again, placed in line with a potential thoracotomy incision) can easily access the underlying tumor under direct vision. Another merit of VATS is the ability to perform talc pleurodesis. Instillation of 4–5 g of sterile medical grade talc is generally sufficient. Pleurodesis does not impact the ability to perform extrapleural pneumonectomy (EPP) or pleurectomy/decortication (PD) at a later stage (indeed it can often facilitate dissection), but can offer significant palliation in patients who are subsequently found not to be surgical candidates. It must be remembered, however, that talc will cause fluorodeoxyglucose (FDG) activity in the pleural distribution and in mediastinal lymph nodes on subsequent positron emission tomography (PET) imaging. For this reason it is ideal that PET imaging be performed prior to talc pleurodesis.

Despite the obvious benefits of VATS as a diagnostic and therapeutic procedure in mesothelioma, it requires general anesthetic and at least an overnight hospital stay. CT-guided core needle biopsy is a more convenient method of establishing a tissue diagnosis. It has a high accuracy for diagnosis of mesothelioma but is probably less sensitive for determination of true histologic subtype as generally only a single tumor site is biopsied. The incidence of tumor seeding may be also less than with thoracoscopic biopsy [1]. At the University of Texas M.D. Anderson Cancer Center CT-guided biopsy is the initial method of diagnosis used for patients with suspected mesothelioma. VATS is reserved for patients in whom there is diagnostic uncertainty or for patients in whom treatment of an associated effusion is indicated.

Thoracotomy, "mini" or otherwise, is to be avoided as a diagnostic method. It not only causes the patient unnecessary trauma but often hampers the performance of subsequent cytoreductive surgery because of disruption of the

7

extrapleural plane and potential contamination of the incision with tumor. The worst situation occurs when a thoracotomy is performed and a partial parietal pleurectomy is undertaken in the mistaken belief that "more is better." In this setting it is virtually impossible to perform an adequate cytoreductive procedure at a later time.

7.4
Staging

The American Joint Commission on Cancer (AJCC)/International Mesothelioma Interest Group (IMIG) staging system is based primarily on pathologic data [56]. As such it has significant limitations when applied to clinical staging. Many of the factors that contribute to stage designation such as pericardial invasion, invasion of the endothoracic fascia, lymph node metastases, and diaphragmatic invasion, to name but a few, are simply not possible to determine accurately with current diagnostic imaging techniques. Though PET can identify occult distant metastatic disease in up to 25% of cases, it is insensitive for determining lymph node involvement or transdiaphragmatic invasion – factors that significantly worsen outcome and generally contraindicate extrapleural pneumonectomy [21, 22].

7.4.1
Laparoscopy

Transdiaphragmatic invasion is a manifestation of advanced disease (Stage IV) and precludes any form of cytoreductive surgery. Involvement may occur either through direct and contiguous invasion of tumor across the diaphragmatic muscle or by lymphatogenous spread via communicating lymphatics between the pleura and the abdomen. This latter form of metastatic spread may lead to peritoneal carcinomatosis

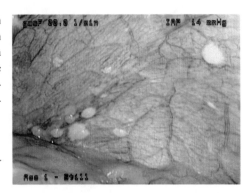

Fig. 7.1 Laparoscopic image showing small volume subdiaphragmatic tumor nodules in a patient with left-sided malignant pleural mesothelioma. Disease of this nature is impossible to detect with current imaging modalities

(Fig. 7.1) and is not necessarily dependent on the degree of tumor bulk within the hemithorax. Because of the inability of axial imaging (MRI, CT or PET) to accurately differentiate transdiaphragmatic from superficial invasion or tumor abutment, Conlon investigated the use of laparoscopy and identified transdiaphragmatic invasion in 6 of 12 patients with equivocal CT findings [15]. Importantly, of the remaining six patients, all underwent thoracotomy and none was found to have transdiaphragmatic invasion. Based on these findings in 1999 we began routinely performing laparoscopy in patients being considered for extrapleural pneumonectomy. Laparoscopy is performed as an outpatient procedure in combination with mediastinoscopy (or, more recently, endobronchial ultrasound (EBUS)), usually utilizing a 10 mm periumbilical port and a 5 mm subcostal port on the same side as the mesothelioma. After initial inspection of both diaphragms and the entire peritoneal cavity the abdomen is irrigated with 1,000 cc normal saline. A 0-degree 5 mm laparoscope is then placed through the subcostal port and advanced beneath the surface of the saline to closely inspect the underside of the ipsilateral diaphragm. The saline helps surrounding organs

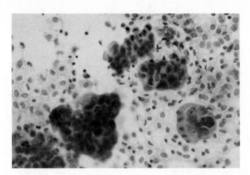

Fig. 7.2 Occult mesothelioma tumor cells obtained from peritoneal lavage during laparoscopic staging

(liver, spleen, and omentum) be atraumatically displaced away from the diaphragmatic surface while preserving visibility. Suspicious lesions are biopsied, which generally requires placement of an additional 5 mm port. The lavage fluid is routinely submitted for cytologic analysis (Fig. 7.2). In 109 patients with potentially resectable mesothelioma 9 (8.3%) patients were found to have transdiaphragmatic extension of tumor, and 1 (0.9%) patient had diffuse peritoneal carcinomatosis [51]. CT scans were suspicious for diaphragmatic invasion in only 3 (33%) of these patients. In addition, of 78 patients who underwent peritoneal lavage, 2 (2.6%) patients were found to have peritoneal micrometastases without obvious diaphragmatic invasion. Thus, 12 (11.0%) patients were identified with unsuspected abdominal involvement and thus were able to avoid futile cytoreductive surgery.

7.4.2
Mediastinoscopy

The high prevalence of lymph node metastases in MPM (up to 50% of patients undergoing trimodality therapy) and the poor prognosis that extrapleural nodal involvement confers, are justifications for preoperative assessment of mediastinal nodal metastases [47, 59]. Unfortunately, current radiographic modalities are inaccurate.

The sensitivity of CT for detecting mediastinal N2 disease in mesothelioma is only 50–60% as there is difficulty in differentiating enlarged mediastinal nodes from adjacent areas of tumor nodularity. Similarly, PET has relatively low accuracy at correctly defining N stage [22]. The efficacy of surgical staging of the mediastinum with cervical mediastinoscopy (CM) is well established for non-small cell lung cancer; however, the utility of the procedure in mesothelioma is less clear. Schouwink and associates performed CM in 43 patients with MPM and compared the staging accuracy of CM with that of CT scanning [62]. Sensitivity, specificity, and accuracy were 80%, 100%, and 93%, respectively, for CM compared with 60%, 71%, and 67% for CT. Mediastinoscopy failed to identify 9 (21%) patients who were found to have positive intrathoracic nodes at thoracotomy, despite the fact that three of these patients had positive nodes in sites that were potentially accessible by CM. We routinely perform mediastinal nodal sampling (now with EBUS) at the time of staging laparoscopy. We reported use of mediastinoscopy in 62 patients with mesothelioma and identified N2 metastases in 10 (16.1%) [51]. Of these, 46 underwent extrapleural pneumonectomy. Fourteen (30.4%) patients were found to have extrapleural (N2) nodes at thoracotomy, of which CM identified only five preoperatively. The sensitivity and accuracy of CM for detecting N2 disease was only 36% and 80%, respectively. One of the reasons for the low sensitivity is that extrapleural nodal metastases in mesothelioma frequently occur in regions that are inaccessible to mediastinoscopy such as the internal mammary artery chain, the aortopulmonary window, the anterior mediastnal fat and thymic tissue, the intercostal spaces and the retrocrural and anterior diaphragmatic regions. Combined laparoscopy and mediastinoscopy identified 15 of 118 patients (12.7%) in whom either contralateral nodal disease (N3) or abdominal involvement precluded further surgical therapy.

7.4.3
Thoracoscopy

More recently, laparoscopy and mediastinoscopy have been combined with bilateral thoracoscopy for surgical staging of patients with
mesothelioma. Alvarez et al identified contralateral chest involvement in 3 of 30 (10%)
patients and five (20%) were upstaged to stage
IV [4]. Additionally, two patients were reclassi-
fied from epithelioid to non-epithelioid histology. Surgical staging identified 26% of patients
who would have received no benefit from
trimodality therapy. Though experience with
bilateral VATS is yet limited, it may have a role
in patients who present with a contralateral
effusion or noncalcified pleural plaques.

7.4.4
Endoscopic Staging

While generally safe, CM requires a cervical
incision and is associated with a small risk of
recurrent nerve injury, pneumothorax, tracheal
injury, hemorrhage, and even death [34]. Endo-
bronchial ultrasound (EBUS) and esophageal
ultrasound (EUS)-guided fine needle aspiration
(FNA) of mediastinal lymph nodes have been
highly effective for staging non-small cell lung
cancer (NSCLC) [18, 20, 28, 85]. Since 2006 we
have replaced mediastinoscopy with EBUS for
assessment of mediastinal nodes in patients being
considered for radical resection of MPM
(Fig. 7.3). We compared 50 consecutive patients
with mesothelioma who underwent CM with 38
patients who underwent EBUS [53]. Sensitivity
and negative predictive value for mediastinoscopy were 28% and 49%, and 59% and 57% for
EBUS. Furthermore, 11 patients had EUS preoperatively, which revealed infradiaphragmatic
nodal metastases in 5 patients (Fig. 7.4). Tournoy
et al performed EUS and FNA in 32 patients with
presumed early stage mesothelioma and identified N2 metastases in 4 (12.5%) [70]. Of the

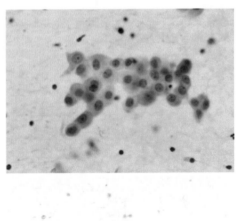
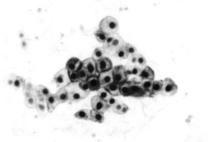

Fig. 7.3 Mesothelioma cells in a lymph node aspirate obtained from a mediastinal node using EBUS

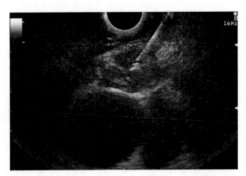

Fig. 7.4 Esophageal ultrasound-guided fine needle aspiration biopsy of a perigastric node in a patient with left-sided malignant pleural mesothelioma

patients who subsequently underwent extrapleural pneumonectomy and mediastinal node
dissection ($n = 17$) there was only one false negative (4.7%). Mediastinoscopy did not identify

additional nodal metastases. The data for EBUS and EUS staging in mesothelioma are preliminary, however, and further studies will be needed to ascertain their benefit. Though these minimally invasive techniques are safe and less traumatic than mediastinoscopy, there is a risk for false positivity because of the danger of mistaking tumor nodules adjacent to the trachea or esophagus as enlarged lymph nodes. Therefore, the procedure should be performed by an operator skilled in endoscopic ultrasound and familiar with mesothelioma and only well-defined, circumscribed nodes should be biopsied. It is also important that there is evidence of lymphoid tissue in any positive aspirate.

7.5
Palliative Surgery

Symptoms in patients with mesothelioma predominately consist of dyspnea, chest pain, cough and constitutional symptoms such as fatigue, fever, and anorexia. Respiratory symptoms are secondary to atelectasis and shunting caused by pleural effusion or lung encasement; or to altered respiratory mechanics secondary to chest wall contraction and impaired movement of the ribs and diaphragm. Surgical palliation is centered around two issues – treatment and prevention of pleural effusion, and tumor debulking to allow lung expansion and improved chest wall mechanics.

7.5.1
Pleural Drainage

Treatment of pleural effusion depends on the size of the effusion, the degree to which it is causing atelectasis and the degree of lung encasement by tumor. Simple thoracentesis is rarely effective in providing long-term relief of mesothelioma-related effusion; however, it is a reasonable initial procedure to establish a diagnosis and to evaluate the degree to which the lung will re-expand. In the absence of complete re-expansion, pleural symphasis is unlikely to occur with sclerotherapy. If the lung is trapped because of tumoral involvement of the visceral pleura (as is most often the case except in Stage I disease) placement of an indwelling pleural catheter such as the PleurX® catherer (CareFusion, San Diego, CA) is preferable. This procedure is most easily performed on an outpatient basis and avoids hospitalization. In addition, complete lung re-expansion is not required to obtain control of the effusion. Tumor progression along the tract of the catheter has been described but is uncommon [30, 63]. VATS is the preferred method for pleurodesis, particularly in cases where the effusion may be loculated, but will ultimately only be successful in cases where expansion of the majority of the lung can be achieved. In addition to drainage of effusion, VATS provides large quantities of tissue for diagnosis and histologic subtyping. Limited visceral decortication can occasionally free entrapped lung, but the case must be taken to limit air leaks as these can lead to the requirement for prolonged chest tube drainage.

7.5.2
Pleurectomy

Pleurectomy and decortication (PD) have long been used for the control of malignant effusions [8, 10]. The aim of palliative PD is to enable lung re-expansion, ameliorate the contracting effect of tumor on the ribs and intercostal muscles, and to create pleural symphasis. Palliative PD is best accomplished via a posterolateral thoracotomy. Although limited PD can be easily accomplished through a muscle sparing incision, if there is significant tumor burden division of the latissimus dorsi muscle and resection of the seventh rib can greatly facilitate exposure and resection. Dissection is begun by establishing a plane between the involved pleura and the endothoracic fascia. This is most easily accomplished using sharp dissection initially followed by blunt finger dissection. Chest wall bleeding may be controlled using gauze pads for tamponade or use of electrocautery, argon beam coagulation, or radiofrequency such as the highly effective AquaMantys® radiofrequency system (Salient Surgical Technologies, Portsmouth, NH). Once the lung and parietal pleura have been completely mobilized, dissection of the visceral pleura away from the underlying lung parenchyma is performed. The tumor rind is incised on the lateral aspect of the mobilized lung and using sharp dissection a plane is created immediately beneath the visceral pleura. Once established, dissection is continued in all directions using a peanut retractor or using a finger and gauze pad. The pericardium and diaphragm are frequently involved, or at least inseparable from tumor. If palliation is the intent of the procedure rather than cytoreduction, these structures should remain intact, leaving tumor in place where necessary.

Quality of life improvements after palliative PD have not been extensively documented and no prospective comparisons between best supportive care and PD exist. Martini et al performed PD on 14 patients with MPM and obtained control of pleural effusion in all patients. Brancatisano et al. performed subtotal parietal pleurectomy in 45 patients and combined this with decortication in 28 patients [10]. There was only one (2%) case of symptomatic recurrence of effusion. In a prospective study evaluating the efficacy of subtotal pleurectomy and intrapleural (i.p.) for MPM, Sauter and colleagues performed pleurectomy only ($n = 7$) or pleurectomy and i.p. cisplatin and cytosine arabinoside ($n = 13$) on 20 patients with early stage MPM [60]. Pleurectomy prevented recurrence of effusion in 80% of patients, with or without chemotherapy, however dyspnea was improved in less than half the patients and pain relief was improved in only 21%. The largest study that

has evaluated symptom outcomes following PD was that reported by Soysal et al who retrospectively reviewed 100 consecutive cases of PD performed for palliation of MPM [64]. Chest pain was the most common presenting feature (71%) followed by pleural effusion (54%) and dyspnea (37%). Pleural effusion was controlled in 52/54 (96%) of patients who presented with symptomatic effusion, chest pain was relieved or improved in 85% and cough and dyspnea improved in all patients. Importantly, symptom relief was achieved for up to 6 months.

Though palliative pleurectomy can achieve excellent control of pleural effusion, it requires a thoracotomy and the associated morbidity may negate some of the potential advantages of pleurectomy, particularly with respect to the control of pain. For this reason video-assisted thoracoscopic surgery (VATS) debulking has emerged as a possible option for palliative pleurectomy. Waller initially described this technique in 19 patients with malignant effusion [79]. At a median follow-up of 12 months, symptomatic recurrent effusion had developed in 3 (16%) patients. It is of concern that tumor seeding at thoracostomy sites developed in 5 of 13 (38%) patients with MPM. The same group later reported their experience with palliative surgical debulking in 51 patients with MPM [36]. Parietal pleurectomy was performed in 17 (34%) patients while pleurectomy and decortication was required in the remainder (3 by VATS and 31 by thoracotomy). Morbidity included prolonged air leaks in 19% and empyema in 2%. Thirty-day mortality was 8% and was 14% by 6 weeks. Significant improvement in dyspnea and pain score was achieved at 6 weeks and 3 months. Patients with epithelial cell type and no weight loss were significantly more likely to retain symptomatic control than those without these features. Symptom relief was found to persist until tumor recurrence, and median survival for patients with non-epithelioid tumors in this study was only 4.4 months, suggesting that surgical palliation may not be appropriate for patients with biphasic or sarcomatoid tumors. There is currently a prospective randomized phase III trial (MESOVATS) ongoing in the UK, which compares VATS pleurectomy with talc pleurodesis in patients with MPM [http://public.ukcrn.org.uk/search/StudyDetail.aspx?StudyID=1352].

7.6
Cytoreductive Surgery

The aim of cytoreductive surgery is to provide a removal of all macroscopic tumor from the hemithorax [65]. It is postulated, though unproven, that R0/R1 cytoreduction may prolong survival in patients particularly those with epithelioid tumors who do not have lymph node metastases. Cytoreductive surgery is usually accomplished in the setting of bi- or tri-modality therapy. Local tumor control appears to be improved with R0/R1 cytoreduction and adjuvant radiation therapy. Because of the high rate of distant recurrences (as high as 50%), systemic therapy is usually also advisable, though the effect of chemotherapy on

reducing distal recurrence is unproven. There are two approaches to cytoreduction: extrapleural pneumonectomy and extended pleurectomy/decortication (or radical pleurectomy/decortication). Each has its merits as well as limitations and will be discussed separately below.

7.6.1
Extrapleural Pneumonectomy (EPP)

7.6.1.1
Technique

Extrapleural pneumonectomy involves the *en-bloc* resection of the parietal and visceral pleura, lung, ipsilateral pericardium and diaphragm (Fig. 7.5). Preoperative placement of defibrillator EKG leads is performed in the event of an intraoperative rapid supraventricular arrhythmia that requires synchronized cardioversion. Because of the potential risk of injury to the superior vena cava during dissection of right-sided tumors, large bore femoral venous access is obtained. A nasogastric tube is placed, which

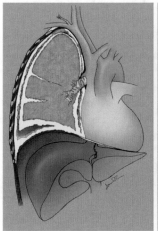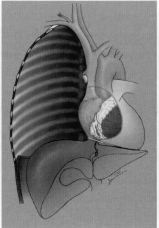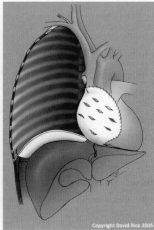

Fig. 7.5 Extrapleural pneumonectomy involves the en bloc resection of the parietal and visceral pleura, lung, ipsilateral pericardium, and diaphragm with reconstruction of the latter two structures, in this case with polytetrafluoroethylene (PTFE) membrane

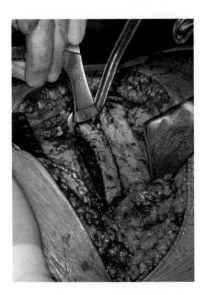

Fig. 7.6 For extrapleural pneumonectomy an extended posterolateral thoracotomy incision is made, resecting the sixth or seventh rib

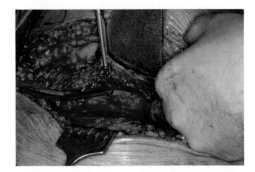

Fig. 7.7 The extrapleural plane is identified using sharp dissection and then developed using blunt dissection

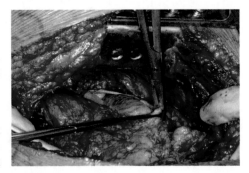

Fig. 7.8 The pericardium is incised sharply anterior to the fused pleura and resected en bloc with the lung

aids in identification of the esophagus during posterior dissection. A generous posterolateral thoracotomy incision is performed, extending the incision anteriorly in line with the underlying ribs. The latissimus dorsi muscle is divided but the serratus anterior muscle should be spared. In the event of a postoperative bronchopleural fistula, an intact serratus muscle is useful for repair. The anterior most attachments of the muscle should be elevated off the underlying chest wall and retracted superiorly. Removal of the seventh rib provides optimal access to the extrapleural plane, which should initially be developed sharply (Fig. 7.6). Once the correct plane is identified it may be extended in all directions using blunt dissection (Fig. 7.7). It is useful to place gauze packs in areas that have been dissected to tamponade oozing from the chest wall. We have found the preoperative intravenous administration of tranexamic acid to be useful to control chest wall oozing. The Aquamantys® radiofrequency system (Salient Surgical Technologies, Portsmouth, NH) or an argon beam coagulator is useful for direct control of chest wall bleeding. Once the extrapleural plane has been dissected to the level of the hilum anteriorly and posteriorly, an incision is made in the pericardium anterior to the phrenic nerve, and the pericardium attached to the overlying pleura and tumor is resected en-bloc with the specimen (Fig. 7.8). Finally, the diaphragm is resected along with the associated overlying lung and tumor. Generally, the diaphragmatic fibers can be bluntly avulsed from their peripheral attachments followed by sharp or cautery dissection of intervening fibers (Fig. 7.9). Once the peripheral attachments are taken down, blunt dissection with sponge forceps allows the

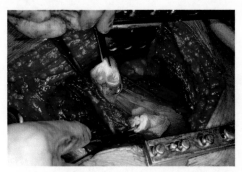

Fig. 7.9 The diaphragm fibers are bluntly avulsed from their lateral attachments and the diaphragm then resected en bloc with the lung. Use of sponge forceps is helpful in preserving the peritoneum. Small defects can later be closed with a running absorbable suture

muscle to be separated from the underlying peritoneum. It can be difficult to keep the peritoneum entirely intact, especially in the region of the central tendon; however, lacerations in the peritoneum can be easily repaired with a fine absorbable suture. The unproven rationale for maintaining the integrity of the peritoneum is that it preserves the integrity of the abdominal cavity from potential contamination with tumor from the chest. In the region of the esophageal hiatus, it is ideal to preserve some of the crural fibers to mitigate against herniation of the stomach into the post-pneumonectomy space. Once the entire specimen has been mobilized the hilar structures can be divided. The pulmonary artery and veins should be divided first. The main bronchus is freed of surrounding tissue to the level of the carina. A firing of the stapling device (generally a TA-30 3.0 mm) is placed on the distal bronchus first. This allows the anesthesiologist to retract the end of the left-sided double lumen endotracheal tube back into the trachea while preventing ventilation of the left lung for left-sided tumors. Additionally, it prevents migration of bronchial secretions into the chest cavity after division of the main bronchus. The stapling device is then placed across the

main stem bronchus at the level of the carina and two separate rows of staples fired before division of the bronchus. Application of the stapler under direct bronchoscopic examination can be useful to ensure that the bronchial stump is flush with the carina and that there is no redundant bronchus left that will retain secretions. Once the specimen is removed from the chest cavity, hemostasis is secured and the cavity irrigated with at least 3 L of weak betadine solution [68]. The anterior and inferior margins of resection are marked with numerous titanium clips to aid in planning of adjuvant radiotherapy (Fig. 7.10).

Reconstruction of the diaphragm is then performed, most often using a large membrane of polytetrafluoroethylene (PTFE, Gore, Flagstaff, AZ). The PTFE patch is secured to the remaining diaphragmatic fibers medially using interrupted 0.0 or 1.0 polypropylene (Fig. 7.11). Laterally, the patch is secured to the chest wall

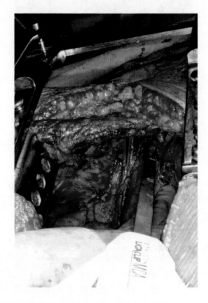

Fig. 7.10 If postoperative radiation is to be administered the anterior and inferior margins of resection should be marked with titanium clips as this will allow more accurate targeting of the entire at-risk area during dosimetry planning

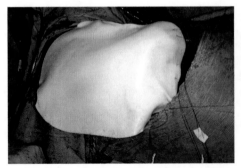

Fig. 7.11 The diaphragm is then reconstructed using nonabsorbable material, in this case 2 mm thick polytetrafluoroethylene mesh (DualMesh, Gore, Flagstaff, AZ)

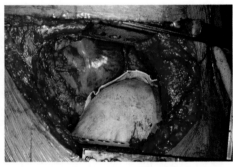

Fig. 7.13 The diaphragm should be reconstructed as low down on the chest wall as possible which facilitates postoperative adjuvant radiation planning and limits surrounding organ toxicity

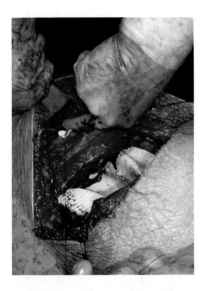

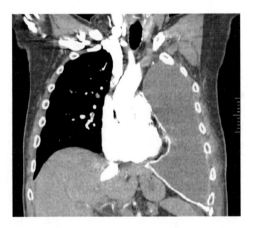

Fig. 7.14 The completed reconstruction of the diaphragm

Fig. 7.12 The diaphragm is secured laterally to the intercostal spaces using nonabsorbable pledgeted horizontal mattress sutures

using pledgeted horizontal mattressed sutures through the intercostal spaces (Fig. 7.12) [68]. Although sutures can be placed around the ribs themselves, there is the risk of nerve entrapment and greater postoperative discomfort with this technique. The patch should be placed as low down as possible in the chest cavity to enable optimal targeting of the entire thoracic cavity, however care must be taken not to place the mesh under undue tension as this can adversely affect ipsilateral movement of the mediastinal structures in the postoperative period, and also lead to suture disruption (Fig. 7.13). Medially, the patch is sewn to the remaining pericardium and care should be taken to ensure that the cut ends of the polypropylene sutures are not at risk for injury to the heart. Use of a softer nonabsorbable suture such as Ethibond may be a better choice in this location (Fig. 7.14). Once the diaphragm has been reconstructed, the pericardium is then replaced using either Dexon mesh or

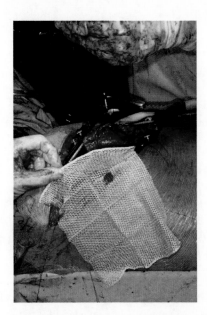

Fig. 7.15 The pericardium is reconstructed using fenestrated mesh, in this case polyglycolic acid (Dexon) mesh

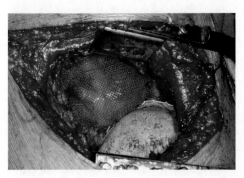

Fig. 7.16 The completed pericardial reconstruction. Care should be taken to ensure that the mesh is placed loosely to avoid compression of the right atrium once the patient is returned to a supine position

fenestrated PTFE membrane (Fig. 7.15). This can be sewn to the edges of the remaining pericardium with interrupted 2.0 or 3.0 polyethyleneglycol sutures. The pericardial patch should be reconstructed loosely to allow for the heart and mediastinum to shift slightly toward the pneumonectomy space (Fig. 7.16). Too tight a patch

can result in hypotension and limit desired ipsilateral mediastinal shift [68]. After reconstruction of the diaphragm and pericardium the chest cavity is irrigated with normal saline and a single large bore thoracostomy tube placed which is connected to a balanced pneumonectomy drain.

7.6.1.2
Postoperative Care

Though postoperative care is similar to that of any pneumonectomy, certain points are worthy of mention. Early mobilization should be encouraged to lessen the risk of contralateral atelectasis and pneumonia. Transient gastroparesis can occur following EPP, especially where one or both vagus nerves have been injured or sacrificed during dissection, therefore nasogastric drainage should be continued during the first 24 h and great care taken when advancing diet. Because of the greater degree of chest wall oozing and drainage after EPP compared to standard pneumonectomy, it is advisable to leave the chest drain in place for at least 48 h. Earlier withdrawal may allow excessive amounts of fluid to accumulate early in the pneumonectomy space which may cause contralateral mediastinal shift and cardiopulmonary dysfunction. Additionally, excellent control of postoperative pain is required not only for patient comfort but also for optimal respiratory function. Epidural analgesia generally provides better control of pain than intravenous narcotics, and because of the extended thoracotomy incision epidural analgesia should be continued for at least 4–5 days after surgery.

7.6.1.3
Adjuvant Therapy

Extrapleural pneumonectomy generally provides a more complete cytoreduction compared to radical P/D since the entire lung is removed, limiting the area at risk for local recurrence to the chest wall and mediastinum contiguous with the resected tumor. As the lung is resected, adjuvant radiation may be administered to the postpneumonectomy space. Hemithoracic radiation following P/D is problematic because it is technically difficult to deliver adequate tumoricidal doses of radiation to the entire at-risk area without causing severe toxicity to the underlying lung. Furthermore, conventional photon/electron beam radiotherapy has not been shown to decrease local recurrence after P/D [26, 33]. EPP is associated with significantly higher postoperative morbidity than P/D, and in most series mortality is also higher (3–8% in experienced centers, Table 7.1) [24, 37, 59, 68, 69, 74].

Extrapleural pneumonectomy is usually performed as part of a multimodality therapeutic regimen (Table 7.2). In the absence of adjuvant therapy local recurrence rates range between 30% and 50%. Two recent studies have demonstrated the efficacy of hemithoracic radiation in reducing local recurrence after EPP. In a phase II multicenter study from Memorial Sloan Kettering Cancer Center (MSKCC), Rusch et al delivered 54 Gy of irradiation to 54 patients who had undergone EPP [59]. Radiotherapy was performed using anteroposterior photon beams, placing specially designed blocks over radiation sensitive structures after threshold doses for those organs had been achieved. The corresponding underdosed areas of the chest wall were then treated with matched electron beams. Local recurrences occurred in only 13% and were mainly in the posteroinferior paravertebral sulcus, areas difficult to adequately treat with this radiotherapy technique. Patients with stages I and II had a median survival of 33.8 months whereas the median survival of patients with stage III or IV was only 10 months. A retrospective study, from the M.D. Anderson Cancer Center (MDACC), evaluated 63 patients treated with intensity modulated radiation therapy (IMRT) (median dose 45 Gy) after EPP [52]. IMRT has advantages over conventional radiation because the entire hemithorax can be more accurately targeted while limiting radiation toxicity to surrounding structures. In-field recurrences occurred in only 5% and overall locoregional recurrence was 13%. It should be kept in mind that the patients treated in both these studies were of advanced stage – 69% stage III/IV in the MSKCC study; 87% stage III/IV in the MDACC study. Despite excellent local control, however, distant metastases occurred in 63% and 54% of patients in each study, respectively, suggesting the need for systemic treatment in addition to local therapy.

Accordingly, trimodality therapy incorporating adjuvant or neoadjuvant chemotherapy is now recommended by most specialist centers. The Brigham and Women's Hospital has utilized trimodality therapy since the early 1980s. The regimen originally included EPP followed by platinum-based chemotherapy and hemithoracic radiation to 30 Gy. In 1999, Sugarbaker reported the results in 183 consecutive patients with MPM treated with this regimen [67]. Although seven patients who died within 30 days were excluded from the final survival analysis, median survival was 19 months and 2-year and 5-year survival was 38% and 15%, respectively. Of 31 (18%) patients with epithelioid, node-negative tumors and negative margins (and who survived surgery), median survival was 51 months, and 2-year and 5-year survival was 68% and 46%, respectively. Local recurrence rates were high, however, most likely due to the lower doses of radiation used and the fact that only regions of the hemithorax thought to be "at risk" for recurrence were targeted rather than the entire hemithorax. Details of the radiation treatment of a subset of these patients who received their radiation treatment at the Brigham and Women's Hospital were reported by Baldini and colleagues [7]. Local recurrence developed in 46% patients. Reasons for failure were likely twofold. First, radiation doses less than 45 Gy are generally not tumoricidal for MPM. Second, diaphragm reconstruction was performed well

Table 7.1 Studies including extrapleural pneumonectomy: tumor characteristics, operative mortality and survival

Author	Year	n	Age (years)	Epithelial (%)	Stage III/IV (%)	N2 (%)	Perioperative Mortality (%)	Survival Median (mo)	1-year (%)	2-year (%)	5-year (%)
Butchart [11]	1976	29	52	38	NR	NR	31	5		10	3.5
Ruffie [55]	1989	23	61	NR	NR	NR	13	9		17	
Rusch [57]	1991	20	60	NR	NR	NR	15	11		33	
Sugarbaker [66]	1991	31	53	53	NR	29	6	21	70	48	
Allen [3]	1994	40	55	64	49	NR	8	13	53	23	10
Sugarbaker [67]	1999	183	57	59	NR	23	4	19		38	15
Aziz [6]	2002	64	57	54	NR	22	9	13–35	84		
Weder [80]	2004	16	57	74	NR	38	0	23	79	37	
dePerot [16]	2007	50	58	72	76	42	8	11			
Rice [52]	2007	100	60	67	87	40	8	10		26	
Weder [81]	2007	45	59	69	25	11	2	23			
Rea [48]	2007	17	59	95	76	24	0	28	82	59	24
Flores [23]	2007	208	NR	69	78	NR	5	14			
Edwards [19]	2007	105	NR	74	85	42	7	15	59	31	
Flores [24]	2008	385	60	69	75	NR	7	12			
Yan [84]	2009	70	55	83	NR	24	6	20	62	41	15
Trousse [74]	2009	83	60	82	53	20	5	15	62	32	14
Tilleman [69]	2009	96	60	55	81	NR	4	13			
Hasani [27]	2009	18	57	67	22	39	11	19	76		
Krug [31]	2009	54	63	82	NR	27	4	22	65	37	
dePerot [17]	2009	45	60	73	58	36	7	14			10

NR Not reported

Table 7.2 Studies incorporating multimodality therapy with extrapleural pneumonectomy in which both survival and recurrence rates were documented

Study	Year	n	Epithelial (%)	Stage III/IV (%)	Chemotherapy	Radiotherapy	Local failure (%)	Distant failure (%)	Median survival (mo)
Baldini [7]	1997	49	71	NR	Adjuvant systemic	Hemithoracic, 31 Gy	46	29	22
Rusch [59]	2001	54	68	69	None	Hemithoracic, 54 Gy	13	56	17
Schouwink [61]	2001	28	61	68	Intra-op PDT	None	31	40	10
Aziz [6]	2002	51	54	All cI-II	Adjuvant systemic	None	17	49	35
Yajnik [83]	2003	35	74	57	None	Hemithoracic, 54 Gy	37	NR	NR
Weder [80]	2004	13	56	80	Adjuvant systemic	Local, 45–60 Gy or hemithoracic, 30 Gy	62	NR	23
Rice [52]	2007	63	71	87	None	Hemithoracic IMRT, 45–50 Gy	13	54	14
Allen [3]	2007	39	64	69	Adjuvant systemic	Hemithoracic, 30 Gy	41	49	19
De Perot [16]	2007	50	72	76	Neoadjuvant systemic	Yes†48%	35	36	11
Miles [41]	2008	13	77	76	Adjuvant systemic	Hemithoracic IMRT, 45 Gy	46	31	NR
Flores [24]	2008	385	69	75	Adjuvant systemic	Type not specified	33	66	12
vanSandick [77]	2008	15	93	NR	None	Hemithoracic, 54 Gy	33	67	29
Tilleman [69]	2009	92	58	84	Intraop hyperthermic chemotherapy	None	17	62	13
Krug [31]	2009	54	82	46	Neoadjuvant systemic	Hemithoracic, 46 Gy	20	28	22

NR Not reported

7

above the original site of insertion of the diaphragmatic fibers. Radiation fields extended to the reconstructed diaphragm, but not below, thereby leaving a large area of the inferior and posterior chest untreated. Not surprisingly it was in this area where most recurrences occurred.

7.6.2
Pleurectomy/Decortication (P/D)

The term "pleurectomy/decortication" can mean different things to different surgeons. It can refer to a partial debulking of tumor from the parietal and visceral pleural surfaces leaving large amounts gross tumor behind, it can be a subtotal resection of the parietal and visceral pleura leaving behind only minimal amounts of macroscopic tumor, or it can include complete removal of all macroscopic tumor, which usually entails resection and reconstruction of the diaphragm and pericardium in addition to total pleurectomy (Fig. 7.17). In terms of cytoreductive surgery, the latter procedure is optimal and is frequently termed "extended" or "radical" pleurectomy/decortication to distinguish it from lesser debulking procedures.

7.6.2.1
Technique

Radical P/D begins with a complete extrapleural mobilization of the lung to the level of the hilar structures similar to that performed during the initial dissection for EPP. If the pleura/tumor is inseparable from the pericardium or diaphragm (as it most often is) these structures are resected and reconstructed in a manner similar to that of EPP. Once the lung and overlying pleura have been completely mobilized, an incision is made in the parietal pleura and taken through the tumor and visceral pleura down to the level of the lung parenchyma. Using sharp dissection a plane is created immediately underneath the visceral pleura. This plane is then further elaborated using blunt dissection with a peanut sponge or a gauzed finger (Fig. 7.3). Paradoxically, this is often more easily accomplished in patients who have a significant tumor rind as it can be difficult to completely remove minimally involved pleura. Although the lung parenchyma often bleeds it will usually abate quickly. In this way the entire visceral pleura and overlying tumor and parietal pleura can be resected down to the hilar

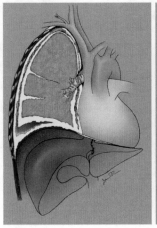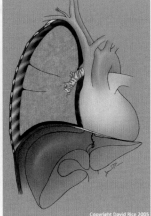

Fig. 7.17 Pleurectomy/decortication involves resection of the tumor involved parietal and visceral pleura, and leaves the lung in situ. If tumor involves the pericardium and diaphragm these structures can be resected and reconstructed in a manner similar to extrapleural pneumonectomy

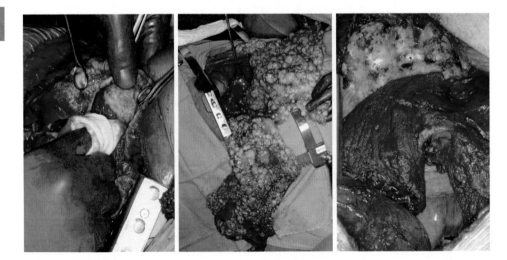

Fig. 7.18 Once the tumor rind is incised down to the level of the underlying parenchyma the lung tissue can be bluntly swept away from the overlying visceral pleura. If the fissures are involved with disease they should be dissected down to the level of the pulmonary vessels to remove all macroscopic tumor

structures. The pleura is traced all the way into the fissures, and the pulmonary artery and veins will usually be encountered and should be completely freed of any overlying pleura or tumor (Fig. 7.18). Occasionally, lung parenchyma that has been atelectatic for lengthy periods from overlying tumor will seldom expand, and these areas are often best resected with a linear stapler. Similarly, portions of lung that have been devitalized during dissection or those with significant lacerations are often best removed. Though usually all tumor can be resected from the underlying lung, occasionally and in particular in early stage disease, there can be a multitude of tiny subpleural tumor deposits that remain adherent to the lung after visceral pleurectomy. These may be directly removed using sharp dissection or may be ablated using thermal energy (argon beam [82], electrocautery, radiofrequency ablation, or cryoablation (personal observation)) (Fig. 7.19). Typically, there are three large-bore chest drains : one over the diaphragm coursing posteriorly to drain the costovertebral recess, one in the posterior sulcus, and one anteriorly.

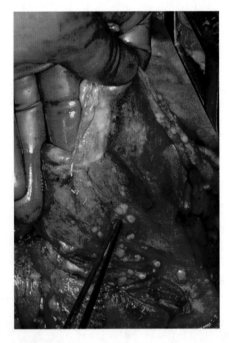

Fig. 7.19 Occasionally multiple small subpleural deposits will be encountered which remain after visceral decortication. These deposits can be individually resected or locally ablated using thermal energy

7.6.2.2
Postoperative Care

Because the chest wall can continue to slowly ooze blood and maximum expansion of the lung is ideal postoperatively, it can be helpful to keep patients intubated overnight following pleu-rectomy/decortications. This ensures maximal expansion of atelectatic lung and the inflated lung aids in tamponading diffuse chest wall oozing. Air leaks are prominent, particularly on positive pressure ventilation, but will usually subside within a week. Chest drains are placed at the lowest amount of suction that is sufficient to maintain complete expansion of the lung, usually negative 10–20 cm H_2O.

7.6.2.3
Adjuvant Therapy

Because the lung is left in situ, P/D offers less complete cytoreduction than EPP but impacts pulmonary function significantly less. This is reflected in the lower perioperative mortal-ity reported in most series compared to EPP (Table 7.3), and also in the higher incidence of local recurrence, which generally ranges from 50% to 100% (Table 7.4). Unlike EPP, the intact lung that remains limits the ability to administer effective radiation postoperatively. Gupta et al reported 123 patients who received hemithoracic radiation therapy (median 43 Gy) similar to the regimen used at MSKCC for EPP [26]. Despite a preponderance of patients with stage I and II (59%) median survival was only 14 months, and local recurrence occurred in 56% of patients. Similarly, Lee and colleagues performed P/D on 26 patients using intraop-erative radiation followed by postoperative 3-dimensional conformal radiation or IMRT [33]. 69% of patients had stage I disease and so it is not surprising that the median survival was reasonably good (18 months). Fifty per-cent of patients had recurred or died by 1 year however, and although the exact frequency of

local recurrences was not reported, the authors stated that most patients died from progressive disease, and that the "site of failure was mostly locoregional."

7.6.3
Intrapleural Therapies

The relatively high local recurrence rate follow-ing cytoreductive surgery alone has prompted use intrapleural therapies after PD or EPP (Table 7.5). These have primarily involved intra-pleural administration of platinum-based chemo-therapy or intracavitary photodynamic therapy (PDT) with preoperatively administered photo-sensitizers. The concept behind intrapleural ther-apy is straightforward – extrapleural dissection of mesothelioma cannot reliably achieve an R0 resection and microscopic tumor deposits are fre-quently left behind. This is evident in local recur-rence rates of up to 30–50% following EPP alone. Because of the even greater propensity for microscopic, and even macroscopic tumor rem-nants following pleurectomy/decortication, local recurrence rates can be as high as 70–100% with this procedure. Intrapleural chemotherapy is the-oretically able to treat the entire at-risk area of the hemithorax and has been shown to permeate up to 5 mm into tissue. Most trials of ip chemo-therapy however have been small phase I and II studies with limited numbers of patients. Rates of local recurrence have varied between 17% and 100% (Table 7.6). Earlier studies tended to rely on the instillation of chemotherapeutic agent into the chest cavity via chest drains in the postopera-tive period. More recently, capitalizing on the tumoricidal effect of hyperthermia, investigators have evaluated intraoperative intrapleural perfu-sion of cytotoxics heated to 42°C. The largest study of this nature was recently reported by Tilleman and colleagues from the Brigham and Women's Hospital [69]. Ninety-two patients were enrolled on a phase II study which included EPP and intraoperative heated chemoperfusion with cisplatin. Renal function was maintained by

7

Table 7.3 Studies including pleurectomy/decortication: tumor characteristics, operative mortality and survival

Author	Year	n	Age (years)	Epithelial (%)	Stage III/IV (%)	Perioperative mortality (%)	Survival Median (mo)	1-year (%)	2-year (%)	5-year (%)
McCormack [39]	1982	33	NR	100	NR	0	21	NR	NR	NR
Hilaris [29]	1984	41	58	68	NR	0	21	65	40	NR
Allen [2]	1994	56	64	50	NR	5	9	30	9	5
Rusch [58]	1994	27	62	70	52	4	18	69	40	NR
Martin- Uncar [36]	2001	51	63	67	NR	8	7	31	NR	NR
Ceresoli [12]	2001	54	60	73	41	NR	12.5–14	50–63	NR	NR
Aziz [6]	2002	47	NR	NR	NR	0	14	NR	NR	NR
Colaut [13]	2004	40	60	NR	23	3	11	NR	28	3
Flores [23]	2007	176	NR	NR	NR	3	16	NR	NR	NR
Flores [24]	2008	278	63	64	65	4	16	NR	NR	NR
Bolukbas [9]	2009	35	65	77	54	3	30	69	50	NR

NR Not reported

Table 7.4 Studies incorporating multimodality therapy with pleurectomy/decortication in which both survival and recurrence rates were documented

Study	Year	n	Epithelial (%)	Stage III/IV (%)	Chemotherapy	Radiotherapy	Local failure (%)	Distant failure (%)	Median survival (mo)
Hilaris [29]	1984	41 PD	68	NR	Adjuvant systemic	Brachytherapy, intrapleural 32P, hemithoracic 45 Gy	71	54	21
Rusch [58]	1994	27 PD	70	52	Adjuvant intrapleural, systemic	None	85	20	18
Lee [32]	1995	15 PD	46	NR	Adjuvant intrapleural, systemic	Type not specified	100	0	12
Monneuse [42]	2003	17 PD	NR	NR	Adjuvant intrapleural	None	59	18	18
Colaut [13]	2004	40 PD	NR	23	Adjuvant systemic	Local, 10 Gy	86	0	11
Matzi [38]	2004	25 PD	56	100	Intraop PDT + hyperbaric O2 (14 pts)	None	48	NR	14
Richards [54]	2006	44 PD	55	39	Intraop hyperthermic chemotherapy	None	57	43	13
Lucchi [35]	2007	49 PD	80	82	Adjuvant intrapleural, systemic	Local 30 Gy	90	14	26
Flores [24]	2008	278 PD	64	65	Adjuvant systemic	Type not specified	65	35	16
Bolukbas [9]	2009	35 PD	77	54	Adjuvant systemic	Local, 21 Gy–50 Gy	36	24	30

NR Not reported

Table 7.5 Studies including intrapleural therapy: tumor characteristics, operative mortality, and survival.

Author	Year	Surgery	Intrapleural therapy	Epithelioid (%)	Stage III/IV (%)	Perioperative Mortality (%)	Survival Median (mo)	2-year (%)	3-year (%)
Rusch [58]	1994	27 PD	Postop ip Cis/MMC	70	52	4	18	40	
Rice [50]	1994	9 PD/10 EPP	Post-op ip Cis/MMC (PD) or Cis (EPP)	NR	NR	5	13		17
Lee [32]	1995	15 PD	Postop ip Cis/cytosine arabinoside	46	NR	0	12		7
Colleoni [14]	1996	20 PD	Postop ip Cis/cytosine arabinoside	50	NR	0	12		
Pass [46]	1997	11 PD/14 EPP	Intraop Porfimer Na PDT	68	84	4	14		
Moskal [43]	1998	33 PD/7 EPP	Intraop Porfimer Na PDT	63	NR	8	15	23	
Schouwink [61]	2001	28 EPP	Intraop Tetrahydroxyphenylchlorin PDT	61	68	11	10		
Aziz [6]	2002	51 EPP	Postop ip Carboplatin	54	All c I-II	9	35		48
Monneuse [42]	2003	17 PD	Intraop ip hyperthermic MMC (7) MMC/Cis (10)	NR	NR	6	18	50	42
Friedberg [25]	2003	19 PD/7 EPP	Intraop Foscan PDT	64	NR	10	12	40	
van Ruth [76]	2004	12 PD/8 EPP	Intraop hyperthermic Cis/Doxorubicin	80	NR	0	11	<20%	NR
Matzi [38]	2004	14 PD	Intraop Porphyrin PDT + hyperbaric O2	56	100	0	14		
Richards [54]	2006	44 PD	Intraop ip hyperthermic Cis	55	39	11	13	30	20
Lucchi [35]	2007	49 PD	IL-2 + Epidoxorubicin	80	82	0	26		
vanSandick [77]	2008	12 PD/8 EPP	Intraop ip hyperthermic Cis	80	NR	0	11	15	10
Tillenam [69]	2009	92 EPP	Intraop ip hyperthermic Cis	58	84	4	13		25

NR Not reported

Table 7.6 Combined series of extrapleural pneumonectomy and pleurectomy/decortication with multimodality intrapleural therapy

Study	Year	n	Epithelial (%)	Stage III/IV (%)	Chemotherapy	Radiotherapy	Local failure (%)	Distant failure (%)	Median survival (mo)
Pass [45]	1997	11 PD/ 14 EPP	68	84	Intraop PDT, Adjuvant systemic	None	76	16	14
Pass [45]	1997	12 PD/ 11 EPP	70	83	Adjuvant systemic, αIFN	None	74	8	14
Friedberg [25]	2003	19 PD/ 7 EPP	64	NR	Intraop PDT	None	15	15	12
van Ruth [76]	2004	12 PD/ 8 EPP	80	NR	Intraop hyperthermic chemotherapy	Local 24 Gy, 3 fx	55	40	11
vanSandick [77]	2008	12 PD/ 8 EPP	80	NR	Intraop hyperthermic chemotherapy	Local, 24 Gy	80	55	11

NR Not reported

the concomitant administration of sodium thiosulfate and amifostine. Though recurrence within the ipsilateral chest was low (17%) and operative mortality 4%, median survival was only 13 months. Admittedly, nearly half of the patients had stage III disease and 42% had non-epithelioid histology. Thirty-two percent recurred in the contralateral chest and 26% in the abdomen, highlighting the need for more effective systemic therapies. The same group previously published their experience using a similar regimen in 44 patients who were ineligible for EPP and who underwent PD instead [54]. Local recurrence was 57% and treatment related mortality was 11%, probably at least somewhat related to the fact that this was an older, higher risk group.

Photodynamic therapy has been evaluated in at least four phase I/II studies [25, 38, 43] and a single phase III trial [45]. Local recurrence rates have varied between 15% and 76% and median survival ranged from 10 to 15 months. Treatment-related toxicity has been an issue and one study reported two deaths, one related to a bronchopleural fistula, and another due to esophageal fistulization [61]. A single randomized study has

been conducted which compared patients who underwent cytoreduction surgery with or without PDT [45]. Adjuvant immunochemotherapy was administered to both groups. No differences in overall or progression free survival was noted between groups.

7.6.4
Extrapleural Pneumonectomy Versus Pleurectomy/Decortication

There is considerable controversy over the selection of which operation is the most appropriate. Some surgeons perform only EPP, others only P/D, and many tailor selection of operation to the patient and the degree of tumor load. As previously mentioned, in addition to the oncologic pros and cons of either operation, selection must also take into account the application of adjuvant therapies as well as patient and tumor-related factors. Clearly, an elderly patient or one with poor cardiopulmonary function is unlikely to tolerate EPP and would be better served with P/D. Patients with non-epithelioid histology

7

(especially sarcomatoid) have poor outcome after EPP and these patients should also probably undergo P/D if surgery is even contemplated at all. The controversy exists mainly around good performance status patients with epithelioid tumors in whom either operation would be technically feasible. There have been no randomized prospective comparisons of these procedures in carefully staged and stratified patients. The largest retrospective comparison of EPP and P/D that exists was performed by Flores and colleagues who reported a combined series from three separate institutions that included 663 patients [24]. Overall median survival was 14 months and was slightly longer for the 278 patients who underwent P/D than for the 385 patients who had EPP (16 vs 12 months, $p<0.001$). However, it should be recognized that significantly more patients in the P/D/ group had early stage tumors (35% vs 25% ($p < 0.001$)). In addition, the institutions involved in this study performed P/D not only for patients who would not medically tolerate EPP, but also for fit patients when there was "minimal visceral involvement" [23] and for patients with low tumor volume [46]. This bias toward performing P/D on patients with biologically more favorable tumors makes it difficult to draw firm conclusions from the data. Furthermore, a previous analysis from one of the institutions revealed no difference in survival among 222 patients with EPP and 126 patients with P/D [23].

Another controversial area relates to whether to offer EPP to patients with known nodal metastases, which are known to occur in up to 50% of patients undergoing EPP. Survival of patients with nodal metastases is significantly reduced compared to that of node negative patients. Nevertheless, there are occasional long-term survivors among patients with N2 disease who have undergone trimodality therapy. A recent retrospective study from the UK compared outcomes of node positive patients who underwent EPP and P/D, and found no survival

benefit for EPP [37]. As survival is limited for this subset of patients (median survival ≈ 10 months) performing a less morbid procedure such as P/D may indeed be justified. There remains the problem, however, of accurately identifying N2 positive patients prior to EPP. As described above, mediastinoscopy has poor sensitivity (≈ 30–40%) and although EBUS and EUS may offer improved accuracy, a large number of positive nodes occur in locations where preoperative histologic sampling is not possible. For this reason we now perform extensive lymph node sampling following the initial extrapleural dissection in patients planned to undergo EPP. If nodal metastases are identified on frozen section, a decision is usually made to perform radical P/D rather than EPP [49].

7.6.5
Does Cytoreductive Surgery Improve Survival?

Both EPP and P/D are extensive surgeries that carry significant risk of morbidity and mortality. The excellent five-year survival of 46% reported by Sugarbaker and colleagues applied to a relatively small fraction of patients (17%), mainly those with epithelioid node negative tumors who could be completely resected [67]. There have been no surgical series that have included internal controls. Survival times in surgical series are of significance only within the context of the surgically treated group and cannot be reliably compared to survival times of patients treated nonoperatively, for the many reasons previously described. Even within non-surgically treated patients, there is wide variation in survival depending on disease stage, tumor burden, and performance status. Though EPP probably results in a more complete cytoreduction compared to P/D, this has not been shown to translate into improved overall survival. The larger issue, however, is whether any form of aggressive cytoreduction actually confers a survival benefit over systemic therapy and symptom control [71]. There are no randomized data available yet, however a prospective randomized trial was commenced in 2005 in the UK and was designed to answer this question. The Mesothelioma and Radical Surgery (MARS) trial enrolled patients with MPM who were deemed eligible for EPP and were without evidence of extrapleural (N2) nodal metastases [72]. All patients received three cycles of platinum-based chemotherapy and were subsequently randomized to either receive EPP and adjuvant radiotherapy, or best supportive care. The trial recently completed a pilot feasibility phase in which 50 patients were successfully randomized [73]. The proposed sample size of the MARS trial was 670 patients; however, the trial has subsequently been closed.[http://public.ukcrn. org.uk/search/StudyDetail.aspx?StudyID=1189]. The survival and recurrence outcomes have not yet been disclosed, however with only 24 and 26 patients in the surgical and nonsurgical arms, any conclusions from the data will likely be of limited clinical significance. At the present time there are no plans to continue the trial in its original form, however, a new trial, MARS II, may be launched in the near future. If a cytoreductive surgical arm is included it will likely not be EPP but rather P/D (personal communication: Dr. Jeremy Steele). Without MARS or trials like it that compare cytoreductive surgery in a randomized fashion to a nonsurgical arm, we will have to continue to base treatment decisions on limited and fundamentally biased data.

7.7
Summary

Controversy remains regarding the optimal therapy for MPM. In fit patients with epithelioid tumors and negative nodes, cytoreductive surgery combined with appropriate adjuvant or neoadjuvant therapy may improve survival compared to best supportive care or chemotherapy alone, though this is unproven. Complete removal of all macroscopic disease should be the goal of any potentially curative surgical procedure, whether EPP or P/D. EPP has been associated with lower rates of local recurrence, particularly when combined with hemithoracic radiation; however, it is also associated with higher perioperative morbidity and mortality in comparison to P/D. Currently, there is no convincing evidence of any survival difference between the two procedures. Distant failure remains a significant issue that limits long-term survival in patients who have undergone EPP. However, it is possible that if micrometastatic disease can be successfully treated in the future with improved chemotherapeutic or immunotherapeutic strategies, then the local control of achievable with cytoreduction might translate into improved survival.

References

1. Agarwal PP et al (2006) Pleural mesothelioma: sensitivity and incidence of needle track seeding after image-guided biopsy versus surgical biopsy. Radiology 241(2):589–594
2. Allen KB, Faber LP, Warren WH (1994) Malignant pleural mesothelioma. Extrapleural pneumonectomy and pleurectomy. Chest Surg Clin N Am 4(1):113–126
3. Allen AM et al (2007) Influence of radiotherapy technique and dose on patterns of failure for mesothelioma patients after extrapleural pneumonectomy. Int J Radiat Oncol Biol Phys 68(5):1366–1374
4. Alvarez JM et al (2009) Bilateral thoracoscopy, mediastinoscopy and laparoscopy, in addition to CT, MRI and PET imaging, are essential to correctly stage and treat patients with mesothelioma prior to trimodality therapy. ANZ J Surg 79(10):734–738
5. Arrossi AV et al (2008) Histologic assessment and prognostic factors of malignant pleural

mesothelioma treated with extrapleural pneumonectomy. Am J Clin Pathol 130(5):754–764

6. Aziz T, Jilaihawi A, Prakash D (2002) The management of malignant pleural mesothelioma; single centre experience in 10 years. Eur J Cardiothorac Surg 22(2):298–305

7. Baldini EH et al (1997) Patterns of failure after trimodality therapy for malignant pleural mesothelioma. Ann Thorac Surg 63(2):334–338

8. Beattie EJ Jr (1963) The treatment of malignant pleural effusions by partial pleurectomy. Surg Clin North Am 43:99–108

9. Bolukbas S et al (2011) Survival after trimodality therapy for malignant pleural Mesothelioma: Radical Pleurectomy, chemotherapy with Cis platin/Pemetrexed and radiotherapy. Lung Cancer 71(1):75–81

10. Brancatisano RP, Joseph MG, McCaughan BC (1991) Pleurectomy for mesothelioma. Med J Aust 154(7):455–457

11. Butchart EG et al (1976) Pleuropneumonectomy in the management of diffuse malignant mesothelioma of the pleura. Experience with 29 patients. Thorax 31(1):15–24

12. Ceresoli GL et al (2001) Therapeutic outcome according to histologic subtype in 121 patients with malignant pleural mesothelioma. Lung Cancer 34(2):279–287

13. Colaut F et al (2004) Pleurectomy/decortication plus chemotherapy: outcomes of 40 cases of malignant pleural mesothelioma. Chir Ital 56(6):781–786

14. Colleoni M et al (1996) Surgery followed by intracavitary plus systemic chemotherapy in malignant pleural mesothelioma. Tumori 82(1): 53–56

15. Conlon KC, Rusch VW, Gillern S (1996) Laparoscopy: an important tool in the staging of malignant pleural mesothelioma. Ann Surg Oncol 3(5):489–494

16. de Perrot M et al (2007) Impact of lymph node metastasis on outcome after extrapleural pneumonectomy for malignant pleural mesothelioma. J Thorac Cardiovasc Surg 133(1): 111–116

17. de Perrot M et al (2009) Trimodality therapy with induction chemotherapy followed by extrapleural pneumonectomy and adjuvant high-dose hemithoracic radiation for malignant pleural mesothelioma. J Clin Oncol 27(9):1413–1418

18. Detterbeck FC et al (2007) Invasive mediastinal staging of lung cancer: ACCP evidence-based clinical practice guidelines (2nd edition). Chest 132(3 Suppl):202S–220S

19. Edwards JG et al (2007) Right extrapleural pneumonectomy for malignant mesothelioma via median sternotomy or thoracotomy? Short- and long-term results. Eur J Cardio Thorac Surg 31(5):759–764

20. Eloubeidi MA et al (2005) Endoscopic ultrasound-guided fine needle aspiration of mediastinal lymph node in patients with suspected lung cancer after positron emission tomography and computed tomography scans. Ann Thorac Surg 79(1):263–268

21. Erasmus JJ et al (2005) Integrated computed tomography-positron emission tomography in patients with potentially resectable malignant pleural mesothelioma: staging implications. J Thorac Cardiovasc Surg 129(6):1364–1370

22. Flores RM et al (2003) Positron emission tomography defines metastatic disease but not locoregional disease in patients with malignant pleural mesothelioma. J Thorac Cardiovasc Surg 126(1):11–16

23. Flores RM et al (2007) Prognostic factors in the treatment of malignant pleural mesothelioma at a large tertiary referral center. J Thorac Oncol 2(10):957–965, Official Publication of the International Association for the Study of Lung Cancer

24. Flores RM et al (2008) Extrapleural pneumonectomy versus pleurectomy/decortication in the surgical management of malignant pleural mesothelioma: results in 663 patients. J Thorac Cardiovasc Surg 135(3):620–626

25. Friedberg JS et al (2003) A phase I study of Foscan-mediated photodynamic therapy and surgery in patients with mesothelioma. Ann Thorac Surg 75(3):952–959

26. Gupta V et al (2005) Hemithoracic radiation therapy after pleurectomy/decortication for malignant pleural mesothelioma. Int J Radiat Oncol Biol Phys 63(4):1045–1052

27. Hasani A et al (2009) Outcome for patients with malignant pleural mesothelioma referred for Trimodality therapy in Western Australia. J Thorac Oncol 4(8):1010–1016, Official Publication of the International Association for the Study of Lung Cancer

28. Herth FJ et al (2006) Real-time endobronchial ultrasound guided transbronchial needle aspiration for sampling mediastinal lymph nodes. Thorax 61(9):795–798

29. Hilaris BS et al (1984) Pleurectomy and intraoperative brachytherapy and postoperative radiation in the treatment of malignant pleural mesothelioma. Int J Radiat Oncol Biol Phys 10(3):325–331

30. Janes SM et al (2007) Catheter-tract metastases associated with chronic indwelling pleural catheters. Chest 131(4):1232–1234

31. Krug LM et al (2009) Multicenter phase II trial of neoadjuvant pemetrexed plus cisplatin followed by extrapleural pneumonectomy and radiation for malignant pleural mesothelioma. J Clin Oncol 27(18):3007–3013

32. Lee JD et al (1995) Intrapleural chemotherapy for patients with incompletely resected malignant mesothelioma: the UCLA experience. J Surg Oncol 60(4):262–267

33. Lee TT et al (2002) Radical pleurectomy/decortication and intraoperative radiotherapy followed by conformal radiation with or without chemotherapy for malignant pleural mesothelioma. J Thorac Cardiovasc Surg 124(6):1183–1189

34. Lemaire A et al (2006) Nine-year single center experience with cervical mediastinoscopy: complications and false negative rate. Ann Thorac Surg 82(4):1185–1189, discussion 1189-90

35. Lucchi M et al (2007) A phase II study of intrapleural immuno-chemotherapy, pleurectomy/decortication, radiotherapy, systemic chemotherapy and long-term sub-cutaneous IL-2 in stage II-III malignant pleural mesothelioma. Eur J Cardiothorac Surg 31(3):529–533, discussion 533-4

36. Martin-Ucar AE et al (2001) Palliative surgical debulking in malignant mesothelioma. Predictors of survival and symptom control. Eur J Cardiothorac Surg 20(6):1117–1121

37. Martin-Ucar AE et al (2007) Case-control study between extrapleural pneumonectomy and radical pleurectomy/decortication for pathological N2 malignant pleural mesothelioma. Eur J Cardiothorac Surg 31(5):765–770, discussion 770-1

38. Matzi V et al (2004) Polyhematoporphyrin-mediated photodynamic therapy and decortication in palliation of malignant pleural mesothelioma: a clinical pilot study. Interact Cardiovasc Thorac Surg 3(1):52–56

39. McCormack PM et al (1982) Surgical treatment of pleural mesothelioma. J Thorac Cardiovasc Surg 84(6):834–842

40. Merritt N et al (2001) Survival after conservative (palliative) management of pleural malignant mesothelioma. J Surg Oncol 78(3):171–174

41. Miles EF et al (2008) Intensity-modulated radiotherapy for resected mesothelioma: the Duke experience. Int J Radiat Oncol Biol Phys 71(4):1143–1150

42. Monneuse O et al (2003) Long-term results of intrathoracic chemohyperthermia (ITCH) for the treatment of pleural malignancies. Br J Cancer 88(12):1839–1843

43. Moskal TL et al (1998) Operation and photodynamic therapy for pleural mesothelioma: 6-year follow-up. Ann Thorac Surg 66(4):1128–1133

44. Muers MF et al (2008) Active symptom control with or without chemotherapy in the treatment of patients with malignant pleural mesothelioma (MS01): a multicentre randomised trial. Lancet 371(9625):1685–1694

45. Pass HI et al (1997) Phase III randomized trial of surgery with or without intraoperative photodynamic therapy and postoperative immunochemotherapy for malignant pleural mesothelioma. Ann Surg Oncol 4(8):628–633

46. Pass HI et al (1997) Surgically debulked malignant pleural mesothelioma: results and prognostic factors. Ann Surg Oncol 4(3):215–222

47. Pilling JE et al (2004) The case for routine cervical mediastinoscopy prior to radical surgery for malignant pleural mesothelioma. Eur J Cardiothorac Surg 25(4):497–501

48. Rea F et al (2007) Induction chemotherapy, extrapleural pneumonectomy (EPP) and adjuvant hemi-thoracic radiation in malignant pleural mesothelioma (MPM): feasibility and results. Lung Cancer 57(1):89–95

49. Rice D (2009) Surgery for malignant pleural mesothelioma. Ann Diagn Pathol 13(1):65–72

50. Rice TW et al (1994) Aggressive multimodality therapy for malignant pleural mesothelioma. Ann Thorac Surg 58(1):24–29

51. Rice DC et al (2005) Extended surgical staging for potentially resectable malignant pleural mesothelioma. Ann Thorac Surg 80(6):1988–1992, discussion 1992-3

52. Rice DC et al (2007) Outcomes after extrapleural pneumonectomy and intensity-modulated radiation therapy for malignant pleural mesothelioma. Ann Thorac Surg 84(5):1685–1692, discussion 1692-3

53. Rice DC et al (2009) Endoscopic ultrasound-guided fine needle aspiration for staging of malignant pleural mesothelioma. Ann Thorac Surg 88(3):862–868, discussion 868-9

54. Richards WG et al (2006) Phase I to II study of pleurectomy/decortication and intraoperative intracavitary hyperthermic cisplatin lavage for mesothelioma. J Clin Oncol 24(10):1561–1567

55. Ruffie P et al (1989) Diffuse malignant mesothelioma of the pleura in Ontario and Quebec: a retrospective study of 332 patients. J Clin Oncol 7(8):1157–1168

56. Rusch VW (1995) A proposed new international TNM staging system for malignant pleural mesothelioma. Chest 108(4):1122–1128

57. Rusch VW, Piantadosi S, Holmes EC (1991) The role of extrapleural pneumonectomy in malignant pleural mesothelioma. A Lung Cancer Study Group trial. J Thorac Cardiovasc Surg 102(1):1–9

58. Rusch V et al (1994) A phase II trial of pleurectomy/decortication followed by intrapleural and systemic chemotherapy for malignant pleural mesothelioma. J Clin Oncol 12(6):1156–1163

59. Rusch VW et al (2001) A phase II trial of surgical resection and adjuvant high-dose hemithoracic radiation for malignant pleural mesothelioma. J Thorac Cardiovasc Surg 122(4):788–795

60. Sauter ER et al (1995) Optimal management of malignant mesothelioma after subtotal pleurectomy: revisiting the role of intrapleural chemotherapy and postoperative radiation. J Surg Oncol 60(2):100–105

61. Schouwink H et al (2001) Intraoperative photodynamic therapy after pleuropneumonectomy in patients with malignant pleural mesothelioma: dose finding and toxicity results. Chest 120(4):1167–1174

62. Schouwink JH et al (2003) The value of chest computer tomography and cervical mediastinoscopy in the preoperative assessment of patients with malignant pleural mesothelioma. Ann Thorac Surg 75(6):1715–1718, discussion 1718-9

63. Sioris T et al (2009) Long-term indwelling pleural catheter (PleurX) for malignant pleural effusion unsuitable for talc pleurodesis. Eur J Surg Oncol 35(5):546–551

64. Soysal O et al (1997) Pleurectomy/decortication for palliation in malignant pleural mesothelioma: results of surgery. Eur J Cardiothorac Surg 11(2):210–213

65. Sugarbaker DJ (2006) Macroscopic complete resection: the goal of primary surgery in multimodality therapy for pleural mesothelioma. J Thorac Oncol 1(2):175–176, Official Publication of the International Association for the Study of Lung Cancer

66. Sugarbaker DJ et al (1991) Extrapleural pneumonectomy, chemotherapy, and radiotherapy in the treatment of diffuse malignant pleural mesothelioma. J Thorac Cardiovasc Surg 102(1):10–14, discussion 14-5

67. Sugarbaker DJ et al (1999) Resection margins, extrapleural nodal status, and cell type determine postoperative long-term survival in trimodality therapy of malignant pleural mesothelioma: results in 183 patients. J Thorac Cardiovasc Surg 117(1):54–63, discussion 63-5

68. Sugarbaker DJ et al (2004) Prevention, early detection, and management of complications after 328 consecutive extrapleural pneumonectomies. J Thorac Cardiovasc Surg 128(1):138–146

69. Tilleman TR et al (2009) Extrapleural pneumonectomy followed by intracavitary intraoperative hyperthermic cisplatin with pharmacologic cytoprotection for treatment of malignant pleural mesothelioma: a phase II prospective study. J Thorac Cardiovasc Surg 138(2):405–411

70. Tournoy KG et al (2008) Transesophageal endoscopic ultrasound with fine needle aspiration in the preoperative staging of malignant pleural mesothelioma. Clin Cancer Res 14(19):6259–6263

71. Treasure T, Sedrakyan A (2004) Pleural mesothelioma: little evidence, still time to do trials. Lancet 364(9440):1183–1185

72. Treasure T et al (2006) The MARS trial: mesothelioma and radical surgery. Interact Cardiovasc Thorac Surg 5(1):58–59

73. Treasure T et al (2009) The Mesothelioma and Radical surgery randomized controlled trial: the Mars feasibility study. J Thorac Oncol 4(10):1254–1258, Official Publication of the International Association for the Study of Lung Cancer

74. Trousse DS et al (2009) Is malignant pleural mesothelioma a surgical disease? A review of

83 consecutive extra-pleural pneumonectomies. Eur J Cardiothorac Surg 36(4):759–763

75. van Meerbeeck JP et al (2005) Randomized phase III study of cisplatin with or without raltitrexed in patients with malignant pleural mesothelioma: an intergroup study of the European Organisation for Research and Treatment of Cancer Lung Cancer Group and the National Cancer Institute of Canada. J Clin Oncol 23(28):6881–6889

76. van Ruth S et al (2003) Pharmacokinetics of doxorubicin and cisplatin used in intraoperative hyperthermic intrathoracic chemotherapy after cytoreductive surgery for malignant pleural mesothelioma and pleural thymoma. Anticancer Drugs 14(1):57–65

77. van Sandick JW et al (2008) Surgical treatment in the management of malignant pleural mesothelioma: a single institution's experience. Ann Surg Oncol 15(6):1757–1764

78. Vogelzang NJ et al (2003) Phase III study of pemetrexed in combination with cisplatin versus cisplatin alone in patients with malignant pleural mesothelioma. J Clin Oncol 21(14): 2636–2644

79. Waller DA, Morritt GN, Forty J (1995) Video-assisted thoracoscopic pleurectomy in the man-agement of malignant pleural effusion. Chest 107(5):1454–1456

80. Weder W et al (2004) Neoadjuvant chemother-apy followed by extrapleural pneumonectomy in malignant pleural mesothelioma. J Clin Oncol 22(17):3451–3457

81. Weder W et al (2007) Multicenter trial of neo-adjuvant chemotherapy followed by extrapleu-ral pneumonectomy in malignant pleural mesothelioma. Ann Oncol 18(7):1196–1202

82. Wolf AS et al (2010) The efficacy of argon beam ablation: Potential role in pleurectomy for mesothelioma (Abstract). In: The 10th interna-tional conference of the international mesothe-lioma interest group, Kyoto, 2010, Japan

83. Yajnik S et al (2003) Hemithoracic radiation after extrapleural pneumonectomy for malig-nant pleural mesothelioma. Int J Radiat Oncol Biol Phys 56(5):1319–1326

84. Yan TD et al (2009) Extrapleural pneumonec-tomy for malignant pleural mesothelioma: out-comes of treatment and prognostic factors. J Thorac Cardiovasc Surg 138(3):619–624

85. Yasufuku K et al (2006) Comparison of endo-bronchial ultrasound, positron emission tomog-raphy, and CT for lymph node staging of lung cancer. Chest 130(3):710–718

Chemotherapy and Radiotherapy for Mesothelioma

8

Xavier Dhalluin and Arnaud Scherpereel

Abstract Previously considered to be rare, malignant pleural mesothelioma (MPM) is a highly aggressive tumor with an increasing incidence linked to asbestos exposure, its main etiological factor. MPM is also a very important issue because patients have usually a short survival (median <12 months) despite current treatments. Moreover an optimal treatment for MPM is not defined yet, even if ERS/ESTS experts recently provided clear and up-to-date guidelines on MPM management. These guidelines on chemotherapy and radiotherapy for mesothelioma, as well as new therapeutic developments, are presented in this chapter.

X. Dhalluin
Service de Pneumologie et d'Oncologie Thoracique, Hôpital Calmette, CHRU de Lille, 59037 Lille Cedex, France and Universite of Lille Nord de France, Medical School Henri Warembourg, Lille, France

A. Scherpereel (✉)
Service de Pneumologie et d'Oncologie Thoracique, Hôpital Calmette, CHRU de Lille, 59037 Lille Cedex, France and University of Lille II, Medical School Henri Warembourg, Lille, France and Unit INSERM 1019, CIIL, Institut Pasteur de Lille, France
e-mail: arnaud.scherpereel@chru-lille.fr

8.1
Introduction

Previously considered to be a rare cancer, malignant pleural mesothelioma (MPM) is a highly aggressive tumor that has become a very important issue over recent years due to its poor prognosis and its increasing incidence of MPM since the 1960s.

An optimal treatment of MPM is not clearly defined, even if guidelines were proposed by several scientific societies such as the French speaking Society for Chest Medicine (SPLF), the British Thoracic Society (BTS), or the European Society of Medical Oncology (ESMO) (2007; [82,87]). More recently, the European Respiratory Society (ERS) in collaboration with the European Society of Thoracic Surgeons (ESTS) brought together experts to draw up recommendations in order to provide clinicians with clear, concise, up-to-date guidelines on management of MPM [84]. These guidelines on chemotherapy and radiotherapy in MPM are detailed in this chapter with an update of the literature.

A. Tannapfel (ed.), *Malignant Mesothelioma*, Recent Results in Cancer Research 189,
DOI: 10.1007/978-3-642-10862-4_8, © Springer-Verlag Berlin Heidelberg 2011

8.2
Radiotherapy

Radiotherapy (RT) can be used in multiple ways for management of patients with mesothelioma: to prevent tumor seeding along interventions sites, adjuvant therapy after surgery, or palliative RT for pain treatment. However, radical RT for the treatment of MPM remains a challenge as the target volume is large with complex shape, and high therapeutic dose may be dangerous due to the proximity of organs at risk (heart, lung, etc.). Development of new techniques and progress in the planning of radiation treatment may lead to a better control of the disease. However, the value of RT still has to be proven in MPM. In this chapter we will review the body of literature that evaluates the efficacy and the safety of the different techniques of RT in MPM.

8.2.1
Radical Radiotherapy

Radical RT is very difficult in MPM due to large radiations fields, a high recommended therapeutic dose (60 Gy), and the proximity of organs at risk with poor tolerance of radiations. For example, the heart can tolerate a maximal dose of 40 Gy; lungs and kidneys, 20 Gy; spinal cord, 45 Gy; and liver, 30 Gy [22].

Most of the time, RT was proposed after surgery, but there are a few old reports of single radical RT.

8.2.1.1
Radical Radiotherapy as a Single Treatment

Ball et al. reviewed 35 MPM including 12 patients receiving RT in a curative intent. Forty grays (Gy) were delivered to the entire hemithorax including spinal cord [6]. Then, spinal cord

was excluded from the radiation fields and a further 10 Gy was given. Radical RT did not significantly affect survival. Moreover, two patients presented severe side effects: one patient developed fatal radiation hepatitis, another had a radiation myelopathy.

Maasilta studied tolerance of RT in 34 patients with unresected mesothelioma [51]. The three different treatment plans were as follows:

- Fifty-five grays to the entire hemithorax in 2.2 Gy fractions/day. After this initial dose, a boost of 70 Gy was given to the gross disease
- Seventy grays in 1.25 twice daily fractions
- Thirty-five grays to the hemithorax in 1.25 Gy twice daily fractions followed by a boost of 36 Gy in 4 Gy fractions to the gross disease

The lung was not shielded. Others organs at risks were shielded after variable doses of radiations. After 1 year, all the patients presented severe radiographic radiation pneumonitis resulting in a total loss of the ipsilateral lung function.

Thus, these reports and others did not show any benefit on survival whereas toxicity was high [2]. Therefore RT alone is not an option for radical treatment of MPM.

8.2.1.2
Radical Radiotherapy as Part of a Multimodal Treatment

There are two potential surgery procedures for MPM: extra-pleural pneumonectomy (EPP) and pleurectomy/decortication (P/D). EPP is an "en bloc" resection of the pleura with ipsilateral lung, associated with resection of the diaphragm and pericardium. P/D is a less aggressive surgery. In this last procedure, after dissection of the parietal pleura from the endothoracic fascia, an incision is made to allow decortication of the visceral pleura. As a single therapy, surgery led to disappointing results. Thus, median survival after EPP alone was less than 1 year whereas inhospital mortality rate varied from 0% to 20%. Because of the diffuse nature of MPM and the difficulty to have clear margins resection, local failure after surgery alone ranged from 30% to 60% [5, 69, 70].

Therefore, RT has been proposed to reduce local relapse after surgery, alone or in association with chemotherapy. Even if to date, there is no published phase III study assessing the benefits of RT in this goal, some reports suggested that RT may reduce local relapse after surgery.

Radiotherapy Following P/D

Pleurectomy/decortication is not a curative surgery. At best, it can relive an entrapped lung and help pain control.

The main limitation for RT after P/D is lung toxicity. As the ipsilateral lung is still in place, implementations of dose are not possible without a significant risk of radiation pneumonitis. The Memorial Sloan-Kettering Cancer Centre (MMSKC) is one of the first centers where P/D and RT were associated. Gupta et al. reported a retrospective series of 123 patients from 1973 to 2004 [29]. The procedure of radiation was complex, associating photons and electrons. Photons were given to the entire hemithorax by anterior and posterior fields with blocks to protect the lung, heart, liver, etc. The areas shielded from the photon's irradiations were treated by electrons. Initially, intraoperative brachytherapy was used. As the surgery became more aggressive and the gross disease remained poor, this technique was abandoned in 1990. Patients underwent fluoroscopic or CT simulations. Median survival was only 13.5 months. Overall survival rate at 2 and 5 years were 23% and 5%, respectively. Survival increased with the dose of RT (more than 40 Gy) and the absence of brachytherapy. Sixty-nine patients experienced local recurrences (1 year rate: 42%). Severe pulmonary symptoms were seen in 10% of the patients; 6% of the patients developed grade 3–4 pericarditis. The authors concluded that conventional RT following P/D did not improve

survival and was associated with high radiation toxicity.

Another series was published including 26 MPM cases treated by P/D followed by an association of intraoperative electrontherapy and external beam RT started within 2 months after surgery [48]. The intraoperative RT was performed on areas difficult to treat by conformal RT, including major fissure, pericardium, and diaphragm. The median dose was 15 Gy and the average number of sites treated by electrontherapy was 3.3. Fourteen patients received 3D conformational RT from January 1995 to November 1997. Then, the last ten patients were treated by intensity modulated radiotherapy (IMRT). Median survival was 18.1 months, and 32% of the patients were alive at 2 years. Progression free survival (PFS) at 1 year was 50%. Most of time, recurrence was locoregional. Radiation pneumonitis was observed in four patients (17%). No comparison was done between the two treatment plans due to the small size of the different subgroups of patients.

There were few other trials again with small samples of patients and heterogeneous treatment plans. Sometimes patients were treated with or without CT, RT regimen was not always described, and surgery procedure was P/D or EPP. These reports cannot preclude any conclusion [52, 59, 95]. Therefore, these studies were not discussed in this review.

In summary, radical RT after P/D does not seem to be efficient with regards to the locoregional control rate of the different studies and the remaining poor survival. Toxicity is frequent as the ipsilateral lung is still in place resulting in poor tolerance to radiations. For this reason, recent guidelines from ERS/ESTS did not recommend RT in a curative attempt after P/D [84].

Radical Radiotherapy After EPP

Even if the absence of the ipsilateral lung after EPP allow higher RT dose, RT remains difficult, essentially due to large size with complex shape of the target volume and the persistence of other organs at risk. As after P/D, the goal of RT after EPP is to increase local control and to enhance survival. Adjuvant therapy after EPP seemed to improve survival as suggested in a review of 231 patients treated by surgery (EPP, P/D or pleurectomy alone) [79].

First studies were mainly retrospective trials aiming at assessing optimal dose and efficiency of RT. Baldini et al. reported a series of 49 patients treated by multimodal treatment combining surgery (EPP), chemotherapy ± RT [5]. Over the 49 patients treated by EPP, 35 subjects received RT, consisting in a median dose of 30 Gy to the entire hemithorax, followed by a boost on previous areas of bulk disease. Total recurrence rate was 54%, including 67% of local recurrences (35% of the total population). In the "RT" group and in the "no RT" group, local failure rate was respectively 9% and 27 % ($p = 0.27$). More recently, another study recruiting 39 patients compared the efficacy and the safety of two dose regimens of RT as part of multimodal therapy [3]. Moderate dose hemithoracic radiotherapy (MDRT) was performed through an anterior posterior field in 1.5 Gy daily fractions, to a total dose of 30 Gy. Mediastinum received 10 additional grays. When positive margins or lymph nodes were present, a boost to 54 Gy was achieved. High dose radiotherapy (HDRT) was CT planned. It consisted in a larger anteroposterior fields treated with a total dose of 39.4 Gy. Then, 14.4 additional Gy were delivered in a field excluding spinal cord and mediastinum. Local recurrence rate was 27% in the HDRT group (4/15 patients) and 50% in the MDRT group (12/24 patients). RT type was not predictive of local failure, diffuse failure, or survival in univariate and multivariate analysis.

Holsti et al. prospectively evaluated different patterns of RT and their effect on survival [34]. Radiations dose range from 20 up to 70 Gy. They could not show any significant difference between treatment plans but sample sizes were small.

Even if there is no relevant clinical proof in the literature, it is suggested that higher dose of radiation may increase local control with acceptable toxicities. Therefore, high dose RT regimens were tested in prospective trials evaluating RT in multimodal treatment of MPM. A phase II trial by Rusch et al. was first designed to assess the feasibility and efficacy of intraoperative and postoperative RT after P/D or EPP [80]. Surgery procedure was essentially chosen with regard to comorbidity. If the patient's comorbidities increased the risk of EPP in unacceptable proportions, P/D was performed. Unfortunately, in the first patients treated by intraoperative RT and EPP, the rate of infections including empyema was important. Study was stopped and redesigned without intraoperative RT. Eighty-eight patients were recruited. EPP was performed in 62 cases. Five patients were treated with P/D and the remaining 21 subjects were excluded after thoracotomy due to an unresectable disease. Among the 62 EPP cases, 54 patients received a median dose of 54 Gy (20–62) in 30 daily fractions of 1.8 Gy through an anterior-posterior field. Liver, heart, stomach, and spinal cord were protected. A complement of radiations using electrons was performed on the blocked areas excluding the spinal cord. For the first time, results were encouraging regarding the local recurrence rate of 13% (seven patients) whereas the toxicity was tolerable, except a nonlethal esophagopleural fistula. For three patients, the recurrence occurred at the edge of the radiations fields. Median survival was 33.8 months in stages I–II patients versus 10 months in stages III–IV patients. Recent reports from the same group found local recurrences rates ranging from 0% to 37% after EPP and RT [25, 30, 101]. Again, local failure occurred in the inferior treatment field, between the levels of T12 and L3 vertebra.

In a prospective phase II trial assessing multimodal treatment by Krug et al., 77 patients received induction chemotherapy followed by EPP in 57 subjects; then only 44 patients out of these 57 subjects had RT (but 4 of them could not achieve this treatment: 1 patient presented a fatal radiation pneumonitis and the last 3 subjects had progressive disease during the treatment) [46]. Median dose was 45.9 Gy (0.28–60). Pulmonary grade 3 toxicity (pneumonitis) was found in two patients. Others grade 3 toxicities were upper gastrointestinal ($n = 2$), larynx ($n = 1$), or skin ($n = 1$) lesions. Out of the 40 patients who completed multimodal treatment, 8 subjects presented local recurrences, 12 subjects had metastases, and 3 patients exhibited relapses in both sites. Median survival in intention to treat population (ITT) was 16.8 versus 21 months in patients benefiting of the full multimodal treatment.

In summary, there is no strong evidence for using radical radiotherapy in the treatment of MPM. It seems that the full cover of the areas at risk, more specifically the lower margins, could improve the control. A dose-effect relation could be present suggesting that the increase of the radiations dose could be relevant. However, to date, there is no published phase III trial that validated this hypothesis. Therefore, considering these results and the high variability of the local recurrence rate, the experts of the ERS/ESTS task force recommend the use of radiotherapy for MPM only in specialized centers, in clinical trials, as a part of multimodal treatment. An ongoing study in the Switzerland by the SAKK group may help to answer the question of the value of RT after surgery in MPM. This phase II study includes only patients with disease stage less than T3 N2 M0. After neoadjuvant chemotherapy and EPP, patients with R0 or R1 disease are randomized to receive or not hemithoracic RT. This is a two part study: first part includes an evaluation of the feasibility and short-term outcome of chemotherapy followed by EPP. Second part will assess the feasibility and long-term outcome of postoperative hemithoracic RT in patients with R0 or R1 resection.

Intensity Modulated Radiotherapy (IMRT)

Large fields, complex target shape, and proximity of organs at risk may limit dose and therefore efficacy of RT in MPM. In this context, IMRT seems to be a relevant alternative as it theoretically allows large irradiations of complex fields.

In 2003, Ahamad and al described the first seven MPM patients treated by IMRT [1]. Radiotherapy started 3–8 weeks after EPP. Definitions of clinical target volume (CTV), boost, and organs at risks were done by a radiation oncologist in association with a thoracic surgeon and a radiation physicist. A dose of 50 Gy with a boost of 60 Gy for positive margins or areas at risk was delivered. Toxicity was tolerable. No recurrence was described. Two patients died of infectious pneumonia. These initial promising results encouraged this team to treat patients using IMRT. In an update from the same group, 100 patients treated with EPP followed by IMRT in 63 cases were reviewed [78]. Local recurrence rate was 13%. Only three patients experienced recurrence within the radiations fields. Another three patients presented marginal recurrences, outlining the difficulty to define the CTV. Two patients died from radiations pneumonia within the 6 months following RT. Pulmonary toxicities could also be incriminated in four other lethal cases.

Allen et al. published the results of 13 patients treated by IMRT following EPP with adjuvant chemotherapy combining pemetrexed and cisplatin. Contouring and target volume delineation were as described by Ahamad et al. [1]. Dose to the CTV was 54 Gy with a 60 Gy boost to gross tumor volume disease defined by surgical and post-chemotherapy PET/CT findings. Of the 13 patients, 6 (46%) developed fatal pneumonitis within 2 months after IMRT. Dose-volume effect of IMRT was the main hypothesis. However, the currently used dosimetric parameters to evaluate toxicity (Volume of lung receiving 20 Gy [V20], mean lung dose received [MLD] and V5) did not seem to predict toxicity, but the number of patients was very limited. This concern leads the MDACC's team to review their experience of IMRT with special regard to dose-volume parameters [78]. There were six pulmonary-related deaths within the 6 months after completion of IMRT. Only V20 was an independent factor to predict pulmonary death. The mean V20 and MLD in their study were significantly lower than those from Allen and al (4.9% for V20 and 8.6 Gy for MLD vs 15.7% and 13.8 Gy, respectively; $p < 0.001$). Based on these results, the authors aimed at keeping V20 lower than 7% and MLD <8.5 Gy. More recently, Kristensen reported the cases of 26 patients treated with IMRT following induction chemotherapy and EPP [45]. Out of these 26 subjects, four patients (15%) developed fatal pneumonitis. Values for MLD and V10 were significantly higher in patients with grade 5 pulmonary toxicity whereas V20, V5, and V30 did not significantly differ. As a result the authors adjusted constraints to the contralateral lung (MLD < 12 Gy and V10 < 50% and V20 < 15%). Even if there is a clear relation between the lung volume receiving low dose radiations, the MLD, V5 and V20 and the development of high grade pulmonary toxicities, there is no clear cutoff values proposed in the literature. However, based on these retrospective results, ERS/ESTS guidelines recommend that the MLD should not exceed 10 Gy and V20 being less than 15% [84].

These constraints could result in an inadequate dose distribution or lower dose to the CTV. Reduction of dose could result in an increase of local recurrence rate with regard to the result of the study by Miles et al., including 13 patients treated by EPP followed by IMRT [56]. Median dose was 45 Gy (40–55 Gy) and local recurrence rate was 46%. One patient died of pulmonary toxicity 6 months after radiations, two other patients developed acute grade ≥2 pulmonary toxicity.

In conclusion, IMRT seems to be a promising procedure in MPM. However, conflicting results about pulmonary toxicity should lead to reserve this technique to experimented team [84]. Recruitment of patients into prospective trials is still needed to prospectively assess efficacy, constraints to contralateral lung, optimal dose, and target volume.

8.2.2
Prophylactic Radiotherapy

Invasive procedures are frequent for the diagnosis and the treatment of MPM patients. Unfortunately, these procedures may induce chest wall tract seeding with various incidence, ranging between 0% and 48% depending on retrospective series. This complication seems to be higher following thoracotomy (24%) than after thoracoscopy (9–16%) or needle biopsy (0-28%). The treatment of these painful tract metastases is difficult, as neither RT nor surgery provides significant results.

Prophylactic RT was proposed to prevent the occurrence of chest wall seeding. Boutin et al. published the first randomized control trial evaluating the efficacy of RT to prevent tract metastases [10]. Forty consecutive MPM patients were randomized between RT or no treatment after pleural puncture, Abram's needle biopsy or thoracoscopy. In the treatment arm, RT was delivered within the 15 days after thoracoscopy, at a dose of 21 Gy in 3 days using electrons. Twenty-eight out of the 40 patients (15 subjects in the treatment arm and 13 patients from the control arm) had chemotherapy later. None of the patients treated by RT developed tract metastases whereas eight patients (40%) of the control arm presented recurrence along intervention sites. The size or the diagnostic procedure type was not predictive of complication. Tolerance of the RT was excellent.

Bydder et al. evaluated another radiations plan using 9 MeV electrons [12]. They delivered a single dose of 10 Gy in the first 2 weeks after diagnostic procedures. Each procedure site was independently randomized. A total of 58 sites from 43 patients were included. Procedure tract metastases were present in three sites in the control arm and in two sites in the treatment arm ($p = 0.23$). Thus, the overall incidence of tract metastases was low in this study, and treatment plan could be critical regarding the energy of electron or total dose delivered. Therefore, no clear conclusion could be obtained.

A third prospective randomized trial was published by O'Rourke et al. [67]. Based on the incidence of tract metastases in the previous study by Boutin et al., the authors tried to demonstrate a reduction of 35% of tract metastases incidence. As 48% of the patient died before complete follow-up, the incidence of tumor seeding was lower than expected, and, therefore, the power of the study fall to 60%. A total of 61 patients were included (one death before treatment). Radiotherapy was performed using the same procedure than Boutin et al. Ten patients only developed tract metastases: seven patients in the treatment arm and three subjects in the control group. Moreover, the authors reported that patients with tumor seeding did not seem to be worried or uncomfortable.

In summary, the methods of these different studies had discrepancies, and their results were conflicting. Therefore, ERS experts were not able to draw any conclusion [84]. However, based on the experience of our reference center for MPM, we decided to continue to use prophylactic RT in our MPM patients.

8.3
Systemic Therapies for Malignant Pleural Mesothelioma

Systemic treatment of malignant pleural mesothelioma (MPM) is an important research area. A numerous of studies have evaluated the value of many different chemotherapy regimens. As a matter of fact, only a few seemed to be relevant with a limited benefit. Only one randomized controlled trial addressed the question of the efficacy of cytotoxic agents versus best supportive Care (BSC) in MPM.

New pathways in MPM pathogenesis have been also identified leading to new targets and innovative therapies. However, the value of these targeted therapies is still under investigation.

8.3.1
Systemic Chemotherapy

There were a few studies assessing the value of intrapleural chemotherapy in MPM. To date, this technique exhibited limited efficiency and high toxicitiy. Intrapleural therapies have not demonstrated clinical benefit for the overall mesothelioma population and should only be considered in the setting of clinical trial [92]. Therefore, this chapter will focus on systemic chemotherapy and other biotherapies.

8.3.1.1
First Line Chemotherapy

A major step in the chemotherapy of the MPM is represented by the two large, prospective and randomized phase III trials reported by Vogelzang et al. in 2003 and by van Meerbeeck et al. in 2005 [94, 99]. In fact, previous clinical trials of chemotherapy in mesothelioma were often little informative because they were most of the time monocentric, nonrandomized, recruiting small series of patients, and bringing discordant conclusions. A systematic review and meta-analysis of the literature between 1965 and June 2001 was published in 2002 by Berghmans et al. from the ELCWP [8]. A total of 83 clinical studies representing 88 treatment arms were included. Four different groups of drug regimens were described by the authors: Studies testing cisplatin-based regimens without doxorubicin ($n = 20$), trials investigating doxorubicin alone or combined with drugs other than cisplatin (eight trials), doxorubicin plus cisplatin trials ($n = 6$), and other drugs regimens including carboplatin, etoposide, vinorelbine, vindesine, epirubicin, ifosfamide, etc. The results showed that the combination of cisplatin with doxorubicin was the best regimen giving an overall response rate of 28% (95% CI [21.3– 35.7]). Associations of cytotoxic drugs did better than any single agent (respectively 22.6% vs 11.6%; $p < 0.001$). Cisplatin seemed to be the most effective single agent. Cisplatin-based regimens gave better response rates than those with carboplatin (24% vs 11.6%; $p = 0.004$). Doxorubicin alone did not induce significantly higher response than other single agents. No other assessment was possible regarding the lack of survival data in 16 studied arms and toxicity data in 49 arms. Due to a various quality, trials included were separated into two groups (low and high quality, regarding the score of validity elaborated by the authors). Results remained the same in the two groups: cisplatin and doxorubicin gave the best response. However, no prospective randomized studies assessing these conclusions were conducted.

Since this meta-analysis, several chemotherapy drugs have been tested in phase II trials as a single agent or in combination. Some drugs, used alone, were ineffective (response rate lower than 10%), such as capacitabine, irinotecan, or docetaxel [7, 43, 68]. Others had only little effect (response rate between 10% and 20%) such as combination of epirubicin and gemcitabine [66, 74], whereas only a few regimens had some significant effect (response rate > 20%) such as oxaliplatin plus vinorelbin, docetaxel plus gemcitabine, or raltitrexed plus oxaliplatin, etc. [23, 24] [91]).

There are only three randomized phase III trials evaluating chemotherapy in MPM. The two first trials compared a combination of cisplatin and an antifolate drug (pemetrexed or raltitrexed) versus cisplatin alone [94, 99]. The third one was a randomized controlled trial assessing the value of different cytotoxic drugs versus best supportive care (BSC) [58]. Muers et al. randomized 406 patients into three arms including BSC alone ($n = 136$), BSC plus vinorelbine alone ($n = 137$) or BSC plus a polycytotoxic regimen (mitomycine, cisplatin and vinblastine – MVP [$n = 136$]). Because of a slow accrual, the study design was changed, the trial stopped earlier and a comparison was made between a merged chemotherapy arm (MVP group plus vinorelbine group) versus the BSC alone arm. Median overall survival was 7.6 months in the BSC arm versus 8.5 months in the treatment arm (HR 0.89 [95% CI: 0.72– 1.10]; $p = 0.29$). If there was no significant difference between the two arms of treatment, a small trend toward a better survival in the vinorelbine arm compared to the BSC arm was found (median survival 9.5 vs 7.6 months; HR 0.80 [0.63–1.02]; $p = 0.08$). Conclusions should be made preciously as several criticisms could be raised about this study. First of all, based on the literature, the drug regimens chosen were not accurate. Second, due to an insufficient enrolment, the study design was changed, resulting in a decrease of the power of the study (76%). Third, the impact of vinorelbine was evocated using an exploratory analysis and therefore has to be confirmed in a prospective phase III trial.

Vogelzang et al. published in 2003 the results of the first large randomized ($n = 456$ patients) phase III trial comparing a combination of cisplatin and pemetrexed (C/P) versus cisplatin alone (C) in the first line treatment of MPM [99]. Due to a high death rate of 7% in the first 43 patients treated with pemetrexed and based on the literature available assessing the hematologic toxicity of pemetrexed, study design was modified with supplementation in B12 vitamin and acid folic before and during treatment in both arms [60]. Median survival was significantly longer in the C/P group than in the C group (12.1 vs 9.3 months; $p = 0.002$). This benefit was associated with an increase of toxicity in the C/P group compared to the C group, including more neutropenia (27.9% vs 2.3% respectively; $p < 0.001$), nausea (14.6% vs 2.6% respectively; $p = 0.005$), vomiting, diarrhea, and stomatitis. In the C/P group, an analysis of neutropenia regarding the supplementation in vitamin was performed. Grade 3 or 4 neutropenia was significantly more frequent in the non-supplemented patients (41.4% vs 23.3%; $p = 0.011$). Moreover, supplementation allowed patients to receive more cycle. It is to be noted that if the difference of survival between the two treatment arms was significant regarding the full or partial supplemented patients, it was not without supplementation. Some criticisms were raised about the study design, and were summarized in the Cochrane review. First, the number of cycle was different in the two arms of treatment as the median of cycles done was six in the C/P arm and four in the C arm. Second, the study was not double blind and study design was modified. Third, population may be not fully representative of usual patients as the lower limit of the Karnoski index was 70% for inclusion. Finally, the choice of the control arm (C) was questionable taking account previous studies' results.

Two years later, the European organization for research and treatment on cancer (EORTC) associated with the National cancer institute (NCI) of Canada confirmed the survival benefit of cisplatin combined with raltitrexed, another antifolate [94]. Two hundred and fifty patients were randomized to receive cisplatin/raltitrexed (C/R; $n = 126$) or cisplatin alone (C; $n = 124$). Out of the 250 patients, 33 (13.2%) had a performance status (PS) of 2. Patients received a median number of cycles of four (range 1–9) in the C arm and five (range 1–10) in the R/C arm. The association of raltitrexed and cisplatin significantly increased median overall survival over cisplatin alone (11.4 vs 8.8 months; $p = 0.048$), whereas toxicities were quite the same except for neutropenia incidence (16% in the patient treated by C/R vs 8% in the C group). There

was no difference in severe toxicity (febrile neutropenia) and no treatment-related death. It is to be noted that no prophylactic vitamin supplementation was recommended.

Therefore, since 2005, the combination of cisplatin plus an antifolate is the standard first line chemotherapy in MPM [84]. However, patients with some comorbidities do not fit into cisplatin-based regimens, leading some authors to investigate alternative drug regimens. One of them is the use of carboplatin instead of cisplatin. Phase II trials evaluating this association found a response rate ranging from 18.5% to 29% with good profile of tolerance even in elderly patients [15, 17, 18, 40, 50]. Moreover, in the pemetrexed expanded access program, the combination of carboplatin and pemetrexed seems to be equivalent to the standard cisplatin-pemetrexed regimen [81]. Other cytotoxic drugs were tried in combination with cisplatin or carboplatin, such as gemcitabine. Response rate ranged between 12% and 48%, precluding any firm conclusion on the value of gemcitabine–platinium combinations [13, 61, 93]. Based on limited literature, other gemcitabine-based regimens seemed to be interesting, such as docetaxel with gemcitabin (RR 28%) [75], pemetrexed plus gemcitabin (RR 26%) [38] or doxorubicin, carboplatin and gemcitabine (RR 32.4%) [33]. In fact, all these results are provided through phase II studies and have to be confirmed in large randomized phase III trials.

8.3.1.2
Optimal Time to Start the Treatment and Duration of Chemotherapy

There are very limited proofs with one randomized pilot study to answer the question of the best time to start the chemotherapy in the MPM patients. O'Brien et al. recruited 43 patients to be randomized to receive immediate chemotherapy after diagnosis ($n = 21$) or initial BSC with the addition of chemotherapy at the time of symptomatic progression [62]. All patients received the same platinum-based chemotherapy regimen: mitomycin C 8 mg/m^2 (cycles 1, 2, 4 and 6), vinblastine 6 mg/m^2, maximum 10 mg, and cisplatin 50 mg/m^2 (or carboplatin AUC 5) (MVP), every 3 weeks for up to six cycles. Eligible patients had a performance status (PS) ≤2, life expectancy >3 months and had stable symptoms for at least 4 weeks prior to randomization. Among the 22 patients included in the "delayed chemotherapy (D)" arm, five subjects died before receiving any treatment. Median time to start chemotherapy was 17 weeks (3–96). Median time to symptomatic progression was longer in the "early chemotherapy (E)" group than in the "D" group (25 vs 11 weeks) although this difference was not significant ($p = 0.1$). When excluding the patients who died before receiving chemotherapy, progression free survival was longer for the "E" patients group ($p = 0.03$). Overall survival seemed to be longer too in the "E" group than in the "D" group (14 vs 10 months) but the study was not powered to show this difference ($p = 0.1$). Other indirect arguments support an early introduction of chemotherapy in MPM. First, chemotherapy improved survival in the two large randomized trials in mesothelioma [94, 99]. Second, chemotherapy seems to be more efficient on small tumor volume [21]. Finally, quality of life was usually better maintained in the "E" group. Based on these considerations, ERS' experts recommended to start chemotherapy as soon as the diagnosis is made, before occurrence of clinical functional signs [84].

Again, limited data assessing the optimal duration of chemotherapy in MPM came from the two phase III randomized controlled trials [94, 99]. In Vogelzang's study, the median number of cycles was six (1–12) cycles and the dose intensity was up to 90%. In the cisplatin-pemetrexed arm, 53.1% of the patients received six cycles and 5.1% of the total continued to receive more than eight cycles. There was no evaluation of this specific group of patient. However, a toxicity analysis of 13 patients who received a median number of four cycles of pemetrexed (range 1–12) as maintenance treatment after induction chemotherapy showed a decrease of creatinin clearance, no grade 4 toxicity but grade 3 neutropenia (15%) and fatigue (15%). It is important to note that the sample size was small; patients could have been included in first or second line treatment. Induction treatment did not include cisplatin but carboplatin pemetrexed or pemetrexed alone. All hematologic toxicities during maintenance occurred for patients receiving carboplatin-pemetrexed as induction treatment. In the second phase III trial (Van meerbeck), patients received a median of five cycles (range 1–10). No data are available about efficiency according to the number of cycles of chemotherapy. Therefore, there are no data to support maintenance therapy in MPM.

In summary, the ERS ETS experts recommend that

- When a decision is made to treat a patient with chemotherapy, subject with good PS (more than 60% of the Karnofsky scale) should be treated with first-line combination chemotherapy consisting of platinum and pemetrexed or raltitrexed (1B). Alternatively, patients could be included in first- and second-line clinical trials.
- Administration of chemotherapy should not be delayed and should be considered before the appearance of functional clinical signs (1 C).
- Chemotherapy should be stopped in case of progressive disease, grade 3–4 toxicities, or cumulative toxic dose (1A), or following up to six cycles in patients who respond or are stable (2 C) [84].

8.3.1.3
Second-Line Treatment

Second-line treatment of MPM has become a reasonable issue because a number of patients progressing after standardized first line chemotherapy are still fit to receive another treatment. Thus, in a retrospective analysis of the patients included in the study of Vogelzang et al., the authors have shown that 42% of the patients received a second-line treatment [53]. Moreover, the use of post-study treatment (PST) was associated with a better survival in the two study arms whatever cytotoxic drugs were used. Although in multivariate analysis PST was associated to better survival (hazard ratio, HR: 0.56 [CI 0.44–0.72]), no clear conclusion could be made as this result could reflect association between decision of PST and a better prognosis. Two approaches emerged depending of the first-line treatment. Pemetrexed-based second-line chemotherapy has been suggested for pemetrexed-naïve patients and non-pemetrexed regimens were used in the other cases.

In second-line treatment, pemetrexed and raltitrexed have been used alone or in association with platin. The Expanded access program (EAP) provided first data about the use of pemetrexed in a second-line setting [37]. The treatment was well tolerated in the 187 patients receiving pemetrexed alone ("P"; $n = 91$) or in association with cisplatin ("C/P"; $n = 96$). No comparison was done between the two types of treatment. Tumor response for combination therapy was 32.5% and disease control rate 68.8% in the 80 assessable patients. For the "P" patients group evaluable for response ($n = 73$), tumor response was lower (5.5%) and disease control rate was about 41.1%. Median overall survival was 7.1 months (95% CI; 6.5–11) with "C/P" versus 4.1 months in the "P" group (95% CI; 3.2- N/A).

A study of 39 patients previously treated with a cisplatin-based combination reported benefit and toxicity of pemetrexed with or without carboplatin in second-line setting [86]. Grade 3 or 4 toxicities were observed for leukocytes (14% with pemetrexed vs 9% with pemetrexed plus carboplatin), thrombocytes (8% vs 18%, respectively) and nausea (only 4% with pemetrexed). Twenty-one percent of the patients experienced

partial response with pemetrexed compared with 18% with carboplatin pemetrexed. No complete response rate was described. Median overall survival was 6 months in both treatment arms.

Raltitrexed has been tested with oxaliplatin in second-line treatment with variable results. In a phase II study of 70 MPM patients including 15 pretreated patients, Fizazi et al. found an objective response rate of 20% in chemonaive and pretreated patients [24]. Overall survival in previously treated patients was 44 weeks (95% CI; 24–40 weeks). Specific toxicity data for the subgroup of previously treated patients were not available. Porta et al. evaluated 14 patients previously treated by chemotherapy (combination with cisplatin for 5 patients, or doxorubicin-based regimens for five other subjects). [73]. After a median of two cycles (range 2–6), there was no objective response but four stable disease. The authors concluded that oxaliplatin and raltitrexed should not be used in a second-line setting. Razak et al. have tested in four selected patients to reintroduce a combination of carboplatin with pemetrexed [77]. All patients had epithelioid MPM subtype and a long period of stability of the disease before relapse (from 2 years up to 6 years). After six cycles of chemotherapy, three patients had stable disease and one presented a partial response. In a retrospective study of 17 patients having relapsed more than 3 months after first line pemetrexed/platinum chemotherapy, the reintroduction of pemetrexed combined or not with platinum permitted a response rate quite low (PR: 6%), but control disease was achieved in 65% of the patients [85].

In 2008, a first randomized phase III trial evaluating the value of pemetrexed in second-line setting after a first line non pemetrexed-based treatment was published [39]. The superiority of pemetrexed over best supportive care (BSC) in second line treatment was not clearly confirmed in this trial. The characteristics of the 243 patients were as following: Karnosfky score <80% in about half of cases, stage IV disease in

60% of patients, and response to prior treatment was as reported in previously published phase II trials. A significant improvement of progression free survival was observed in the pemetrexed group compared to BSC group (PFS 3.6 months 95% CI [3–4.4] vs 1.5 months 95% CI [1.5–1.9]), whereas overall survival did not differ between the two treatment arms. However, this discrepancy could be explained by a higher rate of post-study treatment in the BSC group (51.7% vs 28.5%; $p = 0.0002$). Furthermore, 18.3% of patients in the BSC group received pemetrexed as PST, precluding any firm conclusion.

Other cytotoxics were evaluated in small groups of patients. Gemcitabine value was assessed alone or in combination with different drugs in MPM. Xanthopoulos et al. reported efficacy and safety of gemcitabine and/or oxaliplatin in 29 pemetrexed previously treated patients with good PS (in second line setting [$n = 15$] or more [$n = 14$]) [100]. Twenty-five patients received both drugs whereas the four remaining patients were treated by oxaliplatin alone. Partial response and disease control rates were low (6.9% and 44.8%, respectively). Tolerance was acceptable with no grade 4 toxicity. Time to progression and overall survival were 2.3 and 6 months, respectively. Zucaly et al. published a phase II study evaluating efficacy and toxicity of gemcitabine and vinorelbine combination after failure of a pemetrexed-based chemotherapy [103]. Thirty patients with poor PS (PS ≤ 1 in 83% of cases) and low EORTC prognostic score (73%) were recruited; 29 patients were evaluable for response assessment. Three patients experienced partial response and ten patients had a stable disease. Disease control rate was 43.3%. Median TTP was 2.8 months and median OS was 10.9 months. There was no grade 4 toxicity but three grade 3 neutropenia and one grade 3 thrombocytopenia, fatigue, nausea, and constipation. These results did not justify a phase III study.

A recent study evaluating a docetaxel-gemcitabine regimen provided more promising

results [91]. Response rate in 37 patients was 19% and disease control rate was 81%. Time to progression and mean overall survival were as high as those that may be found in first-line setting (7 months [range: 5.8–8.2] and 16.2 months [13–19.3], respectively). Similar results were achieved with the association of irinotecan, mitomycin, and cisplatin in second-line chemotherapy tested in 13 patients from a phase II open label non-comparative study [23]. All patients but one were previously treated by vinorelbine with or without oxaliplatin. Fifty percent of patients had a PS of 2. Tolerance was acceptable with mainly hematologic toxicity (30% of patients had a grade 3–4 neutropenia). Chemotherapy was associated with quality of life improvement (psycho-social well being). However, all the patients in second-line treatment presented low risk according to the EORTC prognostic score, possibly related to selection bias.

In case of prolonged objective response with first-line chemotherapy, ERS ETS experts recommended to treat patients with the same regimen (2 C). In other cases, inclusion of the patients in clinical trials is encouraged (2 C) [84].

8.3.2
Targeted Therapies

8.3.2.1
Epidermal Growth Factor Receptor (EGFR)

The tyrosine kinase (TK) EGF receptor pathway is involved in angiogenesis, proliferation, survival, and migration of tumor cells. As in many others cancers, EGFR seems to be overexpressed in MPM. However, EGFR TK activating mutations could be rare explaining EGFR TK inhibitors failure in MPM [19, 65, 96]. Govindan et al. evaluated the efficacy of gefitinib in a nonselected population of MPM patients [27]. Forty-three chemonaive patients were recruited. EGFR overexpression or mutations were not required for inclusion, but some biopsies were reviewed with interest for EGFR overexpression. The response rate was low (one partial response, one complete response, and 21 stable diseases). Similar results were obtained with other EGFR TK inhibitors. Erlotinib was tested in 63 unselected chemonaive patients [26]. Although EGFR overexpression was found in 75% of tumor samples, no objective response was observed. Toxicity was acceptable; main side effects were as previously described: skin rash (82%), diarrhea (52%), and fatigue (51%). These negative results could be explained by the absence of activating EGFR mutation in MPM cells.

8.3.2.2
Vascular Endothelial Growth Factor (VEGF) Inhibitors and Other Anti-angiogenic Drugs

There is a strong preclinical rationale supporting the use of VEGF inhibitors in MPM. VEGF and VEGF receptors are highly expressed in MPM; VEGF is an autocrin growth factor in MPM [90]. VEGF has a key role in tumor angiogenesis and lymphangiogenesis in mesothelioma [64]. The increase of VEGF expression plays also a critical role in tumor growth induced by simian virus SV 40 [16]. In murine SCID model of human MPM, the combination of humanized anti-VEGF monoclonal antibodies (bevacizumab) and pemetrexed exhibited antitumor effect on tumors highly expressing VEGF [49]. Several anti-angiogenic drugs were tested alone or in combination with other agents in MPM.

In a phase II trial, bevacizumab (15 mg/kg IV every 3 weeks) was tested in combination with oral erlotinib 150 mg daily in 24 MPM patients with good tolerance but poor results: no objective response, TTP = 2.2 months and median survival time = 5.8 months [36]. In another phase II randomized trial comparing cisplatin plus gemcitabine with or without bevacizumab, the addition of bevacizumab did not result in improved response rate (25% vs 22%) nor survival (MST 15.6 vs 14.7 months; $p = 0.91$) [44]. This may be partly due to second-line chemotherapy (pemetrexed) because this drug permitted a response rate of 12.1% and a stable disease in 46% of cases in pretreated patients, resulting in a 1 year survival rate of 54% and in median time to progression of 4.9 months. Interestingly, overall survival and PFS in both arms, but not response rate, was correlated with serum VEGF level in these patients ($p = 0.008$).

A French phase II randomized clinical trial "MAPS," evaluating a first-line chemotherapy associating cisplatin-pemetrexed versus cisplatin-pemetrexed-bevacizumab in 111 patients, was just achieved on January 2010. Preliminary results will be presented during 2010 meeting (to be updated before publication?).

Thalidomide is another anti-angiogenic drug through inhibition of VEGF, bFGF, and TGFα. In MPM, it was tested alone (two studies) or in combination with chemotherapy (one study) [4, 72]). In a phase I/II trial testing thalidomide alone, 40 patients (half pretreated subjects) were recruited [4]. There was no objective response but 11 patients (27%) had a stable disease more than 6 months; median survival time (MST) was 11 months; TTP was 8 weeks. A smaller Australian study ($n = 22$) had similar results. A last study treated 16 chemonaive patients by cisplatin, gemcitabine, and thalidomide. The authors observed partial response and stable disease rates of 14% and 55%, respectively; MST was 12 months; TTP was 17 weeks. These results did not allow classifying thalidomide as an active drug yet.

There are very limited clinical data in MPM on *multi-target (TK) drugs* such as *sorafenib, vatalanib, pazopanib, or sunitinib*. Although some patients experienced objective response, endpoints of the different studies were never achieved; new trials are ongoing. Four phase II trials assessing *imatinib mesylate* in MPM were deceptive with no response rate in all studies (stable disease: 12–44%) [54, 57, 97]. VEGFR-2 inhibitor *semaxanib* seemed to be efficient (response rate 11%; MST 12.3 months) but was associated with an intolerable risk of thrombosis [41].

Finally, a phase II trial assesses tetrathiomolybdate (TM), a potential anti-angiogenic and anti-VEGF drug through copper depletion and ceruleoplasmin decrease, starting 4–6 weeks after debulking surgery in 30 stage I–III patients compared to a historic series of 164 patients from the same group [71]. Toxicity was low. TM exhibited a potential value in stages I–II disease only, but the control group was a conflicting issue in the methods of the study to raise a firm conclusion.

8.3.2.3
Ribonuclease Inhibitors

Ranpirnase is an enzyme degrading tRNA in the Golgi system resulting in inhibition of proteins synthesis including proteins involved in cell replication and apoptosis. The role of ranpirnase in MPM has been evaluated through one phase II and two phase III trials with quite deceptive results. First, efficacy was evaluated in 105 patients in an open-label single-arm study [55]. Response rate was low (two complete responses and four partial responses, 35 stable diseases). However, regarding the molecule's activity, the use of RECIST criteria could not be the best way to evaluate efficiency of this treatment. There were 21% grade III–IV toxicities, mainly arthralgia, fever, flush, and allergic reactions. A first phase III trial compared doxorubicin (D) versus ranpirnase (R) in a 2:3 randomization of patients [98]. Results were negative as overall survival was not significantly different in the two arms (8.2 vs 8.4 months in D and R groups, respectively) in the intention to treat population. However,

patients with poorer prognostic were more frequent in the R arm. A subset analysis excluding those patients showed an increased survival in the R arm (11.6 vs 9.6 months). Another phase III included 428 chemonaive patients randomized to receive doxorubicin with or without ranpirnase, but failed to demonstrate superiority of the combination.

8.3.2.4
Histone Deacetylase Inhibitors (HDACi)

HDAC are a large group of enzymes; Zn^{2+}-dependent I, II, and IV classes HDAC are the most explored targets in cancer. Inhibition of histone acetylation results in acetylation of histone proteins and in expression of genes associated to cell cycle arrest, apoptosis, and tumor suppression. Moreover, HDACi leads to acetylation of nonhistone proteins leading to other anticancer effects such as inhibition of angiogenesis, motility, and invasion of tumor cells [9]. Many specific or pan HDACi have been tested in different cancers. For example, HDACi such as vorinostat (SAHA), panobinostat or valproic acid (VPA) are evaluated in lung cancer patients in combination with chemotherapy [14, 20, 76]. Vorinostat is already FDA-approved in the treatment of cutaneous T-cell lymphoma.

Vorinostat was first tested in MPM in a phase I study recruiting 13 previously treated patients, and seemed to be safe [41]. Despite unpublished results of a phase II evaluating Vorinostat versus placebo in previously treated MPM patients, a large randomized controlled phase III trial with the same treatment design is ongoing. Six hundred and sixty patients will be recruited until 2011.

Recently, belinostat, a novel HDACi has been tested in MPM patients [76]. Thirteen patients were included; 11 patients had previously pemetrexed-platinum chemotherapy. A median of two cycles was achieved (range 1–6). The study was stopped because no objective response was found; MST in the 13 patients was 1 month and overall survival was 5 months. Main toxicities were fatigue, hyponatremia, hypergly-cemia, and supraventricular tachycardia; all well known to be related to belinostat. The authors concluded that belinostat as a single agent was not effective.

A recent phase II study was reported by Scherpereel et al., evaluating the value and the safety of valproic acid (VPA) combined with doxorubicin in MPM patients after at least one chemotherapy (platinium-pemetrexed) [83]. A total of 45 PS 0–2 patients were evaluated. Response rate was 16% (95% CI 3–25%), dis-ease control rate was 36% (95% CI 22–51%). Overall survival was 6.7 months (95% CI 4.9–8.5 months). Toxicity was acceptable as severe neurological toxicity was seen, main toxicity was leuco-neutropenia induced by doxorubicin.

This was the first phase II suggesting clearly an antitumor effect of HDACi in mesothelioma, associated with an improvement of survival. Results of the ongoing phase III trial 3 assessing vorinostat may provide more information on the potential role of HDACi in MPM.

8.3.3
Immunomodulators, Gene Therapy and Cell Therapy

8.3.3.1
Immunomodulators

Interferons and interleukins are the principal drugs being tested in the treatment of malignant mesothelioma. The dosed, the way of adminis-tration (intrapleural, sub-cutaneous, intramuscu-lar, intravenous) and the type of drug, as well as the disease stage varied greatly from one study to another. Thus the results of these studies must be cautiously analyzed. Monotherapy with interfer-ons or interleukin-2 seemed not effective and is not recommended outside of a clinical trial [84].

Interesting preliminary results were observed after administration of *Mycobacterium vaccae*

in a limited number of patients. This needs to be confirmed before recommending the use of this treatment.

8.3.3.2
Gene Therapy

Gene therapy has shown promising results in mesothelioma in preclinical models and in a phase I trial. An antitumor response in MPM was demonstrated in murine models and in patients during phase I trial when injecting intrapleurally adenoviral vectors (Ad) with thy-midine kinase gene (associated with ganciclovir IV) or IFN-β gene [47, 88, 89]). In this model, CD4+ and CD8+ tumor-specific T cells were the key effector cells for tumor inhibition [63], suggesting a potential benefit to associate cell therapy to this strategy. Significant tumor inhi-bition was also shown in animal models, but not in humans yet, by transfection of p53, Bak, p14^{arf}, or CD40 ligand genes, or using antisens oligonucleotides (ODN) to block the expression of some genes such as growth factors (PDGF α et β, IGF I, TGF-β, etc.) [35, 102].

8.3.3.3
Cell Therapy

Finally, *cell therapy* seems to be another inter-esting treatment in MPM [28, 31]. In fact, if chemotherapy may increase the response rate to treatment and survival in non-resectable patients, there are always some tumor cells, resistant to therapies, that may inactivate the immune system. It is necessary to stimulate and to « educate » the antigen presenting cells (CPA, dendritic cells, etc.) and the effector cells of the immune system: natural killer (NK) cells, cyto-toxic T cells (CTL), etc., how to eliminate these tumor cells. Associated to other standard thera-pies (chemotherapy, etc.), this vaccine strategy may improve the treatment of MPM patients.

8

The results of a promising phase I trial were recently published [32]. The goal of this trial was to assess in ten MPM patients the safety and immunological response induced by the intradermal and intravenous administration of tumor lysate-pulsed dendritic cells (DC) at 2-week intervals after chemotherapy. The treatment was safe with no grade 3 or 4 toxicities associated with the vaccines or any evidence of autoimmunity; moderate fever was the only side effect. Interestingly, local accumulations of infiltrating T cells were found at the site of vaccination. Immunological response to tumor cells was detected in a subgroup of mesothelioma patients.

8.4
Conclusion

Real improvements have been achieved in the systemic treatment of MPM. European scientific societies recently provided clear and up-to-date guidelines for the management of patients with MPM. However, results of the treatment remain quite poor, as MPM exhibits a high resistance to standard chemotherapy, and many questions still have to be answered such as: how long should we give first-line treatment? Which second-line treatment should we use? What is the role of "targeted therapies"? How radiotherapy could improve MPM.

Regarding the incidence of the disease, prospective and randomized international trials are needed to help answer these points and to optimize MPM management. In particular, because of limited data on the best combination treatment, patients who are considered candidates for a multimodal approach should be included in a prospective trial in specialized centers. The continuing collaborations between clinicians and basic science teams are another crucial step to improve the treatment of mesothelioma patients.

References

1. Ahamad A, Stevens CW et al (2003) Intensity-modulated radiation therapy: a novel approach to the management of malignant pleural mesothelioma. Int J Radiat Oncol Biol Phys 55(3): 768–775
2. Alberts AS, Falkson G et al (1988) Malignant pleural mesothelioma: a disease unaffected by current therapeutic maneuvers. J Clin Oncol 6(3):527–535
3. Allen AM, Den R et al (2007) Influence of radiotherapy technique and dose on patterns of failure for mesothelioma patients after extrapleural pneumonectomy. Int J Radiat Oncol Biol Phys 68(5):1366–1374
4. Baas P, Boogerd W et al (2005) Thalidomide in patients with malignant pleural mesothelioma. Lung Cancer 48(2):291–296
5. Baldini EH, Recht A et al (1997) Patterns of failure after trimodality therapy for malignant pleural mesothelioma. Ann Thorac Surg 63(2): 334–338
6. Ball DL, Cruickshank DG (1990) The treatment of malignant mesothelioma of the pleura: review of a 5-year experience, with special reference to radiotherapy. Am J Clin Oncol 13(1):4–9
7. Belani CP, Adak S et al (2004) Docetaxel for malignant mesothelioma: phase II study of the Eastern Cooperative Oncology Group. Clin Lung Cancer 6(1):43–47
8. Berghmans T, Paesmans M et al (2002) Activity of chemotherapy and immunotherapy on malignant mesothelioma: a systematic review of the literature with meta-analysis. Lung Cancer 38(2):111–121
9. Bolden JE, Peart MJ et al (2006) Anticancer activities of histone deacetylase inhibitors. Nat Rev Drug Discov 5(9):769–784
10. Boutin C, Rey F et al (1995) Prevention of malignant seeding after invasive diagnostic procedures in patients with pleural mesothelioma. A randomized trial of local radiotherapy. Chest 108(3):754–758
11. British Thoracic Society (2007) BTS statement on malignant mesothelioma in the UK, 2007. Thorax 62(Suppl 2):ii1–ii19
12. Bydder S, Phillips M et al (2004) A randomised trial of single-dose radiotherapy to prevent

procedure tract metastasis by malignant mesothelioma. Br J Cancer 91(1):9–10

13. Byrne MJ, Davidson JA et al (1999) Cisplatin
and gemcitabine treatment for malignant mesothelioma: a phase II study. J Clin Oncol 17(1):
25–30

14. Candelaria M, Gallardo-Rincon D et al (2007)
A phase II study of epigenetic therapy with
hydralazine and magnesium valproate to over-
come chemotherapy resistance in refractory
solid tumors. Ann Oncol 18(9):1529–1538

15. Castagneto B, Botta M et al (2008) Phase II
study of pemetrexed in combination with carboplatin in patients with malignant pleural mesothelioma (MPM). Ann Oncol 19(2):370–373

16. Catalano A, Romano M et al (2002) Enhanced
expression of vascular endothelial growth factor
(VEGF) plays a critical role in the tumor progression potential induced by simian virus 40
large T antigen. Oncogene 21(18):2896–2900

17. Ceresoli GL, Zucali PA et al (2006) Phase II
study of pemetrexed plus carboplatin in malignant pleural mesothelioma. J Clin Oncol 24(9):
1443–1448

18. Ceresoli GL, Castagneto B et al (2008)
Pemetrexed plus carboplatin in elderly patients
with malignant pleural mesothelioma: combined analysis of two phase II trials. Br J Cancer
99(1):51–56

19. Cortese JF, Gowda AL et al (2006) Common
EGFR mutations conferring sensitivity to gefitinib in lung adenocarcinoma are not prevalent
in human malignant mesothelioma. Int J Cancer
118(2):521–522

20. Crisanti MC, Wallace AF et al (2009) The
HDAC inhibitor panobinostat (LBH589) inhibits mesothelioma and lung cancer cells in vitro
and in vivo with particular efficacy for small cell
lung cancer. Mol Cancer Ther 8(8):2221–2231

21. DeVita VT Jr (1983) The James Ewing lecture.
The relationship between tumor mass and resistance to chemotherapy. Implications for surgical adjuvant treatment of cancer. Cancer
51(7):1209–1220

22. Emami B, Lyman J et al (1991) Tolerance of
normal tissue to therapeutic irradiation. Int J
Radiat Oncol Biol Phys 21(1):109–122

23. Fennell DA, JP CS et al (2005) Phase II trial of
vinorelbine and oxaliplatin as first-line therapy
in malignant pleural mesothelioma. Lung
Cancer 47(2):277–281

24. Fizazi K, Doubre H et al (2003) Combination of
raltitrexed and oxaliplatin is an active regimen
in malignant mesothelioma: results of a phase II
study. J Clin Oncol 21(2):349–354

25. Flores RM, Krug LM et al (2006) Induction chemotherapy, extrapleural pneumonectomy, and
postoperative high-dose radiotherapy for locally
advanced malignant pleural mesothelioma: a
phase II trial. J Thorac Oncol 1(4):289–295

26. Garland LL, Rankin C et al (2007) Phase II
study of erlotinib in patients with malignant
pleural mesothelioma: a Southwest Oncology
Group study. J Clin Oncol 25(17):2406–2413

27. Govindan R, Kratzke RA et al (2005) Gefitinib
in patients with malignant mesothelioma: a
phase II study by the Cancer and Leukemia
Group B. Clin Cancer Res 11(6):2300–2304

28. Gregoire M, Ligeza-Poisson C et al (2003)
Anti-cancer therapy using dendritic cells and
apoptotic tumour cells: pre-clinical data in
human mesothelioma and acute myeloid leu-
kaemia. Vaccine 21(7–8):791–794

29. Gupta V, Mychalczak B et al (2005) Hemithoracic
radiation therapy after pleurectomy/decortica-
tion for malignant pleural mesothelioma. Int J
Radiat Oncol Biol Phys 63(4):1045–1052

30. Gupta V, Krug LM et al (2009) Patterns of local
and nodal failure in malignant pleural mesothelioma after extrapleural pneumonectomy and
photon-electron radiotherapy. J Thorac Oncol
4(6):746–750

31. Hegmans JP, Hemmes A et al (2005)
Immunotherapy of murine malignant mesothe-
lioma using tumor lysate-pulsed dendritic cells.
Am J Respir Crit Care Med 171(10):1168–1177

32. Hegmans JP, Veltman JD et al (2010)
Consolidative dendritic cell-based immunotherapy elicits cytotoxicity against malignant
mesothelioma. Am J Respir Crit Care Med
181(12):1383–90

33. Hillerdal G, Sorensen JB et al (2008) Treatment
of malignant pleural mesothelioma with carboplatin, liposomized doxorubicin, and gemcitabine: a phase II study. J Thorac Oncol 3(11):
1325–1331

34. Holsti LR, Pyrhonen S et al (1997) Altered
fractionation of hemithorax irradiation for pleural mesothelioma and failure patterns after
treatment. Acta Oncol 36(4):397–405

35. Hopkins-Donaldson S, Cathomas R et al (2003)
Induction of apoptosis and chemosensitization

of mesothelioma cells by Bcl-2 and Bcl-xL anti-sense treatment. Int J Cancer 106(2):160–166

36. Jackman DM, Kindler HL et al (2008) Erlotinib plus bevacizumab in previously treated patients with malignant pleural mesothelioma. Cancer 113(4):808–814

37. Janne PA, Wozniak AJ et al (2006) Pemetrexed alone or in combination with cisplatin in previously treated malignant pleural mesothelioma: outcomes from a phase IIIB expanded access program. J Thorac Oncol 1(6):506–512

38. Janne PA, Simon GR et al (2008) Phase II trial of pemetrexed and gemcitabine in chemotherapy-naive malignant pleural mesothelioma. J Clin Oncol 26(9):1465–1471

39. Jassem J, Ramlau R et al (2008) Phase III trial of pemetrexed plus best supportive care compared with best supportive care in previously treated patients with advanced malignant pleural mesothelioma. J Clin Oncol 26(10):1698–1704

40. Katirtzoglou N, Gkiozos I et al (2010) Carboplatin plus pemetrexed as first-line treatment of patients with malignant pleural mesothelioma: a phase II study. Clin Lung Cancer 11(1):30–35

41. Kelly WK, O'Connor OA et al (2005) Phase I study of an oral histone deacetylase inhibitor, suberoylanilide hydroxamic acid, in patients with advanced cancer. J Clin Oncol 23(17): 3923–3931

42. Kindler HL, Vogelzang NJ, Chien K, Stadler WM, Karczmar G, Heimann R, Vokes EE (2001) SU 5416 in malignant mesothelioma: a University of Chicago Phase II Consortium Study. 2001 ASCO meeting. Proc Am Soc Clin Oncol 20:2001 (abstract 1359)

43. Kindler HL, Herndon JE et al (2005) Irinotecan for malignant mesothelioma: a phase II trial by the Cancer and Leukemia Group B. Lung Cancer 48(3):423–428

44. Kindler HL, Karrison T, Gandara DR, Lu C, Guterz TL, Nichols K, Chen H, Stadler WM, Vokes EE (2007) Final analysis of a multi-center, double-blind, placebo-controlled, randomized phase II trial of gemcitabine/cisplatin (GC) plus bevacizumab (B) or placebo (P) in patients with malignant mesothelioma (MM). J Clin Oncol ASCO meeting Proceedings Part I. Vol 25, No. 18S (June 20 Supplement), 2007:7526

45. Kristensen CA, Nottrup TJ et al (2009) Pulmonary toxicity following IMRT after extra-pleural pneumonectomy for malignant pleural mesothelioma. Radiother Oncol 92(1):96–99

46. Krug LM, Pass HI et al (2009) Multicenter phase II trial of neoadjuvant pemetrexed plus cisplatin followed by extrapleural pneumonectomy and radiation for malignant pleural mesothelioma. J Clin Oncol 27(18):3007–3013

47. Kruklitis RJ, Singhal S et al (2004) Immuno-gene therapy with interferon-beta before surgical debulking delays recurrence and improves survival in a murine model of malignant mesothelioma. J Thorac Cardiovasc Surg 127(1):123–130

48. Lee TT, Everett DL et al (2002) Radical pleurectomy/decortication and intraoperative radiotherapy followed by conformal radiation with or without chemotherapy for malignant pleural mesothelioma. J Thorac Cardiovasc Surg 124(6):1183–1189

49. Li Q, Yano S et al (2007) The therapeutic efficacy of anti vascular endothelial growth factor antibody, bevacizumab, and pemetrexed against orthotopically implanted human pleural mesothelioma cells in severe combined immunodeficient mice. Clin Cancer Res 13(19):5918–5925

50. Li L, Razak AR et al (2009) Carboplatin and pemetrexed in the management of malignant pleural mesothelioma: a realistic treatment option? Lung Cancer 64(2):207–210

51. Maasilta P (1991) Deterioration in lung function following hemithorax irradiation for pleural mesothelioma. Int J Radiat Oncol Biol Phys 20(3):433–438

52. Maggi G, Casadio C et al (2001) Trimodality management of malignant pleural mesothelioma. Eur J Cardiothorac Surg 19(3):346–350

53. Manegold C, Symanowski J et al (2005) Second-line (post-study) chemotherapy received by patients treated in the phase III trial of pemetrexed plus cisplatin versus cisplatin alone in malignant pleural mesothelioma. Ann Oncol 16(6):923–927

54. Mathy A, Baas P et al (2005) Limited efficacy of imatinib mesylate in malignant mesothelioma: a phase II trial. Lung Cancer 50(1):83–86

55. Mikulski SM, Costanzi JJ et al (2002) Phase II trial of a single weekly intravenous dose of ranpirnase in patients with unresectable malignant mesothelioma. J Clin Oncol 20(1):274–281

56. Miles EF, Larrier NA et al (2008) Intensity-modulated radiotherapy for resected mesothelioma: the Duke experience. Int J Radiat Oncol Biol Phys 71(4):1143–1150

57. Millward M, Parnis F, Byrne M, Powell A, Dunleavey R, Lynch K, Boyer MJ (2003) Phase II trial of imatinib mesylate in patients with advanced pleural mesothelioma. 2003 ASCO meeting. Proc Am Soc Clin Oncol 22:2003 (abstract 912)

58. Muers MF, Stephens RJ et al (2008) Active symptom control with or without chemotherapy in the treatment of patients with malignant pleural mesothelioma (MS01): a multicentre randomised trial. Lancet 371(9625):1685–1694

59. Nakas A, Trousse DS et al (2008) Open lung-sparing surgery for malignant pleural mesothelioma: the benefits of a radical approach within multimodality therapy. Eur J Cardiothorac Surg 34(4):886–891

60. Niyikiza C, Baker SD et al (2002) Homocysteine and methylmalonic acid: markers to predict and avoid toxicity from pemetrexed therapy. Mol Cancer Ther 1(7):545–552

61. Nowak AK, Byrne MJ et al (2002) A multi-centre phase II study of cisplatin and gemcitabine for malignant mesothelioma. Br J Cancer 87(5):491–496

62. O'Brien ME, Watkins D et al (2006) A randomised trial in malignant mesothelioma (M) of early (E) versus delayed (D) chemotherapy in symptomatically stable patients: the MED trial. Ann Oncol 17(2):270–275

63. Odaka M, Sterman DH et al (2001) Eradication of intraperitoneal and distant tumor by adenovirus-mediated interferon-beta gene therapy is attributable to induction of systemic immunity. Cancer Res 61(16):6201–6212

64. Ohta Y, Shridhar V et al (1999) VEGF and VEGF type C play an important role in angiogenesis and lymphangiogenesis in human malignant mesothelioma tumours. Br J Cancer 81(1):54–61

65. Okuda K, Sasaki H et al (2008) Epidermal growth factor receptor gene mutation, amplification and protein expression in malignant pleural mesothelioma. J Cancer Res Clin Oncol 134(10):1105–1111

66. Okuno SH, Delaune R et al (2008) A phase 2 study of gemcitabine and epirubicin for the treatment of pleural mesothelioma: a North Central Cancer Treatment Study, N0021. Cancer 112(8):1772–1779

67. O'Rourke N, Garcia JC et al (2007) A randomised controlled trial of intervention site radiotherapy in malignant pleural mesothelioma. Radiother Oncol 84(1):18–22

68. Otterson GA, Herndon JE II et al (2004) Capecitabine in malignant mesothelioma: a phase II trial by the Cancer and Leukemia Group B (39807). Lung Cancer 44(2):251–259

69. Pass HI, Kranda K et al (1997) Surgically debulked malignant pleural mesothelioma: results and prognostic factors. Ann Surg Oncol 4(3):215–222

70. Pass HI, Temeck BK et al (1997) Phase III randomized trial of surgery with or without intraoperative photodynamic therapy and postoperative immunochemotherapy for malignant pleural mesothelioma. Ann Surg Oncol 4(8):628–633

71. Pass HI, Brewer GJ et al (2008) A phase II trial of tetrathiomolybdate after surgery for malignant mesothelioma: final results. Ann Thorac Surg 86(2):383–389; discussion 390

72. Pavlakis N, Williams G et al (2002) Thalidomide alone or in combination with cisplatin/gemcitabine chemotherapy for malignant mesothelioma (MM): preliminary results from two phase II studies. Proc Am Soc Clin Oncol 2002;21, 2:p19b, Abstract 1885 38th Annual Meeting, May 18–21, 2002, Orlando FL

73. Porta C, Zimatore M et al (2005) Raltitrexed-Oxaliplatin combination chemotherapy is inactive as second-line treatment for malignant pleural mesothelioma patients. Lung Cancer 48(3):429–434

74. Portalone L, Antilli A et al (2005) Epirubicin and gemcitabine as first-line treatment in malignant pleural mesothelioma. Tumori 91(1):15–18

75. Ralli M, Tourkantonis I et al (2009) Docetaxel plus gemcitabine as first-line treatment in malignant pleural mesothelioma: a single institution phase II study. Anticancer Res 29(8): 3441–3444

76. Ramalingam SS, Belani CP et al (2009) Phase II study of belinostat (PXD101), a histone deacetylase inhibitor, for second line therapy of advanced malignant pleural mesothelioma. J Thorac Oncol 4(1):97–101

77. Razak AR, Chatten KJ et al (2008) Retreatment with pemetrexed-based chemotherapy in malignant pleural mesothelioma (MPM): a second line treatment option. Lung Cancer 60(2):294–297

78. Rice DC, Stevens CW et al (2007) Outcomes after extrapleural pneumonectomy and inten-

sity-modulated radiation therapy for malignant pleural mesothelioma. Ann Thorac Surg 84(5): 1685–1692; discussion 1692-3

79. Rusch VW, Venkatraman ES (1999) Important prognostic factors in patients with malignant pleural mesothelioma, managed surgically. Ann Thorac Surg 68(5):1799–1804

80. Rusch VW, Rosenzweig K et al (2001) A phase II trial of surgical resection and adjuvant high-dose hemithoracic radiation for malignant pleural mesothelioma. J Thorac Cardiovasc Surg 122(4):788–795

81. Santoro A, O'Brien ME et al (2008) Pemetrexed plus cisplatin or pemetrexed plus carboplatin for chemonaive patients with malignant pleural mesothelioma: results of the International Expanded Access Program. J Thorac Oncol 3(7):756–763

82. Scherpereel A (2007) Guidelines of the French Speaking Society for Chest Medicine for management of malignant pleural mesothelioma. Respir Med 101(6):1265–1276

83. Scherpereel A, Berghmans T et al (2011) for the European Lung Cancer Working Party (ELCWP). Valproate-doxorubicin: promising therapy for progressing mesothelioma. A phase II study. Eur Respir J. Jan; 37(1):129–135. Epub 2010 Jun 7

84. Scherpereel A, Astoul P et al (2010) Guidelines of the European Respiratory Society and the European Society of Thoracic Surgeons for the management of malignant pleural mesothelioma. Eur Respir J 35(3):479–495

85. M. Serke, T. Bauer (2007) Pemetrexed in second-line therapy in patients with malignant pleural mesothelioma. J Clin Oncol ASCO Annual Meeting Proceedings Part I. Vol 25, No. 18S (June 20 Supplement), 18198 Chicago, IL 2007 June 1–4

86. Sorensen JB, Sundstrom S et al (2007) Pemetrexed as second-line treatment in malignant pleural mesothelioma after platinum-based first-line treatment. J Thorac Oncol 2(2):147–152

87. Stahel RA, Weder W et al (2009) Malignant pleural mesothelioma: ESMO clinical recommendations for diagnosis, treatment and follow-up. Ann Oncol 20(Suppl 4):73–75

88. Sterman DH, Recio A et al (2007) A phase I clinical trial of single-dose intrapleural IFN-beta gene transfer for malignant pleural mesothelioma and metastatic pleural effusions: high rate of antitumor immune responses. Clin Cancer Res 13(15 Pt 1):4456–4466

89. Sterman DH, Recio A et al (2010) A phase I trial of repeated intrapleural adenoviral-mediated interferon-beta gene transfer for mesothelioma and metastatic pleural effusions. Mol Ther 18(4):852–860

90. Strizzi L, Catalano A et al (2001) Vascular endothelial growth factor is an autocrine growth factor in human malignant mesothelioma. J Pathol 193(4):468–475

91. Tourkantonis I, Makrilia N et al (2010) Phase II Study of Gemcitabine Plus Docetaxel as Second-Line Treatment in Malignant Pleural Mesothelioma: A Single Institution Study. Am J Clin Oncol. May 3. [Epub ahead of print]

92. Tsao AS, Mehran R et al (2009) Neoadjuvant and intrapleural therapies for malignant pleural mesothelioma. Clin Lung Cancer 10(1):36–41

93. van Haarst JM, Baas P et al (2002) Multicentre phase II study of gemcitabine and cisplatin in malignant pleural mesothelioma. Br J Cancer 86(3):342–345

94. van Meerbeeck JP, Gaafar R et al (2005) Randomized phase III study of cisplatin with or without raltitrexed in patients with malignant pleural mesothelioma: an intergroup study of the European Organisation for Research and Treatment of Cancer Lung Cancer Group and the National Cancer Institute of Canada. J Clin Oncol 23(28):6881–6889

95. van Sandick JW, Kappers I et al (2008) Surgical treatment in the management of malignant pleural mesothelioma: a single institution's experience. Ann Surg Oncol 15(6):1757–1764

96. Velcheti V, Kasai Y et al (2009) Absence of mutations in the epidermal growth factor receptor (EGFR) kinase domain in patients with mesothelioma. J Thorac Oncol 4(4):559

97. Villano JL, Husain AM, Stadler WM, Hanson LL, Vogelzang NJ, Kindler HL (2004) A phase II trial of imatinib mesylate in patients with malignant mesothelioma. J Clin Oncol 22(14S):663

98. Vogelzang N, Taub RN, Shin D, Costanzi J, Pass H, Gutheil J, Georgiadis M, McAndrew P, Kelly K, Chun H, Mittelman A, McCachren S, Shogen K, Mikulski S (2000) Phase III Randomised Trial of Onconase (ONC) vs. Doxorubicin (DOX) in Patients (Pts) with Unresecable Malignant Mesothelioma (UMM): analysis of survival. 2000 ASCO meeting. Proc Am Soc Clin Oncol 19:2000 (abstract 2274)

99. Vogelzang NJ, Rusthoven JJ et al (2003) Phase III study of pemetrexed in combination with cisplatin versus cisplatin alone in patients with malignant pleural mesothelioma. J Clin Oncol 21(14):2636–2644

100. Xanthopoulos A, Bauer TT et al (2008) Gemcitabine combined with oxaliplatin in pretreated patients with malignant pleural mesothelioma: an observational study. J Occup Med Toxicol 3:34

101. Yajnik S, Rosenzweig KE et al (2003) Hemithoracic radiation after extrapleural pneumonectomy for malignant pleural mesothelioma. Int J Radiat Oncol Biol Phys 56(5):1319–1326

102. Yang CT, You L et al (2003) A comparison analysis of anti-tumor efficacy of adenoviral gene replacement therapy (p14ARF and p16INK4A) in human mesothelioma cells. Anticancer Res 23(1A):33–38

103. Zucali PA, Ceresoli GL et al (2008) Gemcitabine and vinorelbine in pemetrexed-pretreated patients with malignant pleural mesothelioma. Cancer 112(7):1555–1561

Genetics and Molecular Biology of Mesothelioma

9

Dean A. Fennell

9.1
Apoptosis as a Tumor Suppressor Mechanism

Mesothelioma remains an incurable cancer due to the ineffectiveness of conventional cytotoxic chemotherapy. This is reflected in the preponderance of mostly negative phase II clinical trials over the last 30 years [32]. Resistance to apoptosis is a hallmark of cancer in general [48], accounts for multidrug resistance [58], and is a signature of mesothelioma [31]. During tumorigenesis, it is now understood that as in common with other solid cancers, somatic genetic alteration is a frequent event predisposing to apoptosis resistance. These changes include the activation of oncogenic cell survival pathways, and the inactivation of tumor suppressors.

This chapter will focus on how apoptosis susceptibility in mesothelioma is, in general, inhibited by the acquisition of multiple somatic alterations in oncogenic and tumor suppressor

D.A. Fennell
Thoracic Oncology Research Group,
Drug Resistance Laboratory,
Centre for Cancer Research and Cell Biology,
Queen's University Belfast, 97 Lisburn Road,
Belfast BT9 7BL, Northern Ireland, UK
e-mail: d.fennell@qub.ac.uk

protein expression. Growing knowledge of these key genetic changes and their requirement for sustaining the malignant mesothelioma phenotype provide insights into potential vulnerabilities that may be successfully exploited using new therapeutic strategies. I will first of all, summarize our understanding of how the core death machinery is altered in mesothelioma (summarized in Fig. 9.1). This will be followed by a summary of the most frequent genetic alterations driving oncogenic pathways or leading to dysfunction of tumor suppressors (summarized in Fig. 9.2). Translational research opportunities arising from this knowledge of mesothelioma pathobiology will then be highlighted.

9.2
Key Alterations in the Core Apoptosis Signaling in Mesothelioma

9.2.1
Regulation of the Intrinsic (Mitochondrial) Apoptosis Pathway in Mesothelioma

The BCL-2 family of proteins constitutes the pivotal molecular regulators of the core cell death machinery. This family is subdivided into proapoptotic and antiapoptotic proteins. BCL-2, the prototypical member of the BCL-2 family

A. Tannapfel (ed.), *Malignant Mesothelioma*, Recent Results in Cancer Research 189,
DOI: 10.1007/978-3-642-10862-4_9, © Springer-Verlag Berlin Heidelberg 2011

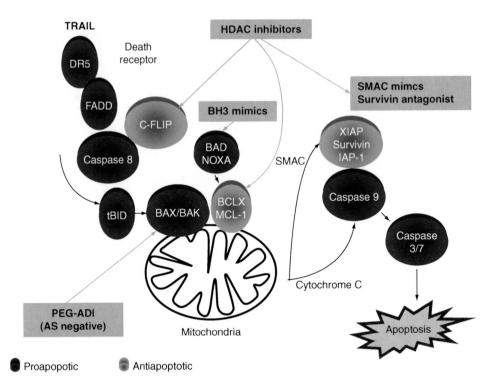

Fig. 9.1 Altered regulation of the core apoptosis pathway in mesothelioma. Upregulated antiapoptotic proteins are highlighted (*green*)

was identified as a proto-oncogene associated with the t(14;18) translocation in follicular lymphoma [129]. The antiapoptotic protein subgroup now includes five additional proteins, MCL-1, BCL-X, BCL-W, A1 and BCL-B. Prosurvival BCL-2 family proteins regulate apoptosis at the level of the mitochondrial and endoplasmic reticulum outer membranes. The canonical cell death pathway involves mitochondria; organelles responsible for generating ATP, the cell's energy currency, through oxidative phosphorylation.

Prosurvival BCL-2 family proteins function to block a critical death switch which is responsible for making the all-or-none decision to commit a cell irreversibly to death [4,24]. This switch is the permeabilization of the outer mitochondrial membrane, induced by oligomerization and pore formation by the tumor suppressors and multidomain proapoptotic proteins BAK and BAX [99,115,146,147]. Mitochondrial outer membrane permeabilization or MOMP is a rapid,

kinetically invariant event that results in the release several proteins from the mitochondria into the cytosol. These proteins include cytochrome C [77], SMAC [27], OMI/HtrA2 [82] and apoptosis-inducing factor [122]. Cytochrome C in conjunction with APAF-1 [149] and dATP, triggers the activation of a family of zymogens called caspases, which cooperate in mediating cellular demolition by cleaving hundreds of substrates. Bax and Bak are genetically redundant tumor suppressors [140]; prosurvival BCL-2 proteins heterodimerize to prevent BAX and BAK activation, functioning as a rheostat that is dependent on the ratio of pro- to antiapoptotic proteins.

In common with other tumor suppressors, BAX deficiency has been identified in primary malignancies [84]. However, low bcl-2/bax ratio has been reported in mesothelioma cells despite their apoptosis resistance, implicating a mechanism other than BCL-2 in regulating apoptosis. In vivo, MCL-1 is more commonly

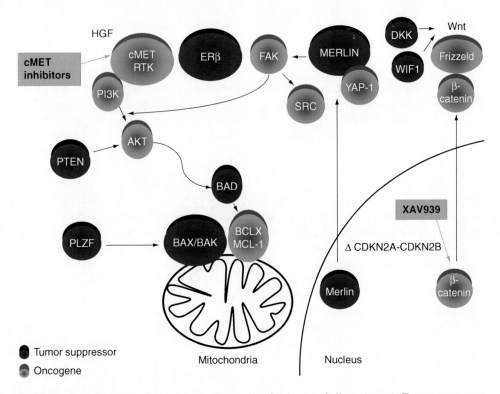

Fig. 9.2 Key proteins involved in survival pathway signaling in mesothelioma (*green*). Tumor suppressors are shown in *blue*

expressed whereas BCL-2 expression is less frequent [96,119]. BAX and BAK require a subset of proapoptotic BCL-2 family proteins for activation which share homology in a death-inducing BCL-2 homology 3 (BH3) domain, but do not contain other BH domains. Two such BH3 domain-only proteins, BID [136] and BIM [95] can directly induce the oligomerization and activation of BAX. Interestingly, in mesothelioma, loss of expression of BH3-only proteins has been reported in vivo, namely, BID (37%) and BIM (18%). In addition, loss of BAX expression has been reported in one series in 42% of primary mesotheliomas [96].

Prosurvival BCL-2 family proteins are inhibited by a subset of BH3-only proteins, which are incapable of direct BAX/BAK activation, but bind directly to prosurvival counterparts. These so-called dissociator BH3-only proteins reflect a growing family and include BAD,

NOXA, PUMA, BMF, BIK and HRK. Because dissociator BH3-only proteins are endogenous prosurvival BCL-2 family inhibitors, they represent a prototype for small molecule drug development, most notably ABT737 [76,98]. BH3 mimetics are a promising class of mitochondria targeted therapy with potential for treating mesothelioma. This is suggested by studies in which silencing BCl-2 and BCL-XL was sufficient to induce apoptosis and chemosensitization [52]. However, target specificity is likely to be important for therapeutic efficacy. MCL-1 is highly expressed in mesothelioma and is one of the most commonly amplified oncogenes in human cancer [9]. It is also a resistance biomarker for ABT737 [68,132]. Nevertheless, other prosurvival BCL-2 family targeted agents such as obatoclax [92] are currently in clinical development, and may exhibit efficacy in mesothelioma.

9

9.2.2
Extrinsic Apoptosis Pathway Regulation in Mesothelioma

Apoptosis can be efficiently induced in mesothelioma cell lines by ligation of cell surface death receptors. Activation of death receptors by their ligands (which include TNF and FAS) leads to recruitment of FADD through a conserved death domain [22], followed by recruitment of caspase 8 [10] activating complex known as the death-inducing signaling complex or DISC [127]. Caspase 8 cleaves BID, leading to activation of BAX/BAK, mitochondrial apoptosis, and therefore signal amplification [78]. Tumor necrosis factor-related apoptosis inducing ligand (TRAIL) or TRAIL receptor agonists are currently in clinical development but have yet to be evaluated in mesothelioma. Upon interaction, its receptors (TRAIL R1 or R2) can induce apoptosis in vitro. TRAIL also synergizes with DNA damage induced by etoposide in a manner that requires c-jun N terminal kinase [135].

FLIP is an inhibitor of TRAIL-induced apoptosis and is recruited to the DISC [90], where it inhibits caspase 8 recruitment and activation. Mesothelioma cells overexpress FLIP resulting in inhibition of death receptor-induced apoptosis [112]. Silencing of FLIP in mesothelioma and other cancer models re-establishes sensitivity to TRAIL [112,141]. Novel, clinically applicable approaches for downregulating FLIP in the clinical setting will be highlighted later in this chapter.

9.2.3
Inhibitors of Apoptosis in Mesothelioma

Inhibitors of apoptosis (IAPs) comprise a family of structurally related proteins, which share a common 70 amino acid baculovirus IAP (BIR) repeat. IAPs interact with and inhibit caspases 9, 3 and 7. Mesotheliomas have been shown to overexpress the IAPs survivin, XIAP and IAP-1

in vivo using immunohistochemistry [43,65]. IAP-1 has been shown to be associated with shorter survival [44]. RNAi-mediated silencing of IAP-1 is sufficient to reduce mesothelioma cell viability and induce apoptosis by activating the mitochondrial pathway [43]. Conversely, IAP-1, IAP-2 and XIAP are upregulated by tumor necrosis factor alpha, whereas survivin and livin are not [45]. Survivin is overexpressed in mesothelioma and its silencing in vitro is associated with induction of apoptosis suggesting that it might be a potential molecular target [29,144,152].

IAP proteins are inhibited by Smac, which is released from the mitochondria following outer membrane permeabilization by BAX/BAK. Small molecule smac mimetics offer one way of targeting IAPs and are currently in early development, for example, AT406 and TL32711; these compounds also downregulate IAP-1 and IAP-2 [137]. Selective inhibitors of survivin, for example, YM155 are currently in clinical development in other cancers. Other approaches capable of modulating IAP proteins include histone deacetylase inhibition, which is discussed in more detail later in this chapter.

9.3
Tumor Suppressor Loss in Mesothelioma

9.3.1
Loss of nf2 Is Frequent in Mesothelioma

The short arm of chromosome 9 (9p) is a region associated with frequent cytogenetic abnormalities in mesothelioma [19,21,91,100,125]. Loss of the CDKN2b-CDKN2a locus on chromosome 9p21 in humans is a common event in cancer, in general, including mesothelioma. This locus includes the tumor suppressor p16ink4a, which is encoded by CDKN2A and is one of the most frequently silenced tumor suppressors in mesothelioma [53]. This tumor suppressor is an inhibitor of the Rb1 pathway involved in cell cycle progression, and its loss whether by deletion (75–85%) or methylation is associated with poor prognosis [67,72]. There is frequently co-deletion of p16inka and p15ink4b, occurring in 75% of mesotheliomas [145]. It has been recently shown that p15ink4b, which is encoded by CDKN2b, can substitute for loss of p16ink4a, and that this back-up function could account for the frequently observed loss of the complete CDKN2b-CDKN2a locus [70].

Loss of expression has been shown to be associated with homozygous deletion of exons 1–3 [91,102], and this is more frequently associated with exposure to asbestos even in non-small cell lung cancer, compared with tobacco exposure (which is associated with hypermethylation) [3]. In mesothelioma, hypermethylation occurs in the first exon [142]. Re-expression in mesothelioma cells is sufficient to induce cell cycle arrest, as well as reduced tumor growth and spread in vivo [40,41]. Because hypermethylation silences p16ink4a in approximately 20% of mesotheliomas [142], re-expression can be achieved using demethylating agents such as cytidine analog dihydro-5-azacytidine (DHAC). Analysis of tissue samples from CALGB 8833 and 9031 clinical trials employing DHAC-based therapy identified 4/20 tumors with methylation of p16ink4a. Although there was a trend to improved survival in this clinical trial associated with p16ink4a methylation, this was not statistically significant, probably as a result of the small sample size [69].

Around 40% mesotheliomas harbor somatic mutations in the neurofibromatosis type 2 gene (NF2) located at chromosome 22q12 [116]. Treatment of Nf2 ($\pm$) knockout mice with asbestos causes accelerated development of mesothelioma, with biallelic inactivation of the wild-type Nf2 allele, and loss of the CDKN2A locus [1]. Conditional knockout of nf2/p16ink4a in a murine model has been shown to exhibit more invasive, aggressive mesothelioma compared with conditional nf2/p53 knockout, with shorter survival [59]. Together, this implicates an important role in mesothelioma [59]. Mutation of NF2 is frequent in mesothelioma but not observed in non-small cell lung cancer [116]. Somatic mutation of NF2 is conserved across mesothelioma in different species, being frequently detected in murine mesothelioma [73].

9.3.2
NF2 Encodes the Tumor Suppressor Merlin

Merlin, the gene product of NF2 is a FERM domain protein that functions at the plasma membrane where it inhibits mitogenic signaling. It functions as a growth inhibitor, and accumulates in the nucleus where it interacts with and inhibits the E3 ligase CRL4 (DCAF1) [79]. Loss of merlin has a pro-mitogenic effect, and this is lost when DCAF1 is depleted, or if a merlin insensitive mutant is expressed. Mutations of merlin disrupt the direct interaction with CRL4(DCAF1).

When Merlin expression is restored in NF2 deficient mesothelioma cells, there is a marked inhibition of cell motility, spreading and invasiveness. Focal adhesion kinases (FAK) play a critical role in regulating invasive phenotype, and are negatively targeted by merlin. This mechanism of inhibition involves merlin dependent FAK phosphorylation at a critical residue on tyrosine 397, resulting in a block of its interaction with binding partners src and the PI3kinase regulatory subunit p85 [106].

The transcriptional coactivator YAP1 [88] is an oncogene that is commonly amplified at the 11q22 locus in mesotheliomas, and physically interacts with merlin, contributing to the promitogenic effects of NF2 deletion [148]. RNAi-mediated suppression of YAP1 suppresses growth of mesothelioma cells with NF2 homozygous deletion through induction of apoptosis and cell cycle arrest. Conversely, overexpression of YAP1 in immortalized mesotheliomal cells is mitogenic. Merlin inhibits YAP1 through the induction of its phosphorylation and cytoplasmic retention.

9

9.3.3
PLZF Is a Novel Tumor Suppressor in Mesothelioma

Focal deletion of 11q23 has been identified in mesothelioma, and involves a locus encompassing promyelocytic leukemia zinc finger (PLZF), a transcriptional repressor gene. Loss of PLZF confirmed by analysis of transcript levels, and loss of protein expression has been observed in mesothelioma compared with mesothelial cells. Ectopic expression of PLZF causes reduced clonogenicity and initiation of apoptosis involving caspase activation; together, with the loss of PLZF implicates a potentially important role in regulating mesothelioma cell survival.

9.4
Therapeutic Inhibition of Survival Pathways

9.4.1
PI3K/AKT/mTOR Axis in Mesothelioma

Mesothelioma cells, which have been grown in three dimensions to more closely resemble solid tumors, acquire multidrug resistance, including resistance to TRAIL and chemotherapy [6,62]. The molecular basis underlying acquisition of multidrug resistance has not been fully delineated, but involves activation of the phosphatidylinositol-3-kinase (PI3K)/Akt/mammalian target of rapamycin (mTOR) pathway since rapamycin or RNAi silencing of the mTOR target, S6K, can restore TRAIL sensitivity. This effect requires BID, since silencing using RNAi implicates mTOR/S6K as a major contributor of resistance to TRAIL in three-dimensional but not two-dimensional tumors. TRAIL sensitivity is also enhanced by inhibition of the PI3K/AKT pathway following heat stress, supporting a role for this pathway in blocking apoptosis [104]. Mesotheliomas exhibit an elevated level of activity in the PI3K/AKT/mTOR pathway both in mouse and human models, and its inhibition

is associated with potentiation of cisplatin-induced apoptosis [2].

AKT is antagonized by the endogenous inhibitor, phosphatase and tensin analog (PTEN), which acts to inhibit phosphorylation. When overexpressed in mesothelioma, PTEN induces loss of viability [87]. Not surprisingly, given the survival function of PTEN in regulating PI3K/AKT/mTOR signaling, the expression is lost in a significant proportion of mesotheliomas [101]. Recently it has been shown that PTEN is required for maintaining the integrity of chromosomes [117]. Loss of PTEN confers a defect in homologous repair which can be exploited by inhibition of poly ADP ribose polymerase (PARP) [85]. Given the recent evidence that PARP inhibitors are very effective in inducing tumor responses under conditions of defective DNA double strand break repair due to BRCA1 mutation [30,37], the possibility exists that a subset of PTEN deficient mesotheliomas may be sensitive to PARP inhibitors.

9.4.2
HGF/cMET Pathway Is Activated in Mesothelioma

C-met receptor tyrosine kinase is overexpressed in mesothelioma by 82% compared with normal tissues, and in 90% of serous effusions [153]. It is associated with high circulating levels of its ligand scatter factor/HGF [57], which in turn is overexpressed in 40–85% of mesotheliomas. HGF stimulates mesothelioma cell motility in vitro via the c-met receptor [49,50,66,128], and has been shown to mediate cell survival by upregulating BCL-XL. The mechanism involves mitogen-activated protein kinase-dependent phosphorylation and activation of the ETS family of transcription factors, which bind to the promoter of BCL-XL [17]. Because phosphorylated c-met and BCL-XL expression are correlated in vivo, it has been proposed that the HGF/met axis mediates survival in part through this interaction at the transcriptional level [17].

The early-response proto-oncogene, fos-related antigen or fra-1 transcriptionally regulates c-met and is upregulated in preclinical models of mesothelioma, as evidenced by expression microarray analysis [109]. Accordingly, HGF-dependent phosphorylation is inhibited by Fra-1 silencing [111]. Fra-1 is a component of the dimeric transcription factor, activator protein-1 or AP-1 and is regulated by phosphatidyl-inositol-3-kinase, extracellular signal-regulated kinases ERK1 and 2, and Src-associated pathways [110]. In addition to c-met being a target of Fra-1, it also directly regulates expression of CD44, the predominant hyaluronic receptor in mesothelioma expression, and thus potentially contributes to control of migration and invasive behavior.

The small molecule c-met inhibitors SU 11274 or PHA-665752, as well as RNAi silencing of c-met, inhibits migration of mesothelioma cells. Susceptibility to c-met inhibition has been reported to depend on the presence of a Met/HGF autocrine loop as evidenced by PHA-665752 [89]. Specific c-met mutations have been identified in two domains; N375S, M431V, and N454I mutations in the semaphorin domain; T1010I and G1085X in the juxtamembrane domain. Interestingly, two mesothelioma cell lines H513 and H2596, which harbor the T1010I mutation, are highly sensitive to SU11274. In addition to c-met mutations, deletion of exon 10 resulting in a splice variant of c-met has been identified in some mesothelioma specimens.

Although activation of the epidermal growth receptor family is observed in mesothelioma, activating mutations of the epidermal growth factor receptor (EGFR) have not been identified in patients with mesothelioma [134]. Targeting EGFR alone in mesothelioma cells has little effect, whereas simultaneous targeting of c-met and EGFR is associated with strong inhibition of proliferation and invasion, suggesting that blocking the coactivation of these two pathways may be more effective than targeting c-met alone [60].

9.4.3
WNT Pathway Activation in Mesothelioma

The Wnt signaling pathways play an important role in homeostasis and development [39]. It suppresses apoptosis through activation of beta-catenin/Tcf-mediated transcription, and is constitutively activated in mesothelioma cells [130]. The canonical Wnt signaling pathway cooperates with loss of NF2 to promote the loss of contact inhibition during proliferation [12]. Gene expression analysis of rat peritoneal mesothelioma induced by o-nitrotoluene or bromochloroacetic acid demonstrates an upregulation of the Wnt/beta-catenin pathway compared with non-transformed mesothelial cells [63]. Using Wnt specific microarray analysis of normal pleura versus mesothelioma, Wnt2 upregulation has been found to be the most common event in mesothelioma [83]. Knockdown of Wnt using RNAi or anti-Wnt2 antibody is sufficient to induce apoptosis, suggesting that Wnt2 could be a potential molecular target [83].

The beta-catenin gene is deleted at 3p21.3 in NCI-H28 cell line [14,118], and this model has been useful in determining the role of beta-catenin-independent Wnt signaling in mesothelioma, via the so-called noncanonical pathway. Wnt inhibitory factor (WIF-1) is a secreted protein that inhibits Wnt signaling and is downregulated in mesotheliomas compared with adjacent pleura [8]. The mechanism of downregulation involves promoter hypermethylation which is seen in malignant, but not adjacent normal pleural tissue. This suggests that epigenetic silencing of WIF-1 could be an important mechanism driving Wnt activation [8]. Similarly, RNAi-mediated knockdown has been shown to suppress cell growth, and colony formation [131]. Secreted Frizzled-related proteins (SFRPs) and the secreted protein dickopf-1 (Dkk-1) are negative regulators of Wnt signaling. SFRPs are silenced by promoter hypermethylation in mesothelioma [74] and re-expression of SFRP4 or Dkk-1 is sufficient to block Wnt signaling in beta-catenin deficient mesothelioma cells. This implicates a beta-catenin-independent, noncanonical Wnt pathway as a key regulator of cell survival in mesothelioma [51,75,150].

Given the potential importance of Wnt in maintaining mesothelioma cell survival, as well as other cancers (e.g., 80% of colorectal cancers are driven by Wnt mutations [42]), targeting Wnt is a promising strategy. However, no agents have yet entered clinical development. This is because drugging the Wnt pathway has proved difficult. Nevertheless, some small molecules have been identified with the potential to become experimental agents for future clinical studies [20,81]. One promising, but alternative strategy has been to target beta-catenin-mediated transcription. The small molecule XAV939 has been identified by genetic screening. It induces degradation of beta catenin via mechanism involving inhibition of the poly-ADP ribosylating enzymes tankyrase 1 and 2 [54]. This approach might provide a novel strategy for targeting the Wnt pathway in mesothelioma and other cancers.

9.4.4
Estrogen Receptor Beta

Female gender is associated with a favorable prognosis and estrogen receptor beta (ER beta) has been previously shown to be lost in other cancers. This loss is associated with poor prognosis, implicating ER beta as a putative tumor suppressor [7,120]. In mesothelioma, ER beta is downregulated in tumor tissues compared with normal pleura, whereas ER alpha is not expressed [105]. ER beta was recently shown to be an independent prognostic factor for better survival. Activation of ER beta in vitro with 17 beta-estradiol reduces cell proliferation associated with G2/M cell cycle arrest, downregulation of p27, p21, and survivin. These findings suggest that selective estrogen receptor modulators may have a potential role in controlling mesotheliomas.

9.5
Therapeutic Reactivation of Tumor Suppressors

9.5.1
Epigenomic Dysregulation in Mesothelioma

Transformation of normal mesothelium into mesothelioma involves changes to the epigenome. In a study interrogating 1505 CpG loci associated with 803 cancer-associated genes in 158 mesothelioma specimens and 18 normal pleura, the methylation profile was able to effectively discriminate normal pleura from mesothelioma, and was an independent predictor of shorter survival [23]. In an independent study that examined 6157 CpG islands in 20 mesotheliomas in parallel with comparative genomic hybridization and chromatin immunoprecipitation arrays [47], 6.3% of genes were found to be hypermethylated in mesothelioma including MAPK13, KAZALD1, and TMEM30B; 11% of heterozygously deleted genes were affected by DNA methylation and/or H3K27me3. Furthermore, a group of genes silenced by histone H3 lysine 27 methylation (H3K27me3) could be reactivated by histone deacetylation.

Combined epigenetic alterations in mesothelioma are linked with poor prognosis, and these epigenetic alterations may interact cooperatively. In a study, which used nested methylation specific PCR to interrogate the promoter methylation status of nine genes from serum DNA, high incidence of methylation of E-cadherin (71.4%) and FHIT (78%) [36] was measured, whereas intermediate methylation is associated with p16(INK4a) (28.2%), APC1B (32.5%), p14(ARF) (44.2%), and RARbeta (55.8%). Low methylation frequencies were seen for ACP1A (14.3%), RASSF1A (19.5%), and DARK (20%). Interestingly, although no single gene alone predicted survival, combination of RARbeta with either RASSF1A or DARK was associated with significantly shorter survival. This implicates that silencing of multiple genes can cooperate to influence prognosis in contrast to the effects of these single genes alone.

MicroRNAs are associated with epigenetic regulation. In a study in which 98 mesothelioma specimens were studied using a custom micro-RNA platform, a training set of 44 tumors and a test set of 98 tumors were analyzed [103]. The microRNA, hsa-miR-29c was shown to be a favorable independent predictor of time to progression and survival after surgical cytoreduction, and was selectively overexpressed in the epithelioid histological subtype. Overexpression of hsa-miR-29c in cell lines was associated with a reduction in clonogenicity associated with reduced proliferation, as well as invasiveness and motility. Epigenetic regulation by hsa-miR-29c was evidenced by its downregulation of DNA methyltransferases and upregulation of demethylating genes, suggesting its role as a prognostic biomarker could relate to its ability to depress transcription of tumor suppressors.

9.5.2
Targeting the Mesothelioma Epigenome via Inhibition of Histone Deacetylases

Histone deacetylases (HDACs) are a class of enzymes that repress genes by inhibiting transcription. As such, they function opposite to histone acetyltransferase which promotes transcription. HDACs remove acetyl groups from ε-N-acetyl lysine amino acid on a histone; the effect is to remove the positive charge required for electrostatic interaction with the negatively charged phosphate/DNA backbone, leading to remodeling of chromatin (also termed chromatin expansion), resulting in increased transcription.

HDACs can be selectively inhibited by small molecules [35], and are an active molecular target for clinical development. Mesothelioma cells are sensitive to HDAC inhibition, which can directly modify signaling through the core apoptosis pathway; HDAC inhibition, for example, by sodium

butyrate [15,114], causes the downregulation of BCL-XL and induces apoptosis [16]. XIAP is downregulated by HDAC inhibition, and results in increased apoptosis when mesothelioma cells are treated with TRAIL [123]. The HDAC inhibitor Panobinostat (LBH589) is active against mesothelioma cell lines and xenografts [25]. Using a mouse model of B cell lymphoma to explore the proapoptotic pharmacodynamics of vorinostat (suberoylanilide hydroxamic acid or SAHA), the BH3- only proteins BID and BIM were identified as key regulators of intrinsic apoptosis signaling [80]. HDAC inhibition directly downregulates FLIP [18,86,126], with potential to synergize with death receptor agonists [18].

Valproate is an HDAC inhibitor, and has been shown to synergistically interact with cisplatin and pemetrexed in both cell lines, and a xenograft model of mesothelioma [133]. In cells, its cytotoxic activity is associated with activation of both the extrinsic apoptosis pathway, and the intrinsic pathway. Hyperacetylation of histone H3 is induced by valproate consistent with its pharmacodynamics as an HDAC inhibitor. Induction of cell death involves the generation of reactive oxygen species; accordingly, cells can be rescued by the antioxidant N-acetylcysteine.

HDAC inhibition may be a promising new development in the treatment of mesothelioma. Although a phase II trial of belinostat (PXD101) which targets class I and II HDACs was shown to be inactive [108], vorinostat exhibited significant activity in a phase I trial, in which monotherapy achieved partial responses [71]. A randomized phase II/III comparing oral vorinostat versus placebo is currently enrolling patients who have relapsed following first line therapy [143]. Given the lack of standard therapy in this clinical setting, this large randomized trial has potential to change practice if it is positive. Recent evidence implicates HR23B as a resistance biomarker of HDAC inhibitors, albeit in cutaneous T cell lymphoma, an indication for which vorinostat has received FDA approval. HR23B shuttles ubiquitinated proteins to the proteasome. Loss of expression confers resistance to HDAC inhibitors as originally identified by genome-wide RNAi screen. As such, HR23B may represent a potential biomarker for vorinostat in other indications such as treatment of mesothelioma [38,61,113,121,138,151].

9.5.3
Targeting the Ubiquitin Proteasome Pathway

Protein degradation is an essential cellular process which involves tagging with ubiquitin by enzymes called ubiquitin ligases. Proteins are then ferried to the proteasome where degradation to peptides occurs. Small molecule proteasome inhibitors such as bortezomib (velcade) activates BCL-2 family tumor suppressors, leading to induction of apoptosis [33]. These include myc-dependent upregulation of the MCL-1 inhibitor NOXA [34,93,107,139], and other BH3 only proteins such as BIK and BIM [94]. Gene expression studies have implicated dysregulation of the ubiquitin proteasome pathway in mesothelioma [11], and preclinical studies have demonstrated proapoptotic efficacy of proteasome inhibitors in vitro and in vivo [46,113,121,138,151]. This promising activity has led to completion of phase II trials of bortezomib in mesothelioma; EORTC 08052 exploring combination with cisplatin in the first-line setting, and bortezomib monotherapy in the relapsed setting. Mutation and overexpression of proteasome subunit B5 (PSMB5) has been previously identified as a cause of resistance to bortezomib. However, the existence of such mutations in mesothelioma has not yet been established [97].

9.6
Synthetic Lethal Strategies

Mutation of a putative tumor suppressor gene may expose vulnerabilities in a cancer that can be exploited therapeutically. This has been most dramatically demonstrated in the case of somatic BRCA1/BRCA2 mutations, which through inactivation of DNA repair render cancers vulnerable to DNA damage resulting from PARP inhibition [30,85]. Two examples of synthetic lethality associated with dysfunctions in tumor metabolism in mesothelioma will now be considered, where loss of function due to genetic or epigenetic alterations may be exploited, with translation into the clinical setting.

Homozygous codeletion of CDKN2A is frequently associated (90%) with loss of methylthioadenosine phosphorylase (MTAP) [55]. MTAP deficient tumors are responsive to inhibitors of de novo AMP synthesis in the preclinical setting, suggesting a strategy for mediating synthetic lethality. In a multicenter phase II trial to test this concept, patients with MTAP deficient tumors including mesothelioma (as well as non-small cell lung cancer, soft tissue sarcoma, osteosarcoma or pancreatic cancer) were treated with L-alanosine at a dose of 180 mg/m^2 by continuous intravenous infusion daily for 5 out of 21 days. However, no objective responses to therapy were observed leading the investigators to conclude a lack of efficacy [64].

The gene encoding argininosuccinate synthetase (AS), a rate-limiting enzyme involved in arginine metabolism is epigenetically silenced in mesotheliomas, implicating it as a tumor suppressor and highlighting a potential vulnerability which may be exploited therapeutically [26]. AS was shown to be downregulated both in mesothelioma cell lines and a high proportion (63%) of primary mesothelioma specimens [124]. Cell lines lacking AS were unable to synthesize arginine following depletion of arginine from the medium, and underwent apoptosis associated with activation of BAX and mitochondrial depolarization. Silencing of AS was associated with gene methylation.

Induction of apoptosis in AS negative cells following withdrawal of arginine is selective, and not observed in AS positive cell lines, reflecting arginine auxotrophy of AS deficient cells. Accordingly, lack of AS presents a potential metabolic Achilles' heel in mesothelioma. This phenotype can be targeted pharmacologically, by removing arginine from the circulation using pegylated arginine deiminase, an agent that has received orphan drug status from the FDA for the treatment of hepatocellular carcinoma, and has shown efficacy in melanoma [5,13,28,56]. Because of the high frequency of AS deficiency in mesothelioma, a phase II trial will be evaluating this strategy in patients, tailoring treatment to patients with AS negative mesothelioma [26,124].

9.7
Summary

In recent years, it has become clear that mesothelioma is characterized by frequent activation of survival pathways and inactivation of tumor suppressors. This has opened the door to a growing number of new, rational treatment strategies for targeting vulnerabilities in mesothelioma, that for the first time have real potential for significantly improving treatment response in this chemoresistant cancer, and improving survival outcomes, particularly in the relapsed setting where it is still an unmet clinical need.

References

1. Altomare DA, Vaslet CA, Skele KL, De Rienzo A, Devarajan K, Jhanwar SC, McClatchey AI, Kane AB, Testa JR (2005) A mouse model recapitulating molecular features of human mesothelioma. Cancer Res 65(18):8090–8095
2. Altomare DA, You H, Xiao GH, Ramos-Nino ME, Skele KL, De Rienzo A, Jhanwar SC, Mossman BT, Kane AB, Testa JR (2005) Human and mouse mesotheliomas exhibit elevated AKT/PKB activity, which can be targeted pharmacologically to inhibit tumor cell growth. Oncogene 24(40):6080–6089
3. Andujar P, Wang J, Descatha A, Galateau-Salle F, Abd-Alsamad I, Billon-Galland MA, Blons H, Clin B, Danel C, Housset B et al (2010) p16INK4A inactivation mechanisms in non-small-cell lung cancer patients occupationally exposed to asbestos. Lung Cancer (Amsterdam, Netherlands 67(1):23–30
4. Antonsson B, Conti F, Ciavatta A, Montessuit S, Lewis S, Martinou I, Bernasconi L, Bernard A, Mermod JJ, Mazzei G et al (1997) Inhibition of Bax channel-forming activity by Bcl-2. Science (New York) 277(5324):370–372
5. Ascierto PA, Scala S, Castello G, Daponte A, Simeone E, Ottaiano A, Beneduce G, De Rosa V, Izzo F, Melucci MT et al (2005) Pegylated arginine deiminase treatment of patients with metastatic melanoma: results from phase I and II studies. J Clin Oncol 23(30):7660–7668
6. Barbone D, Yang TM, Morgan JR, Gaudino G, Broaddus VC (2008) Mammalian target of rapamycin contributes to the acquired apoptotic resistance of human mesothelioma multicellular spheroids. J Biol Chem 283(19):13021–13030
7. Batistatou A, Kyzas PA, Goussia A, Arkoumani E, Voulgaris S, Polyzoidis K, Agnantis NJ, Stefanou D (2006) Estrogen receptor beta (ERbeta) protein expression correlates with BAG-1 and prognosis in brain glial tumours. J Neurooncol 77(1):17–23
8. Batra S, Shi Y, Kuchenbecker KM, He B, Reguart N, Mikami I, You L, Xu Z, Lin YC, Clement G et al (2006) Wnt inhibitory factor-1, a Wnt antagonist, is silenced by promoter hypermethylation in malignant pleural mesothelioma. Biochem Biophys Res Commun 342(4):1228–1232
9. Beroukhim R, Mermel CH, Porter D, Wei G, Raychaudhuri S, Donovan J, Barretina J, Boehm JS, Dobson J, Urashima M et al (2010) The landscape of somatic copy-number alteration across human cancers. Nature 463(7283):899–905
10. Boldin MP, Goncharov TM, Goltsev YV, Wallach D (1996) Involvement of MACH, a novel MORT1/FADD-interacting protease, in Fas/APO-1- and TNF receptor-induced cell death. Cell 85(6):803–815
11. Borczuk AC, Cappellini GC, Kim HK, Hesdorffer M, Taub RN, Powell CA (2007) Molecular profiling of malignant peritoneal mesothelioma identifies the ubiquitin-proteasome pathway as a therapeutic target in poor prognosis tumors. Oncogene 26(4):610–617
12. Bosco EE, Nakai Y, Hennigan RF, Ratner N, Zheng Y (2010) NF2-deficient cells depend on the Rac1-canonical Wnt signaling pathway to

promote the loss of contact inhibition of proliferation. Oncogene 29(17):2540–2549

13. Bowles TL, Kim R, Galante J, Parsons CM, Virudachalam S, Kung HJ, Bold RJ (2008) Pancreatic cancer cell lines deficient in argininosuccinate synthetase are sensitive to arginine deprivation by arginine deiminase. Int J Cancer 123(8):1950–1955

14. Calvo R, West J, Franklin W, Erickson P, Bemis L, Li E, Helfrich B, Bunn P, Roche J, Brambilla E et al (2000) Altered HOX and WNT7A expression in human lung cancer. Proc Natl Acad Sci USA 97(23):12776–12781

15. Candido EP, Reeves R, Davie JR (1978) Sodium butyrate inhibits histone deacetylation in cultured cells. Cell 14(1):105–113

16. Cao XX, Mohuiddin I, Ece F, McConkey DJ, Smythe WR (2001) Histone deacetylase inhibitor downregulation of bcl-xl gene expression leads to apoptotic cell death in mesothelioma. Am J Respir Cell Mol Biol 25(5):562–568

17. Cao X, Littlejohn J, Rodarte C, Zhang L, Martino B, Rascoe P, Hamid K, Jupiter D, Smythe WR (2009) Up-regulation of Bcl-xl by hepatocyte growth factor in human mesothelioma cells involves ETS transcription factors. Am J Pathol 175(5):2207–2216

18. Carlisi D, Lauricella M, D'Anneo A, Emanuele S, Angileri L, Di Fazio P, Santulli A, Vento R, Tesoriere G (2009) The histone deacetylase inhibitor suberoylanilide hydroxamic acid sensitises human hepatocellular carcinoma cells to TRAIL-induced apoptosis by TRAIL-DISC activation. Eur J Cancer 45(13): 2425–2438

19. Center R, Lukeis R, Dietzsch E, Gillespie M, Garson OM (1993) Molecular deletion of 9p sequences in non-small cell lung cancer and malignant mesothelioma. Genes Chromosomes Cancer 7(1):47–53

20. Chen B, Dodge ME, Tang W, Lu J, Ma Z, Fan CW, Wei S, Hao W, Kilgore J, Williams NS et al (2009) Small molecule-mediated disruption of Wnt-dependent signaling in tissue regeneration and cancer. Nat Chem Biol 5(2):100–107

21. Cheng JQ, Jhanwar SC, Klein WM, Bell DW, Lee WC, Altomare DA, Nobori T, Olopade OI, Buckler AJ, Testa JR (1994) p16 alterations and deletion mapping of 9p21-p22 in malignant mesothelioma. Cancer Res 54(21):5547–5551

22. Chinnaiyan AM, O'Rourke K, Tewari M, Dixit VM (1995) FADD, a novel death domain-containing protein, interacts with the death domain of Fas and initiates apoptosis. Cell 81(4):505–512

23. Christensen BC, Houseman EA, Godleski JJ, Marsit CJ, Longacker JL, Roelofs CR, Karagas MR, Wrensch MR, Yeh RF, Nelson HH et al (2009) Epigenetic profiles distinguish pleural mesothelioma from normal pleura and predict lung asbestos burden and clinical outcome. Cancer Res 69(1):227–234

24. Cory S, Adams JM (2005) Killing cancer cells by flipping the Bcl-2/Bax switch. Cancer Cell 8(1):5–6

25. Crisanti MC, Wallace AF, Kapoor V, Vandermeers F, Dowling ML, Pereira LP, Coleman K, Campling BG, Fridlender ZG, Kao GD et al (2009) The HDAC inhibitor panobinostat (LBH589) inhibits mesothelioma and lung cancer cells in vitro and in vivo with particular efficacy for small cell lung cancer. Mol Cancer Ther 8(8):2221–2231

26. Delage B, Fennell DA, Nicholson L, McNeish I, Lemoine NR, Crook T, Szlosarek PW (2010) Arginine deprivation and argininosuccinate synthetase expression in the treatment of cancer. Int J Cancer 126(12):2762–2772

27. Du C, Fang M, Li Y, Li L, Wang X (2000) Smac, a mitochondrial protein that promotes cytochrome c-dependent caspase activation by eliminating IAP inhibition. Cell 102(1):33–42

28. Ensor CM, Holtsberg FW, Bomalaski JS, Clark MA (2002) Pegylated arginine deiminase (ADI-SS PEG20, 000 mw) inhibits human melanomas and hepatocellular carcinomas in vitro and in vivo. Cancer Res 62(19):5443–5450

29. Falleni M, Pellegrini C, Marchetti A, Roncalli M, Nosotti M, Palleschi A, Santambrogio L, Coggi G, Bosari S (2005) Quantitative evaluation of the apoptosis regulating genes Survivin, Bcl-2 and Bax in inflammatory and malignant pleural lesions. Lung Cancer (Amsterdam, Netherlands) 48(2):211–216

30. Farmer H, McCabe N, Lord CJ, Tutt AN, Johnson DA, Richardson TB, Santarosa M, Dillon KJ, Hickson I, Knights C et al (2005) Targeting the DNA repair defect in BRCA mutant cells as a therapeutic strategy. Nature 434(7035):917–921

31. Fennell DA, Rudd RM (2004) Defective core-apoptosis signalling in diffuse malignant pleural mesothelioma: opportunities for effective drug development. Lancet Oncol 5(6):354–362

32. Fennell DA, Gaudino G, O'Byrne KJ, Mutti L, van Meerbeeck J (2008) Advances in the

systemic therapy of malignant pleural mesothelioma. Nat Clin Pract 5(3):136–147
33. Fennell DA, Chacko A, Mutti L (2008) BCL-2 family regulation by the 20S proteasome inhibitor bortezomib. Oncogene 27(9):1189–1197
34. Fernandez Y, Verhaegen M, Miller TP, Rush JL, Steiner P, Opipari AW Jr, Lowe SW, Soengas MS (2005) Differential regulation of noxa in normal melanocytes and melanoma cells by proteasome inhibition: therapeutic implications. Cancer Res 65(14):6294–6304
35. Finnin MS, Donigian JR, Cohen A, Richon VM, Rifkind RA, Marks PA, Breslow R, Pavletich NP (1999) Structures of a histone deacetylase homologue bound to the TSA and SAHA inhibitors. Nature 401(6749):188–193
36. Fischer JR, Ohnmacht U, Rieger N, Zemaitis M, Stoffregen C, Kostrzewa M, Buchholz E, Manegold C, Lahm H (2006) Promoter methylation of RASSF1A, RARbeta and DAPK predict poor prognosis of patients with malignant mesothelioma. Lung Cancer (Amsterdam, Netherlands) 54(1):109–116
37. Fong PC, Boss DS, Yap TA, Tutt A, Wu P, Mergui-Roelvink M, Mortimer P, Swaisland H, Lau A, O'Connor MJ et al (2009) Inhibition of poly(ADP-ribose) polymerase in tumors from BRCA mutation carriers. N Engl J Med 361(2):123–134
38. Fotheringham S, Epping MT, Stimson L, Khan O, Wood V, Pezzella F, Bernards R, La Thangue NB (2009) Genome-wide loss-of-function screen reveals an important role for the proteasome in HDAC inhibitor-induced apoptosis. Cancer Cell 15(1):57–66
39. Fox S, Dharmarajan A (2006) WNT signaling in malignant mesothelioma. Front Biosci 11:2106–2112
40. Frizelle SP, Grim J, Zhou J, Gupta P, Curiel DT, Geradts J, Kratzke RA (1998) Re-expression of p16INK4a in mesothelioma cells results in cell cycle arrest, cell death, tumor suppression and tumor regression. Oncogene 16(24):3087–3095
41. Frizelle SP, Rubins JB, Zhou JX, Curiel DT, Kratzke RA (2000) Gene therapy of established mesothelioma xenografts with recombinant p16INK4a adenovirus. Cancer Gene Ther 7(11):1421–1425
42. Garber K (2009) Drugging the Wnt pathway: problems and progress. J Natl Cancer Inst 101(8):548–550
43. Gordon GJ, Appasani K, Parcells JP, Mukhopadhyay NK, Jaklitsch MT, Richards WG, Sugarbaker DJ, Bueno R (2002) Inhibitor of apoptosis protein-1 promotes tumor cell survival in mesothelioma. Carcinogenesis 23(6):1017–1024
44. Gordon GJ, Mani M, Mukhopadhyay L, Dong L, Edenfield HR, Glickman JN, Yeap BY, Sugarbaker DJ, Bueno R (2007) Expression patterns of inhibitor of apoptosis proteins in malignant pleural mesothelioma. J Pathol 211(4):447–454
45. Gordon GJ, Mani M, Mukhopadhyay L, Dong L, Yeap BY, Sugarbaker DJ, Bueno R (2007) Inhibitor of apoptosis proteins are regulated by tumour necrosis factor-alpha in malignant pleural mesothelioma. J Pathol 211(4):439–446
46. Gordon GJ, Mani M, Maulik G, Mukhopadhyay L, Yeap BY, Kindler HL, Salgia R, Sugarbaker DJ, Bueno R (2008) Preclinical studies of the proteasome inhibitor bortezomib in malignant pleural mesothelioma. Cancer Chemother Pharmacol 61(4):549–558
47. Goto Y, Shinjo K, Kondo Y, Shen L, Toyota M, Suzuki H, Gao W, An B, Fujii M, Murakami H et al (2009) Epigenetic profiles distinguish malignant pleural mesothelioma from lung adenocarcinoma. Cancer Res 69(23):9073–9082
48. Hanahan D, Weinberg RA (2000) The hallmarks of cancer. Cell 100(1):57–70
49. Harvey P, Warn A, Newman P, Perry LJ, Ball RY, Warn RM (1996) Immunoreactivity for hepatocyte growth factor/scatter factor and its receptor, met, in human lung carcinomas and malignant mesotheliomas. J Pathol 180(4):389–394
50. Harvey P, Warn A, Dobbin S, Arakaki N, Daikuhara Y, Jaurand MC, Warn RM (1998) Expression of HGF/SF in mesothelioma cell lines and its effects on cell motility, proliferation and morphology. Br J Cancer 77(7):1052–1059
51. He B, Lee AY, Dadfarmay S, You L, Xu Z, Reguart N, Mazieres J, Mikami I, McCormick F, Jablons DM (2005) Secreted frizzled-related protein 4 is silenced by hypermethylation and induces apoptosis in beta-catenin-deficient human mesothelioma cells. Cancer Res 65(3):743–748
52. Hopkins-Donaldson S, Cathomas R, Simoes-Wust AP, Kurtz S, Belyanskaya L, Stahel RA, Zangemeister-Wittke U (2003) Induction of apoptosis and chemosensitization of mesothelioma cells by Bcl-2 and Bcl-xL antisense treatment. Int J Cancer 106(2):160–166
53. Hu Q, Akatsuka S, Yamashita Y, Ohara H, Nagai H, Okazaki Y, Takahashi T, Toyokuni S

9

(2010) Homozygous deletion of CDKN2A/2B is a hallmark of iron-induced high-grade rat mesothelioma. Lab Invest: A Journal of Technical Methods and Pathology 90(3): 360–373

54. Huang SM, Mishina YM, Liu S, Cheung A, Stegmeier F, Michaud GA, Charlat O, Wiellette E, Zhang Y, Wiessner S et al (2009) Tankyrase inhibition stabilizes axin and antagonizes Wnt signalling. Nature 461(7264): 614–620

55. Illei PB, Rusch VW, Zakowski MF, Ladanyi M (2003) Homozygous deletion of CDKN2A and codeletion of the methylthioadenosine phosphorylase gene in the majority of pleural mesotheliomas. Clin Cancer Res 9(6): 2108–2113

56. Izzo F, Marra P, Beneduce G, Castello G, Vallone P, De Rosa V, Cremona F, Ensor CM, Holtsberg FW, Bomalaski JS et al (2004) Pegylated arginine deiminase treatment of patients with unresectable hepatocellular carcinoma: results from phase I/II studies. J Clin Oncol 22(10):1815–1822

57. Jagadeeswaran R, Ma PC, Seiwert TY, Jagadeeswaran S, Zumba O, Nallasura V, Ahmed S, Filiberti R, Paganuzzi M, Puntoni R et al (2006) Functional analysis of c-Met/hepatocyte growth factor pathway in malignant pleural mesothelioma. Cancer Res 66(1):352–361

58. Johnstone RW, Ruefli AA, Lowe SW (2002) Apoptosis: a link between cancer genetics and chemotherapy. Cell 108(2):153–164

59. Jongsma J, van Montfort E, Vooijs M, Zevenhoven J, Krimpenfort P, van der Valk M, van de Vijver M, Berns A (2008) A conditional mouse model for malignant mesothelioma. Cancer Cell 13(3):261–271

60. Kawaguchi K, Murakami H, Taniguchi T, Fujii M, Kawata S, Fukui T, Kondo Y, Osada H, Usami N, Yokoi K et al (2009) Combined inhibition of MET and EGFR suppresses proliferation of malignant mesothelioma cells. Carcinogenesis 30(7):1097–1105

61. Khan O, Fotheringham S, Wood V, Stimson L, Zhang C, Pezzella F, Duvic M, Kerr DJ, La Thangue NB (2010) HR23B is a biomarker for tumor sensitivity to HDAC inhibitor-based therapy. Proc Natl Acad Sci USA 107(14): 6532–6537

62. Kim KU, Wilson SM, Abayasiriwardana KS, Collins R, Fjellbirkeland L, Xu Z, Jablons DM, Nishimura SL, Broaddus VC (2005) A novel in vitro model of human mesothelioma for studying tumor biology and apoptotic resistance. Am J Respir Cell Mol Biol 33(6): 541–548

63. Kim Y, Ton TV, DeAngelo AB, Morgan K, Devereux TR, Anna C, Collins JB, Paules RS, Crosby LM, Sills RC (2006) Major carcinogenic pathways identified by gene expression analysis of peritoneal mesotheliomas following chemical treatment in F344 rats. Toxicol Appl Pharmacol 214(2):144–151

64. Kindler HL, Burris HA III, Sandler AB, Oliff IA (2009) A phase II multicenter study of L-alanosine, a potent inhibitor of adenine biosynthesis, in patients with MTAP-deficient cancer. Invest New Drugs 27(1):75–81

65. Kleinberg L, Lie AK, Florenes VA, Nesland JM, Davidson B (2007) Expression of inhibitor-of-apoptosis protein family members in malignant mesothelioma. Hum Pathol 38(7): 986–994

66. Klominek J, Baskin B, Liu Z, Hauzenberger D (1998) Hepatocyte growth factor/scatter factor stimulates chemotaxis and growth of malignant mesothelioma cells through c-met receptor. Int J Cancer 76(2):240–249

67. Kobayashi N, Toyooka S, Yanai H, Soh J, Fujimoto N, Yamamoto H, Ichihara S, Kimura K, Ichimura K, Sano Y et al (2008) Frequent p16 inactivation by homozygous deletion or methylation is associated with a poor prognosis in Japanese patients with pleural mesothelioma. Lung Cancer (Amsterdam, Netherlands) 62(1):120–125

68. Konopleva M, Contractor R, Tsao T, Samudio I, Ruvolo PP, Kitada S, Deng X, Zhai D, Shi YX, Sneed T et al (2006) Mechanisms of apoptosis sensitivity and resistance to the BH3 mimetic ABT-737 in acute myeloid leukemia. Cancer Cell 10(5):375–388

69. Kratzke RA, Wang X, Wong L, Kratzke MG, Green MR, Vokes EE, Vogelzang NJ, Kindler HL, Kern JA (2008) Response to the methylation inhibitor dihydro-5-azacytidine in mesothelioma is not associated with methylation of p16INK4a: results of cancer and leukemia group B 159904. J Thorac Oncol 3(4):417–421

70. Krimpenfort P, Ijpenberg A, Song JY, van der Valk M, Nawijn M, Zevenhoven J, Berns A (2007) p15Ink4b is a critical tumour suppressor in the absence of p16Ink4a. Nature 448(7156):943–946

71. Krug LM, Curley T, Schwartz L, Richardson S, Marks P, Chiao J, Kelly WK (2006) Potential

role of histone deacetylase inhibitors in mesothelioma: clinical experience with suberoylanilide hydroxamic acid. Clin Lung Cancer 7(4):
257–261

72. Ladanyi M (2005) Implications of P16/CDKN2A
deletion in pleural mesotheliomas. Lung Cancer
(Amsterdam, Netherlands) 49(Suppl 1):S95–S98

73. Lecomte C, Andujar P, Renier A, Kheuang L,
Abramowski V, Mellottee L, Fleury-Feith J,
Zucman-Rossi J, Giovannini M, Jaurand MC
(2005) Similar tumor suppressor gene alteration profiles in asbestos-induced murine and
human mesothelioma. Cell Cycle (Georgetown,
TX) 4(12):1862–1869

74. Lee AY, He B, You L, Dadfarmay S, Xu Z,
Mazieres J, Mikami I, McCormick F, Jablons DM
(2004) Expression of the secreted frizzled-related
protein gene family is downregulated in human
mesothelioma. Oncogene 23(39):6672–6676

75. Lee AY, He B, You L, Xu Z, Mazieres J, Reguart N,
Mikami I, Batra S, Jablons DM (2004) Dickkopf-1
antagonizes Wnt signaling independent of beta-
catenin in human mesothelioma. Biochem Biophys
Res Commun 323(4):1246–1250

76. Letai A, Bassik MC, Walensky LD, Sorcinelli
MD, Weiler S, Korsmeyer SJ (2002) Distinct
BH3 domains either sensitize or activate mitochondrial apoptosis, serving as prototype cancer therapeutics. Cancer Cell 2(3):183–192

77. Li P, Nijhawan D, Budihardjo I, Srinivasula
SM, Ahmad M, Alnemri ES, Wang X (1997)
Cytochrome c and dATP-dependent formation
of Apaf-1/caspase-9 complex initiates an apoptotic protease cascade. Cell 91(4):479–489

78. Li H, Zhu H, Xu CJ, Yuan J (1998) Cleavage of
BID by caspase 8 mediates the mitochondrial
damage in the Fas pathway of apoptosis. Cell
94(4):491–501

79. Li W, You L, Cooper J, Schiavon G, Pepe-
Caprio A, Zhou L, Ishii R, Giovannini M,
Hanemann CO, Long SB et al (2010) Merlin/
NF2 suppresses tumorigenesis by inhibiting
the E3 ubiquitin ligase CRL4(DCAF1) in the
nucleus. Cell 140(4):477–490

80. Lindemann RK, Newbold A, Whitecross KF,
Cluse LA, Frew AJ, Ellis L, Williams S,
Wiegmans AP, Dear AE, Scott CL et al (2007)
Analysis of the apoptotic and therapeutic activi-
ties of histone deacetylase inhibitors by using a
mouse model of B cell lymphoma. Proc Natl
Acad Sci USA 104(19):8071–8076

81. Lu J, Ma Z, Hsieh JC, Fan CW, Chen B,
Longgood JC, Williams NS, Amatruda JF,

Lum L, Chen C (2009) Structure-activity relationship studies of small-molecule inhibitors of
Wnt response. Bioorg Med Chem Lett 19(14):
3825–3827

82. Martins LM, Iaccarino I, Tenev T, Gschmeissner S,
Totty NF, Lemoine NR, Savopoulos J, Gray CW,
Creasy CL, Dingwall C et al (2002) The serine
protease Omi/HtrA2 regulates apoptosis by bind-
ing XIAP through a reaper-like motif. J Biol
Chem 277(1):439–444

83. Mazieres J, You L, He B, Xu Z, Twogood S,
Lee AY, Reguart N, Batra S, Mikami I, Jablons
DM (2005) Wnt2 as a new therapeutic target in
malignant pleural mesothelioma. Int J Cancer
117(2):326–332

84. Meijerink JP, Mensink EJ, Wang K, Sedlak TW,
Sloetjes AW, de Witte T, Waksman G,
Korsmeyer SJ (1998) Hematopoietic malignan-
cies demonstrate loss-of-function mutations of
BAX. Blood 91(8):2991–2997

85. Mendes-Pereira AM, Martin SA, Brough R,
McCarthy A, Taylor JR, Kim JS, Waldman T,
Lord CJ, Ashworth A (2009) Synthetic lethal
targeting of PTEN mutant cells with PARP
inhibitors. EMBO Mol Med 1(6–7):315–322

86. Mitsiades CS, Poulaki V, McMullan C, Negri J,
Fanourakis G, Goudopoulou A, Richon VM,
Marks PA, Mitsiades N (2005) Novel histone
deacetylase inhibitors in the treatment of thyroid
cancer. Clin Cancer Res 11(10):3958–3965

87. Mohiuddin I, Cao X, Ozvaran MK, Zumstein L,
Chada S, Smythe WR (2002) Phosphatase and
tensin analog gene overexpression engenders
cellular death in human malignant mesothelioma cells via inhibition of AKT phosphorylation. Ann Surg Oncol 9(3):310–316

88. Moye-Rowley WS, Harshman KD, Parker CS
(1989) Yeast YAP1 encodes a novel form of the
jun family of transcriptional activator proteins.
Genes Dev 3(3):283–292

89. Mukohara T, Civiello G, Davis IJ, Taffaro ML,
Christensen J, Fisher DE, Johnson BE, Janne PA
(2005) Inhibition of the met receptor in mesothelioma. Clin Cancer Res 11(22):8122–8130

90. Muzio M, Chinnaiyan AM, Kischkel FC,
O'Rourke K, Shevchenko A, Ni J, Scaffidi C,
Bretz JD, Zhang M, Gentz R et al (1996) FLICE,
a novel FADD-homologous ICE/CED-3-like
protease, is recruited to the CD95 (Fas/APO-1)
death–inducing signaling complex. Cell 85(6):
817–827

91. Neragi-Miandoab S, Sugarbaker DJ (2009)
Chromosomal deletion in patients with malignant

9

pleural mesothelioma. Interact Cardiovasc Thorac Surg 9(1):42–44

92. Nguyen M, Marcellus RC, Roulston A, Watson M, Serfass L, Murthy Madiraju SR, Goulet D, Viallet J, Belec L, Billot X et al (2007) Small molecule obatoclax (GX15-070) antagonizes MCL-1 and overcomes MCL-1-mediated resistance to apoptosis. Proc Natl Acad Sci USA 104(49):19512–19517

93. Nikiforov MA, Riblett M, Tang WH, Gratchouck V, Zhuang D, Fernandez Y, Verhaegen M, Varambally S, Chinnaiyan AM, Jakubowiak AJ et al (2007) Tumor cell-selective regulation of NOXA by c-MYC in response to proteasome inhibition. Proc Natl Acad Sci USA 104(49):19488–19493

94. Nikrad M, Johnson T, Puthalalath H, Coultas L, Adams J, Kraft AS (2005) The proteasome inhibitor bortezomib sensitizes cells to killing by death receptor ligand TRAIL via BH3-only proteins Bik and Bim. Mol Cancer Ther 4(3):443–449

95. O'Connor L, Strasser A, O'Reilly LA, Hausmann G, Adams JM, Cory S, Huang DC (1998) Bim: a novel member of the Bcl-2 family that promotes apoptosis. EMBO J 17(2):384–395

96. O'Kane SL, Pound RJ, Campbell A, Chaudhuri N, Lind MJ, Cawkwell L (2006) Expression of bcl-2 family members in malignant pleural mesothelioma. Acta Oncol (Stockholm, Sweden) 45(4):449–453

97. Oerlemans R, Franke NE, Assaraf YG, Cloos J, van Zantwijk I, Berkers CR, Scheffer GL, Debipersad K, Vojtekova K, Lemos C et al (2008) Molecular basis of bortezomib resistance: proteasome subunit beta5 (PSMB5) gene mutation and overexpression of PSMB5 protein. Blood 112(6):2489–2499

98. Oltersdorf T, Elmore SW, Shoemaker AR, Armstrong RC, Augeri DJ, Belli BA, Bruncko M, Deckwerth TL, Dinges J, Hajduk PJ et al (2005) An inhibitor of Bcl-2 family proteins induces regression of solid tumours. Nature 435(7042):677–681

99. Oltvai ZN, Milliman CL, Korsmeyer SJ (1993) Bcl-2 heterodimerizes in vivo with a conserved homolog, Bax, that accelerates programmed cell death. Cell 74(4):609–619

100. Onofre FB, Onofre AS, Pomjanski N, Buckstegge B, Grote HJ, Bocking A (2008) 9p21 Deletion in the diagnosis of malignant mesothelioma in serous effusions additional to immunocytochemistry, DNA-ICM, and AgNOR analysis. Cancer 114(3):204–215

101. Opitz I, Soltermann A, Abaecherli M, Hinterberger M, Probst-Hensch N, Stahel R, Moch H, Weder W (2008) PTEN expression is a strong predictor of survival in mesothelioma patients. Eur J Cardiothorac Surg 33(3):502–506

102. Papp T, Schipper H, Pemsel H, Bastrop R, Muller KM, Wiethege T, Weiss DG, Dopp E, Schiffmann D, Rahman Q (2001) Mutational analysis of N-ras, p53, p16INK4a, p14ARF and CDK4 genes in primary human malignant mesotheliomas. Int J Oncol 18(2):425–433

103. Pass HI, Goparaju C, Ivanov S, Donington J, Carbone M, Hoshen M, Cohen D, Chajut A, Rosenwald S, Dan H et al (2010) hsa-miR-29c* is linked to the prognosis of malignant pleural mesothelioma. Cancer Res 70(5): 1916–1924

104. Pespeni MH, Hodnett M, Abayasiriwardana KS, Roux J, Howard M, Broaddus VC, Pittet JF (2007) Sensitization of mesothelioma cells to tumor necrosis factor-related apoptosis-inducing ligand-induced apoptosis by heat stress via the inhibition of the 3-phosphoinositide-dependent kinase 1/Akt pathway. Cancer Res 67(6):2865–2871

105. Pinton G, Brunelli E, Murer B, Puntoni R, Puntoni M, Fennell DA, Gaudino G, Mutti L, Moro L (2009) Estrogen receptor-beta affects the prognosis of human malignant mesothelioma. Cancer Res 69(11):4598–4604

106. Poulikakos PI, Xiao GH, Gallagher R, Jablonski S, Jhanwar SC, Testa JR (2006) Re-expression of the tumor suppressor NF2/merlin inhibits invasiveness in mesothelioma cells and negatively regulates FAK. Oncogene 25(44):5960–5968

107. Qin JZ, Ziffra J, Stennett L, Bodner B, Bonish BK, Chaturvedi V, Bennett F, Pollock PM, Trent JM, Hendrix MJ et al (2005) Proteasome inhibitors trigger NOXA-mediated apoptosis in melanoma and myeloma cells. Cancer Res 65(14):6282–6293

108. Ramalingam SS, Belani CP, Ruel C, Frankel P, Gitlitz B, Koczywas M, Espinoza-Delgado I, Gandara D (2009) Phase II study of belinostat (PXD101), a histone deacetylase inhibitor, for second line therapy of advanced malignant pleural mesothelioma. J Thorac Oncol 4(1): 97–101

109. Ramos-Nino ME, Scapoli L, Martinelli M, Land S, Mossman BT (2003) Microarray analysis and RNA silencing link fra-1 to cd44 and c-met expression in mesothelioma. Cancer Res 63(13):3539–3545

110. Ramos-Nino ME, Blumen SR, Pass H, Mossman BT (2007) Fra-1 governs cell migration via modulation of CD44 expression in human mesotheliomas. Mol Cancer 6:81

111. Ramos-Nino ME, Blumen SR, Sabo-Attwood T, Pass H, Carbone M, Testa JR, Altomare DA, Mossman BT (2008) HGF mediates cell proliferation of human mesothelioma cells through a PI3K/MEK5/Fra-1 pathway. Am J Respir Cell Mol Biol 38(2): 209–217

112. Rippo MR, Moretti S, Vescovi S, Tomasetti M, Orecchia S, Amici G, Catalano A, Procopio A (2004) FLIP overexpression inhibits death receptor-induced apoptosis in malignant mesothelial cells. Oncogene 23(47): 7753–7760

113. Sartore-Bianchi A, Gasparri F, Galvani A, Nici L, Darnowski JW, Barbone D, Fennell DA, Gaudino G, Porta C, Mutti L (2007) Bortezomib inhibits nuclear factor-kappaB dependent survival and has potent in vivo activity in mesothelioma. Clin Cancer Res 13(19):5942–5951

114. Sealy L, Chalkley R (1978) The effect of sodium butyrate on histone modification. Cell 14(1):115–121

115. Sedlak TW, Oltvai ZN, Yang E, Wang K, Boise LH, Thompson CB, Korsmeyer SJ (1995) Multiple Bcl-2 family members demonstrate selective dimerizations with Bax. Proc Natl Acad Sci USA 92(17):7834–7838

116. Sekido Y, Pass HI, Bader S, Mew DJ, Christman MF, Gazdar AF, Minna JD (1995) Neurofibromatosis type 2 (NF2) gene is somatically mutated in mesothelioma but not in lung cancer. Cancer Res 55(6):1227–1231

117. Shen WH, Balajee AS, Wang J, Wu H, Eng C, Pandolfi PP, Yin Y (2007) Essential role for nuclear PTEN in maintaining chromosomal integrity. Cell 128(1):157–170

118. Shigemitsu K, Sekido Y, Usami N, Mori S, Sato M, Horio Y, Hasegawa Y, Bader SA, Gazdar AF, Minna JD et al (2001) Genetic alteration of the beta-catenin gene (CTNNB1) in human lung cancer and malignant mesothelioma and identification of a new 3p21.3 homozygous deletion. Oncogene 20(31):4249–4257

119. Soini Y, Kinnula V, Kaarteenaho-Wiik R, Kurttila E, Linnainmaa K, Paakko P (1999) Apoptosis and expression of apoptosis regulating proteins bcl-2, mcl-1, bcl-X, and bax in malignant mesothelioma. Clin Cancer Res 5(11):3508–3515

120. Sumi K, Matsuyama S, Kitajima Y, Miyazaki K (2004) Loss of estrogen receptor beta expression at cancer front correlates with tumor progression and poor prognosis of gallbladder cancer. Oncol Rep 12(5):979–984

121. Sun X, Gulyas M, Hjerpe A, Dobra K (2006) Proteasome inhibitor PSI induces apoptosis in human mesothelioma cells. Cancer Lett 232(2):161–169

122. Susin SA, Lorenzo HK, Zamzami N, Marzo I, Snow BE, Brothers GM, Mangion J, Jacotot E, Costantini P, Loeffler M et al (1999) Molecular characterization of mitochondrial apoptosis-inducing factor. Nature 397(6718):441–446

123. Symanowski J, Vogelzang N, Zawel L, Atadja P, Pass H, Sharma S (2009) A histone deacetylase inhibitor LBH589 downregulates XIAP in mesothelioma cell lines which is likely responsible for increased apoptosis with TRAIL. J Thorac Oncol 4(2):149–160

124. Szlosarek PW, Klabatsa A, Pallaska A, Sheaff M, Smith P, Crook T, Grimshaw MJ, Steele JP, Rudd RM, Balkwill FR et al (2006) In vivo loss of expression of argininosuccinate synthetase in malignant pleural mesothelioma is a biomarker for susceptibility to arginine depletion. Clin Cancer Res 12(23):7126–7131

125. Taguchi T, Jhanwar SC, Siegfried JM, Keller SM, Testa JR (1993) Recurrent deletions of specific chromosomal sites in 1p, 3p, 6q, and 9p in human malignant mesothelioma. Cancer Res 53(18):4349–4355

126. Takada Y, Gillenwater A, Ichikawa H, Aggarwal BB (2006) Suberoylanilide hydroxamic acid potentiates apoptosis, inhibits invasion, and abolishes osteoclastogenesis by suppressing nuclear factor-kappaB activation. J Biol Chem 281(9):5612–5622

127. Tartaglia LA, Ayres TM, Wong GH, Goeddel DV (1993) A novel domain within the 55 kd TNF receptor signals cell death. Cell 74(5): 845–853

128. Thirkettle I, Harvey P, Hasleton PS, Ball RY, Warn RM (2000) Immunoreactivity for cadherins, HGF/SF, met, and erbB-2 in pleural malignant mesotheliomas. Histopathology 36(6):522–528

129. Tsujimoto Y, Finger LR, Yunis J, Nowell PC, Croce CM (1984) Cloning of the chromosome breakpoint of neoplastic B cells with the t(14;18) chromosome translocation. Science (New York 226(4678):1097–1099

130. Uematsu K, Kanazawa S, You L, He B, Xu Z, Li K, Peterlin BM, McCormick F, Jablons DM

(2003) Wnt pathway activation in mesothelioma: evidence of Dishevelled overexpression and transcriptional activity of beta-catenin. Cancer Res 63(15):4547–4551

131. Uematsu K, Seki N, Seto T, Isoe C, Tsukamoto H, Mikami I, You L, He B, Xu Z, Jablons DM et al (2007) Targeting the Wnt signaling pathway with dishevelled and cisplatin synergistically suppresses mesothelioma cell growth. Anticancer Res 27(6B):4239–4242

132. van Delft MF, Wei AH, Mason KD, Vandenberg CJ, Chen L, Czabotar PE, Willis SN, Scott CL, Day CL, Cory S et al (2006) The BH3 mimetic ABT-737 targets selective Bcl-2 proteins and efficiently induces apoptosis via Bak/Bax if Mcl-1 is neutralized. Cancer Cell 10(5):389–399

133. Vandermeers F, Hubert P, Delvenne P, Mascaux C, Grigoriu B, Burny A, Scherpereel A, Willems L (2009) Valproate, in combination with pemetrexed and cisplatin, provides additional efficacy to the treatment of malignant mesothelioma. Clin Cancer Res 15(8): 2818–2828

134. Velcheti V, Kasai Y, Viswanathan AK, Ritter J, Govindan R (2009) Absence of mutations in the epidermal growth factor receptor (EGFR) kinase domain in patients with mesothelioma. J Thorac Oncol 4(4):559

135. Vivo C, Liu W, Broaddus VC (2003) c-Jun N-terminal kinase contributes to apoptotic synergy induced by tumor necrosis factor-related apoptosis-inducing ligand plus DNA damage in chemoresistant, p53 inactive mesothelioma cells. J Biol Chem 278(28):25461–25467

136. Wang K, Yin XM, Chao DT, Milliman CL, Korsmeyer SJ (1996) BID: a novel BH3 domain-only death agonist. Genes Dev 10(22): 2859–2869

137. Wang L, Du F, Wang X (2008) TNF-alpha induces two distinct caspase-8 activation pathways. Cell 133(4):693–703

138. Wang Y, Rishi AK, Puliyappadamba VT, Sharma S, Yang H, Tarca A, Ping Dou Q, Lonardo F, Ruckdeschel JC, Pass HI et al (2009) Targeted proteasome inhibition by Velcade induces apoptosis in human mesothelioma and breast cancer cell lines. Cancer Chemother Pharmacol 10:1235–1244

139. Wang Q, Mora-Jensen H, Weniger MA, Perez-Galan P, Wolford C, Hai T, Ron D, Chen W, Trenkle W, Wiestner A et al (2009) ERAD inhibitors integrate ER stress with an epigenetic mechanism to activate BH3-only protein NOXA in cancer cells. Proc Natl Acad Sci USA 106(7):2200–2205

140. Wei MC, Zong WX, Cheng EH, Lindsten T, Panoutsakopoulou V, Ross AJ, Roth KA, MacGregor GR, Thompson CB, Korsmeyer SJ (2001) Proapoptotic BAX and BAK: a requisite gateway to mitochondrial dysfunction and death. Science (New York) 292(5517):727–730

141. Wilson TR, Redmond KM, McLaughlin KM, Crawford N, Gately K, O'Byrne K, Le-Clorrenec C, Holohan C, Fennell DA, Johnston PG et al (2009) Procaspase 8 overexpression in non-small-cell lung cancer promotes apoptosis induced by FLIP silencing. Cell Death Differ 16(10):1352–1361

142. Wong L, Zhou J, Anderson D, Kratzke RA (2002) Inactivation of p16INK4a expression in malignant mesothelioma by methylation. Lung Cancer (Amsterdam, Netherlands) 38(2): 131–136

143. www.cancer.gov: Suberoylanilide hydroxamic acid (Vorinostat, MK0683) versus placebo in advanced malignant pleural mesothelioma. In www.http://clinicaltrials.goc/ct2/show/ NCT00128102.

144. Xia C, Xu Z, Yuan X, Uematsu K, You L, Li K, Li L, McCormick F, Jablons DM (2002) Induction of apoptosis in mesothelioma cells by antisurvivin oligonucleotides. Mol Cancer Ther 1(9):687–694

145. Xio S, Li D, Vijg J, Sugarbaker DJ, Corson JM, Fletcher JA (1995) Codeletion of p15 and p16 in primary malignant mesothelioma. Oncogene 11(3):511–515

146. Yin XM, Oltvai ZN, Korsmeyer SJ (1994) BH1 and BH2 domains of Bcl-2 are required for inhibition of apoptosis and heterodimerization with Bax. Nature 369(6478):321–323

147. Yin C, Knudson CM, Korsmeyer SJ, Van Dyke T (1997) Bax suppresses tumorigenesis and stimulates apoptosis in vivo. Nature 385 (6617):637–640

148. Yokoyama T, Osada H, Murakami H, Tatematsu Y, Taniguchi T, Kondo Y, Yatabe Y, Hasegawa Y, Shimokata K, Horio Y et al (2008) YAP1 is involved in mesothelioma development and negatively regulated by Merlin through phosphorylation. Carcinogenesis 29(11):2139–2146

149. Yoshida H, Kong YY, Yoshida R, Elia AJ, Hakem A, Hakem R, Penninger JM, Mak TW (1998) Apaf1 is required for mitochondrial pathways of apoptosis and brain development. Cell 94(6):739–750

150. You L, He B, Uematsu K, Xu Z, Mazieres J, Lee A, McCormick F, Jablons DM (2004) Inhibition of Wnt-1 signaling induces apoptosis in beta-catenin-deficient mesothelioma cells. Cancer Res 64(10):3474–3478

151. Yuan BZ, Chapman JA, Reynolds SH (2008) Proteasome inhibitor MG132 induces apoptosis and inhibits invasion of human malignant pleural mesothelioma cells. Transl Oncol 1(3): 129–140

152. Zaffaroni N, Costa A, Pennati M, De Marco C, Affini E, Madeo M, Erdas R, Cabras A, Kusamura S, Baratti D et al (2007) Survivin is highly expressed and promotes cell survival in malignant peritoneal mesothelioma. Cell Oncol 29(6):453–466

153. Zimmerman RL, Fogt F (2001) Evaluation of the c-Met immunostain to detect malignant cells in body cavity effusions. Oncol Rep 8(6):1347–1350

Early Stages of Mesothelioma, Screening and Biomarkers

10

Sonja Klebe and Douglas W. Henderson

Abstract The early diagnosis of mesothelioma is notoriously difficult, both from a clinical and pathological perspective. Patients often undergo several medical investigations without definitive diagnosis. The discovery of biomarkers that can be assessed in pleural effusions, histological samples, and serum may assist with the difficult early diagnosis of mesothelioma. In this chapter we focus on those markers that have been examined in the setting of either early diagnosis of mesothelioma in symptomatic individuals or that have been proposed as suitable for screening of asbestos-exposed individuals, with an emphasis on cytology and histology.

10.1 Early-Stage Malignant Mesothelioma, Including the Concept of Mesothelioma In Situ and the Distinction from Reactive Mesothelial Hyperplasia

A subserosal multipotential fibroblastoid cell (SMFC) has been invoked in the past as the stem cell for mesothelial renewal following injury resulting in destruction of the surface mesothelium and as the progenitor cell for the development of malignant mesothelioma (MM) [16,17]. According to this theory, an origin of MM from such SMFCs could explain the observation that the time required for mesothelial regeneration remains constant, irrespective of the area of the injury, and also the biphasic differentiation characteristic of approximately 30% of MMs, within a range of about 25–35% [54,59]. (If this model is correct, it follows that MM is an invasive neoplasm ab initio, with no in situ phase of development.) Based, in part, on experimental models of mesothelial healing following injury without disruption of the submesothelial basal lamina [177,178,181], and on detection of early-stage MMs of epithelial type – where mesothelial atypia appeared to be predominantly in situ, in the absence of any radiological or gross anatomical evidence of pleural thickening or nodularity – Whitaker et al. [180]

S. Klebe (✉) and D.W. Henderson
Department of Anatomical Pathology,
Flinders University of South Australia,
Bedford Park, Adelaide SA, Australia and
SA Pathology, Flinders Medical Centre,
3 Flinders Drive, Bedford Park,
Adelaide SA, Australia
e-mail: sonja.klebe@health.sa.gov.au

A. Tannapfel (ed.), *Malignant Mesothelioma*, Recent Results in Cancer Research 189,
DOI: 10.1007/978-3-642-10862-4_10, © Springer-Verlag Berlin Heidelberg 2011

refocused upon the mesothelium itself as the reserve cell for "normal" mesothelial cell turnover and for healing, and as the progenitor cell for MM, advancing the concept of mesothelioma in situ (MMIS). (For a detailed discussion of mesothelial cell turnover and renewal, see Whitaker et al. [181]; the constancy of the time for mesothelial healing according to this model is largely explicable by detachment of mesothelial cells from viable mesothelium and their random reimplantation over the denuded area.) These authors [180,183] defined MMIS as the replacement of benign surface mesothelium by mesothelial cells with markers of malignancy – with the consequent problem of identifying an acceptable and consistently reproducible marker of neoplastic change. Whitaker et al. [180] described 22 cases of mesothelial proliferation that had presented in a "conventional" fashion, in the form of a pleural effusion with either no identifiable pleural tumor or only tiny nodules at thoracoscopy (Fig. 10.1). The diagnosis in a number of cases was established by existing cytologic criteria. Whitaker et al. [180] suggested that the markers for MMIS in pleural biopsies included the following [60,61] (Figs. 10.2–10.5):

- *Abnormal architecture of the mesothelium at the surface of the affected pleural tissue.* Such architectural abnormalities included noninvasive, linear, papillary, and tubulopapillary patterns, sometimes with a complex exophytic architecture (Figs. 10.2–10.4).
- *Substantial cytological atypia* (Fig. 10.5). However, these authors [183] also considered that other cases might occur where there is substantially less cytological atypia, so that such cases would be diagnosable (if at all) only by ancillary techniques: among those techniques they included strong linear labeling for epithelial membrane antigen (EMA) – see later discussion on *Diagnostic Biomarkers.*
- *Absence of background inflammation* as an incitement for mesothelial hyperplasia.

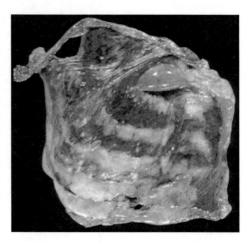

Fig. 10.1 Pleurectomy specimen from a patient who presented with a massive pleural effusion. No distinctive abnormality was seen at thoracoscopy but multiple random biopsies revealed an extensive atypical mesothelial proliferation, in situ in most areas of the biopsies, but with small foci of invasion. A pleurectomy was subsequently carried out, and in the surgical specimen, small foci of white invasive tumour were found, some of which extended into sub-pleural adipose tissue (From Battifora and McCaughey [11], Fig. 4-6. ; figure originally contributed by Dr. Douglas Henderson, Adelaide, Australia)

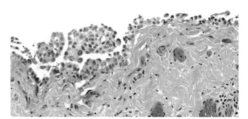

Fig. 10.2 Atypical mesothelial proliferation at the surface of a pleural biopsy, with the formation of at least two small papillary structures. Invasive mesothelioma was found in other areas of the same biopsy

The major problem in translating this concept into diagnosis in practice is that there is overlap in the degree of cytological atypia between benign reactive mesothelial proliferations (RMPs) versus mesothelioma [20,26,27,61]. In the

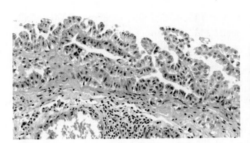

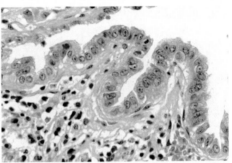

Fig. 10.3 Atypical mesothelial proliferation in a pleural biopsy, with an exophytic papillary architecture at the surface. The lesion is entirely in situ in distribution in this field, but superficial invasion into the submesothelial fibrous tissue was found in other areas of this biopsy (Reproduced from Hammar et al. [54], p 643; Fig. 43.95A. ©Springer Science+Business Media 2008. With kind permission of Springer Science+Business Media)

Fig. 10.5 Same pleural biopsy shown in Fig. 10.3, depicting the mesothelial atypia at higher magnification (Reproduced from Hammar et al. [54], p 643; Fig 43.95B. ©Springer Science+Business Media 2008. With kind permission of Springer Science+Business Media)

only consistently reliable marker for mesothelioma as opposed to RMP is the presence of acceptable neoplastic invasion (Fig. 10.6) – as

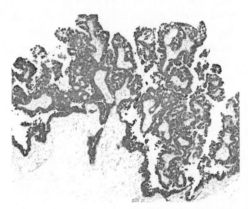

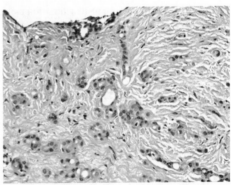

Fig. 10.4 Exophytic in situ mesothelial atypia: superficial but undoubted invasion was found in other areas of the same biopsy. Positive labeling of the lesional cells for CK5/6 (Reproduced from Hammar et al. [54], p 620; Fig. 43.61. ©Springer Science+Business Media 2008. With kind permission of Springer Science+Business Media)

Fig. 10.6 Early-stage invasive mesothelioma of epithelial type, with infiltration into the submesothelial fibrous tissue. This pattern is considered inconsistent with benign mesothelial entrapment as part of a fibro-inflammatory process, although there was no evidence of invasion into subpleural adipose tissue. There is only low-grade cytological atypia. This biopsy showed no evidence of exudative inflammation (Reproduced from Hammar et al. [54], p 645; Fig. 43.100. ©Springer Science+Business Media 2008. With kind permission of Springer Science+Business Media)

absence of any consistently reliable immunohistochemical or molecular biomarker for discrimination between benign and malignant applicable to everyday diagnosis, Whitaker et al. [180] and Henderson et al. [60,61] emphasized that the

10

opposed to benign entrapment of mesothelium within pleural fibrous tissue as a consequence of inflammation – either in the same biopsy, a different biopsy taken at a different time, or at autopsy (see also [54]). Accordingly, Henderson et al. [60] commented in 1997:

> We caution against rash or premature diagnosis of mesothelioma in situ from conventional light microscopy examination of biopsy tissue, taking into account the overlap in the cytologic abnormalities that occur in reactive mesothelioses versus mesothelioma. However, [findings suggestive of a component of MMIS] (especially in conjunction with effusion fluid cytology) may delineate "at risk" patients with "early" stage disease who require further investigation and follow-up. Because of the minimal and perhaps predominantly in situ tumor burden, the mesotheliomas may also be amenable to new modalities of therapy, and some of our "in situ" patients have had prolonged survivals.

Some authorities [27], including the International Mesothelioma Panel [20] consider that noninvasive atypical mesothelial proliferations should be designated simply as an *atypical mesothelial proliferation (AMP)*. We would discourage use of the term *atypical mesothelial hyperplasia*, because by definition *hyperplasia* denotes a benign process and in effusion fluid cytology specimens invasion cannot be assessed and it often cannot be assessed in small or superficial biopsies. Even so, complex exophytic mesothelial proliferations (Figs. 10.3 and 10.4) do not usually occur as part of benign inflammation-induced mesothelial proliferations; such appearances (Figs. 10.2–10.4) raise a suspicion of MM where an invasive component (if present) has not been sampled by the biopsy. Hammar et al. [54] consider that such complex and exophytic AMPs should not be dismissed as benign; they require close clinical follow-up and/or further cytologic or biopsy investigation. That is, a noninvasive AMP in biopsy tissue or an effusion fluid cytology specimen does not by itself represent a treatable disorder – unless carefully correlated with the clinical and in particular the radiological findings or in exceptional circumstances where biopsy is contraindicated – instead, it is a finding that requires follow-up and/or further investigation.

Although it has been claimed that there is no direct proof that in situ mesothelial atypia together with areas of invasive MM represents a single neoplastic lesion [27], Simon et al. [151] reported a single case of "mesothelioma in situ" in association with focal early-stage invasive MM. They investigated the lesion by laser microdissection and comparative genomic hybridization and found similar chromosomal alterations in both the areas of in situ mesothelial atypia and in the foci of early invasive mesothelioma. Accordingly, in the areas of "mesothelioma in situ" they recorded losses at 3p, 5q, 6q, 8p, 9p, 15q, 22q, and Y, with a gain on 7q; in the area of early invasive mesothelioma there were losses at 3p, 5pq, 6q, 8p, 9p, 15q, and 22q with no gains; more advanced mesothelioma showed losses at 1p, 4pq, 6q, 9p, 13q, 14q, and 22q, with gains at 1q, 7pq, and 15q. In a study of 31 cases of MM for EMA, p53 and bcl-2 expression, Cury et al. [34] reported that the seven cases of MM with "… both in situ and invasive mesothelioma, the in situ elements showed similar staining patterns to the invasive epithelioid elements" (see following discussion).

Hammar et al. [54] continue to regard "mesothelioma in situ" as a useful concept for the development of MM. By refocussing attention on the mesothelium itself as the target for neoplastic transformation, this model foreshadows the potential for diagnosis of noninvasive mesotheliomas, with the hope of more effective therapy in the future. They [54] continue to believe that the expression "mesothelioma in situ" represents a valid retrospective diagnosis in cases where at least early-stage invasive MM has been demonstrated.

Hammar et al. [54] set forth the following guidelines and caveats as useful in the differential diagnosis of mesothelial lesions where the discrimination between MM and hyperplasia is problematic:

- *Correlation of the histologic appearances with the findings on pleural effusion fluid cytology and with any abnormalities revealed by imaging studies, such as chest radiographs or CT scans*: in this context, the radiologic investigations in some cases can constitute a surrogate for the histological identification of invasion, in a patient with an AMP as shown by cytological examination of effusion fluid [22] (see later discussion).

- *Invasion of subpleural adipose tissue (or deeper chest wall structures) or invasion into peripheral lung parenchyma by either an epithelioid or sarcomatoid mesothelial proliferation is usually a decisive indicator of malignancy*, for either epithelial or sarcomatoid MM respectively (provided that benign displacement by antecedent procedures such as thoracentesis or biopsy can be ruled out). Immunohistochemical staining for cytokeratins can often highlight genuine neoplastic invasion (especially for desmoplastic MMs [54,98], for assessment of invasion into subpleural adipose tissue).

- *Even in the absence of infiltration into subpleural tissues, MM is still diagnosable from superficial invasion within the pleural fibrous layer, provided that the pattern of infiltration is characteristic or diagnostic of neoplastic invasion*, as opposed to a tangential plane of section through pleural tissue folded upon itself, artefact or benign entrapment of mesothelial cells as part of an organizing fibroinflammatory process (please see below). In our experience this problem represents one of the frequent reasons for referral of biopsy tissue for further opinion: "it looks like it

ought to be a mesothelioma, but I can't find invasion into fat."

- *Hammar et al. [54] emphasize the importance of correct orientation for pleural biopsy tissue as a prelude to histological sectioning*, so that the tissue is embedded on edge with *en profile* sectioning (*en face* sections are frequently problematical as to what represents true invasion as contrasted to a tangential plane of section). Whenever sufficient pleural membrane is available (for example, pleurectomy/decortication specimens and some video-assisted thoracoscopy [VAT] biopsies) and especially when the tissue is received unfixed, it is useful to prepare a *Swiss Roll* from the biopsy, followed by fixation and then slicing of the *Swiss Roll* like a loaf of bread, so that the pleural membrane is sectioned *en profile*. This exercise has the added benefit that large areas of the pleura can be sampled, with a minimal number of tissue blocks. Whenever there is any doubt as to whether the histological appearances represent pseudo-invasion versus genuine neoplastic invasion, the appearances should be considered inconclusive [54].

- *Is it benign inflammation-induced entrapment of mesothelium or MM?* Most inflammation-driven reactive mesothelial hyperplasias are noninvasive, but hyperplastic mesothelial cells can become entrapped within some organizing serosal inflammatory processes – an occurrence that requires distinction from genuine invasion. A florid fibrinous or neutrophilic inflammatory reaction is one marker for the likelihood of benign entrapment (but cases of proven invasive MM with prominent associated exudative inflammation are encountered occasionally). Hammar et al. [54] suggest that such benign entrapment results from burying of the plane where the surface mesothelium is normally located, by a layer of inflammatory exudate that extends over the surface of the membrane, with subsequent organization; in other words, it is the surface of the pleura that has moved inward, into the lumen of the serosal cavity – a process that they [54] sometimes liken to the shrinking of the Aral Sea (the *Aral Sea Effect*). For the distinction between entrapment and invasion, immunohistochemical staining for cytokeratins (or calretinin) is often of value, because it delineates a clear linear boundary between the entrapped mesothelial cells versus the deeper tissues [54].

- *There is a consensus that neoplastic invasion remains the mainstay for diagnosis of early-stage MMs of epithelial type* [20,26,27,54,61,180] (Fig. 10.6): whenever there is any doubt as to whether genuine invasion is present or not, Hammar et al. [54] assign a less-than-definite confidence index for a diagnosis of MM (for example, "possible," "probable," or "highly probable," depending on the degree of doubt) – on the principle that if the lesion is MM "it will declare itself as such soon enough, whereas, inappropriate overdiagnosis of mesothelioma can lead to erroneous cytotoxic chemotherapy or even radical surgery, together with the anguish that a diagnosis of mesothelioma usually entails" (*primum non nocere*).

- *Even when invasion cannot be found in a biopsy sample, there are several findings in combination that are suspicious of MM – requiring clinical follow-up or further investigation – although each is nondiagnostic by itself* [54]. Such findings include:

  - The extent of the mesothelial proliferation
  - A complex exophytic or papillary architecture at the surface of the pleura, in the absence of exudative inflammation
  - Prominent cytological atypia
  - Focal necrosis within sheets of proliferative mesothelial cells in the pleura
  - Prominent intracytoplasmic vacuoles devoid of mucin-like content

- Strong thick linear labeling for EMA with antibodies based on the E29 clone (see later discussion)

A consensus document from the International Mesothelioma Interest Group (IMIG) states that a diagnosis of MM "… has to be made with certainty …", so "that a cytologic suspicion of MM is followed by tissue confirmation that must be supported by both clinical and radiological data" [69]. However, the 2007 statement on MM from the British Thoracic Society (BTS) [22] takes a less restrictive approach to diagnosis: "If the clinical, radiological, and cytological results … support a diagnosis of mesothelioma, then this can be accepted.… A biopsy is required if the diagnosis is not clear after the pleural tap and a CT scan."

10.2
Biomarkers for Early-Stage Epithelioid Malignant Mesothelioma Versus Reactive Mesothelial Hyperplasia

As indicated in the preceding discussion, there is a consensus at present that neoplastic invasion represents the only consistently reliable marker for the discrimination between benign versus malignant mesothelial proliferations. Nonetheless, the potential of several biomarkers has been investigated, for the diagnosis of epithelioid MM as opposed to RMPs, for example, in effusion fluid cytology preparations – with mixed results.

10.2.1
Epithelial Membrane Antigen (EMA)

In their paper emphasizing the concept of mesothelioma in situ, Whitaker et al. [180] observed thick linear labeling of the mesothelial cells for EMA in 17 of 22 such cases (see also Wolanski et al. [183] and Segal et al. [144]); in contrast, proven benign reactive mesothelial proliferations usually showed no significant labeling or only patchy weak labeling [60]. These findings seem to be applicable only to EMA antibodies based upon the E29 clone. In this context, Saad et al. [134] studied EMA expression in 20 cases of reactive mesothelial proliferation (RMP) and 20 cases of MM, using antibodies based on the Mc5 and E29 clones: for the Mc5 clone, 14/20 cases of MM (70%) and 12/20 cases of RMP (60%) showed positive staining. However, for the E29 clone, the corresponding results were 15/20 for MM (75%) and 0/20 for RMP. Saad et al. [134] concluded that EMA antibodies based on the E29 clone are a reliable discriminator between RMP and MM, and Simon et al. [151] commented along similar lines.

Cury et al. [34] investigated EMA, p53 and bcl-2 expression among 31 cases of MM (plus four biopsies initially reported as suspicious, from patients who later developed overt MM) and 20 cases of RMP, as well as 14 cases of benign pleural fibrosis (BPF). Thirty-four out of 35 cases of MM showed diffuse linear staining for EMA (97%). Of the 20 cases of RMP, 5 (25%) showed "focal weak staining" for EMA, and 6/14 cases of BPF also stained for EMA (43%). They [34] concluded that "… strong diffuse linear staining for EMA is a good marker of malignancy when differentiating epithelioid malignant mesothelioma and mesothelioma in situ from reactive mesothelial hyperplasia, although weak focal staining may occur in reactive conditions."

Attanoos et al. [6] investigated 60 cases of pleural MM and 40 cases of RMP for desmin, EMA), p53, bcl-2, P-glycoprotein and platelet-derived growth factor receptor (PDGF-R) β-chain: 48/60 MMs were positive for EMA (80%) in comparison to 8/40 RMPs (20%); 6/60 MMs (10%) showed expression of desmin, versus 34/40 RMPs (85%). These authors [6] concluded: "Desmin and EMA appear to be the most useful markers in distinguishing benign from malignant mesothelial proliferations. Desmin appears to be preferentially expressed in reactive mesothelium and EMA appears to be preferentially expressed in neoplastic mesothelium."

In summarizing the usefulness of EMA immunostaining for the distinction between MM and RMP, the following points and caveats seem to be worth emphasis: [144]:

- Diffuse strong thick linear staining of single cells and cell groups for EMA is a useful pointer on a probability basis for mesothelial neoplasia – especially in effusion cytology – but it is not decisively diagnostic in isolation. In some studies [164,179,180,183], about 75–90% of MMs *or more* showed this pattern of EMA labeling [69], whereas labeling in RMPs is usually undetectable or weak [40,90,99,150,151,164,174,179,182].
- EMA staining can be used as a cytology screening test for patients with a pleural effusion and a past history of asbestos exposure or for effusions that appear to contain "reactive" mesothelial cells [144] – that is, as an indicator for further investigation and follow-up of the patient.
- Negative EMA staining does not exclude a diagnosis of MM, and in biopsy tissue undetectable EMA expression is not uncommon in the deep zones of invasive MMs [54].
- Lymphoplasmacytic cells often show positive EMA staining, so that it is imperative to show that the cell proliferation is mesothelial in character [144].

10.2.2
GLUT-1

GLUT-1 is one of a family of 14 glucose transmembrane transporters that facilitate the entry of glucose into cells [77]. Although immunohistochemically undetectable in normal epithelial tissues and benign tumors, GLUT-1 is expressed in a variety of malignant neoplasms.

In one study on pleural effusion fluids [2], GLUT-1 was expressed in 28/39 of cases of malignant effusion (72%) – 100% from the ovary, 91% from the lung, 67% from the gastrointestinal tract, and 12% from the breast – but none (0/25) of the benign effusions expressed GLUT-1.

Kato et al. [77] studied GLUT-1 expression in 48 cases of MM, 40 RMPs, and 58 cases of carcinoma of lung. GLUT-1 expression as demonstrated by linear membrane-related staining was observed in all 48 epithelioid, biphasic, and sarcomatoid MMs, whereas GLUT-1 was undetectable in all 40 RMPs: in the 11 biphasic MMs, staining for GLUT-1 was found in the epithelioid areas in 10 (91%) and in the sarcomatoid areas in 7 (64%). GLUT-1 staining was also found in 56/58 carcinomas of lung (96.5%). The authors [77] concluded that GLUT-1 is a sensitive and specific discriminator between MM and RMP, but it cannot distinguish MM from lung carcinomas. Husain et al. [69] also refer to the abstract for a study carried out by Acurio et al. [1], which revealed negative reactions in all 40 benign mesothelial tissues (20 normal and 20 RMPs); of the 45 MMs, 9 were negative (20%), 34 showed weak positivity (53%) and 12 were strongly positive (27%). Husain et al. [69] concluded that GLUT-1 staining when positive is a helpful marker for MM in comparison to RMP, but it is unhelpful when negative.

Shen et al. [147] compared EMA with GLUT-1 (both monoclonal and polyclonal antibodies) and the X-linked inhibitor of apoptosis protein (XIAP) in 35 MMs and 38 cases of "benign effusion" and they concluded that EMA "… is a better marker than XIAP or GLUT-1 for the diagnosis of MM."

10.2.3
Bcl-2

Bcl-2 is a proto-oncogene that inhibits apoptosis and thereby promotes survival of individual cells. Detectable overexpression [42] and direct mutations of bcl-2 in MM are rare [110] (unlike many other tumors, including follicular lymphoma and even lung carcinoma [12,44,111], where overexpression is common and may be predictive of a poor prognosis). Segers et al. [145] investigated bcl-2 expression in 62 cases of MM and 44 cases of non-neoplastic mesothelium: cytoplasmic staining was found in 5 MMs (8%) and the benign cases were "… not immunoreactive." All 15 pleural MMs and 15 RMPs studied by Attanoos et al. [6] were negative for bcl-2, and these authors concluded that bcl-2 is of "… no use in distinguishing reactive from neoplastic mesothelium, although more formal evaluation of these markers is required."

10.2.4
p53

The tumor suppressor gene p53 is an inducer of cell cycle arrest and is maintained at low levels in normal unstressed cells, whereas "stress" can induce increased levels of p53 and result in cell cycle arrest and apoptosis. P53 is rarely detectable in normal cells (related to its short half-life) but increased expression of p53 is common in malignant tumors, related to mutations that render p53 nonfunctional and resistant to degradation, as opposed to an increase in functional p53. In MM, such mutations of p53 are rare [121], but the p53 pathway is affected by numerous mutations.

The presence of p53 has been reported in between 25% and 97% of MMs, whereas p53 was found in between 0% and 82% of reactive mesothelial lesions examined [6,23,39,71,83,101,102,109,128,143]. For example, Cury et al. [34] found positive nuclear staining for p53 in 30/31 cases of MM (97%), with greater frequency of positivity in epithelioid than in sarcomatoid tissue, and "occasional nuclear positivity" was found in 13/20 RMPs (65%). Therefore, this antibody does not appear to be useful for the distinction of benign from malignant mesothelial lesions. A relationship between p53 expression and prognosis has not been identified.

10.2.5
X-Linked Inhibitor of Apoptosis Proteins (XIAP)

Wu et al. [184] reported that labeling for XIAP (a member of a family of inhibitors of apoptosis proteins: IAPs) also shows promise in distinguishing benign from reactive pleural effusions. In a study of 116 samples of cell block material from 82 pleural effusions, 22 ascites, 11 pelvic/peritoneal washes, and 1 pericardial effusion, these authors [184] found positive particulate cytoplasmic staining for XIAP in 4/5 MMs, as well as variable positivity in 33–100% of carcinomas according to the site of origin – for example, in all 13 ovarian carcinomas and 9/11 carcinomas of lung (82%) – but all 4 colonic carcinomas were negative and the 35 benign effusions were "virtually XIAP-negative except for two cases (6%)." In a further study on XIAP, Wu et al. [186] found that all nine samples of normal mesothelium were negative, and only one of 13 RMPs showed weak positivity in less than 10% of cells; of 31 MMs, 25 (81%) displayed XIAP positivity. Wu et al. [186] concluded that strong staining for XIAP allowed a distinction between MM and RMPs, especially for small samples and problematical cases.

Lyons-Boudreaux et al. [96] investigated XIAP (and other markers that included calretinin, D2-40, WT1 and MOC31) in five MMs, 48 adenocarcinomas, and 19 benign effusions and found that most MMs stained for XIAP (80%) as well as some adenocarcinomas (51%) and rare benign effusions (11%). They [96] concluded that XIAP is not a sensitive marker for malignancy and has limited value in cytology.

As indicated above, Shen et al. [147] found EMA to be a better marker than XIAP for MM versus RMP.

Based on studies of mesothelial cell lines, XIAP has been mooted (along with IAP-1 and IAP-2, and p21/WAF1, p27/KIP1 and survivin) as a potential target for treatment of MM using the proteasome inhibitor bortezomib alone or in combination with standard chemotherapy [48].

10.2.6
P-Glycoprotein (P-170)

P-glycoprotein plays a role in cell membrane transport, and its expression has been associated with resistance to chemotherapy [146]. Expression of P-170 glycoprotein has not been identified in normal mesothelium, but it has been found in a high proportion of MMs [146], albeit with no apparent effect on patient survival [152]. Ramael et al. [129] detected P-170 in most cases of MM studied, whereas it was not found in normal mesothelium, and Segers et al. [146] found that 54/57 mesothelioma cases showed immunoreactivity for P-170. In a study of 36 cases of MM in comparison to normal mesothelium, Soini et al. [152] detected P-170 in 61% of the MMs but not in normal mesothelial cells. However, in a later study of 15 MMs and 15 RMPs, Attanoos et al. [6] reported that P-glycoprotein was expressed in only 2/15 of the MMs (13%) and none of the RMPs: they [6] concluded that P-glycoprotein (as well as bcl-2 and PDGF-R β-chain) appeared to be of no value for the distinction of MM from RMP, although further studies were required.

10.2.7
Neural Cell Adhesion Molecules (NCAMs): CD56

Neural cell adhesion molecules (NCAMs) corresponding to CD56 antigen are a family of closely related cell surface glycoproteins, thought to play a role in the development of neural cells and the interactions between them. Lantuéjoul et al. [89] studied 26 cases of epithelial, biphasic,

10

and sarcomatoid MM for NCAM reactivity using the 123C3 antibody, in comparison to normal mesothelium and 50 non-small cell lung carcinomas divided evenly between adenocarcinomas and squamous cell carcinomas. Although normal mesothelium was "negative," staining for NCAM was recorded in 19 of the 26 MMs of all histological subtypes (73%). Although this finding raises the possibility that CD56 may be useful for discrimination between RMPs versus MM, there appears to be too little data on NCAM/CD56 expression in MM and mesothelial hyperplasia to justify inclusion of NCAM/CD56 antibodies in everyday diagnostic practice, until further and more extensive studies become available.

10.3
Screening for Malignant Mesothelioma and Prognostic Biomarkers: Serum Levels of Soluble Mesothelin-Related Proteins (SMRPs), Osteopontin (OPN), Megakaryocyte Potentiating Factor (MKPF) and CA125

10.3.1
Introductory Remarks on Screening for Malignant Mesothelioma

As a matter principle and logic, screening for any disease such as cancer is justifiable only when a certain set of circumstances prevail, apart from any considerations of cost [142]:

- The disease occurs with reasonable frequency in the population for which screening is proposed (i.e., it must not be one of great rarity). Because MM is rare in the general population – with an annual incidence of about one case or less per million of the population without identifiable asbestos exposure [22] – screening would be justifiable only for high-risk populations such as middle-aged to older men with substantial (usually occupational) exposure to asbestos.

- The disease in question must result in substantial morbidity or mortality (clearly the case for MM).

- The screening procedure(s) must have reasonable specificity and sensitivity for the detection of the cancer at early presymptomatic stage; in other words, the procedure should have a reasonable positive predictive value for the detection of the cancer in question.

- Ideally, the screening procedure(s) should be noninvasive or only minimally invasive: as a follow-on to this principle, the morbidity and even mortality from the screening test(s) – and any subsequent test(s) necessary to establish a definitive diagnosis for those who test positively for the initial screening – must be taken into consideration and balanced against the potential benefits of therapy for any early-stage disease so detected.

- One or more effective therapeutic interventions exist for the early-stage cancer, with substantially improved outcomes in comparison to the prognosis for those whose cancer is diagnosed at a later and symptomatic stage. (Apart from radical pleuropneumonectomy – applicable for only a minority of MM patients, even when the disease is detected at an early stage – this is not the case for MM and present-day chemotherapy results in only a slight improvement in medial/mean survival times [142], but this situation may change).

Therefore, screening specifically for MM, even in high-risk groups, seems unjustifiable at present [21,51,52,123,142,165] – although groups with past occupational asbestos exposure may be under intermittent clinical and radiological surveillance (or screening) for other asbestos-related disorders such as asbestosis and lung cancer [35,37,43,62,63,85,86,127,153,162,192], (even so, the value of screening programs for lung cancer among former asbestos workers remains debatable [100]). The anguish that can result from a false-positive screening result for MM and the consequent requirement for further investigative procedures also needs to be taken into account [13].

10.3.2
Radiological Screening for MM

The radiographic appearances of pleural MM can vary from essentially normal with early-stage disease, to complete opacification of the affected hemithorax, with confluent nodular pleural thickening sometimes accompanied by extension along interlobar fissures and encasement of the lung, often with contraction of the hemithorax; depending on the size of the MM and its associated effusion, the mediastinum may be displaced to one side or the other [22,92,104]. A pleural effusion of variable volume without pleural thickening is often the only detectable radiological abnormality in cases of symptomatic early-stage MM [180], and as such the finding of an effusion by itself lacks specificity.

Conventional chest x-rays (CXRs) and computerized tomography (CT) have not been shown to be effective screening procedures for early-stage MM [142]. For example, Fasola et al. [43] studied 1,045 asbestos-exposed workers aged 40–75 years (median 58 years), using CXRs and low-dose CT (LDCT) scans. Pleural abnormalities were identified in 70% by LDCT (44% by CXR); ten non-small cell lung carcinomas and one thymic carcinoid tumor were found (1%) but no case of pleural MM was diagnosed. There were "11 false-positive results."

10.3.3
Soluble Mesothelin-Related Proteins (SMRPs)

A significant recent development for the investigation of MM has been the demonstration of elevated serum SMRP levels in MM patients

[29,31,131,132], and a commercially marketed test for SMRP is now available in the form of a two-step immunoenzymatic assay in an ELISA format (MESOMARK™) [14].

Mesothelin is a cell-surface glycoprotein on normal mesothelial cells and can be found in several cancers [105,114,188], including mesotheliomas with an epithelioid component [87,105,114,188], ovarian adenocarcinomas [32,133,188,189], squamous and large cell carcinomas and adenocarcinomas of lung [64,87,105], pancreatic adenocarcinomas [9,55], and some gastrointestinal cancers [133]. The protein product of the mesothelin gene appears to be a 69–71 kDa polypeptide anchored to the cell membrane by a glycosyl-phosphatidyl-inositol (GPI) linkage [97,133,139]; this anchored protein can be cleaved by a protease to yield a 31 kDa soluble protein called megakaryocyte potentiating factor (MKPF) secreted into the blood [97,133,139], and a 40 kDa protein named mesothelin, attached to the cell membrane [139]. The normal biological function of mesothelin is unclear and mice with a knock-out of the mesothelin gene(s) show no obvious phenotypic abnormality [189]. Although attached to the cell membrane, mesothelin can be shed like other cell membrane proteins and Robinson et al. [29,31,131,132] have described a 42–44 kDa soluble mesothelin/MKPF-related protein (SMRP) in sera from patients with pleural MM and also ovarian carcinoma. The process underlying the release of SMRP from cell membranes may be related to an abnormal splicing event that leads to synthesis of a secreted protein (release) or to enzymatic cleavage of membrane-bound mesothelin (ectodomain shedding), and Sapede et al. [139] found evidence that both mechanisms are implicated.

Robinson et al. [31,131] detected SMRP using the OV569 monoclonal antibody – which is used together with another monoclonal antibody, 4H3, for the commercially marketed MESO-MARK™ test [14]. However, others [56,148,149] appear to have used different antibodies to mesothelin, making it difficult to compare their results with those for other studies where the MESO-MARK™ test [14] was used, for example, Scherpereel et al. [141] and Park et al. [122]. Robinson et al. [131] found elevated blood SMRP levels in 37/44 patients previously diagnosed with MM (sensitivity = 84%) as opposed to one of 22 lung cancers (histologic types not specified) and seven out of 40 asbestos-exposed control patients (three of these subjects developed MM 15–19 months after the SMRP sample had been taken). In a more recent (2006) publication from the same laboratory, Creaney et al. [31] reported the results as nanoMoles (nM), with a mean value of about 15.3 ± 20.5 nM in the mesothelioma group, in comparison to a level of approximately 0.9 ± 0.8 nM for healthy controls.

Beyer et al. [14] investigated serum SMRP levels in 409 apparently healthy individuals, 177 patients with nonmalignant disorders and 500 cancer patients (88 of whom had pleural MM). The 99th percentile level for the reference group was 1.5 nM/L, in comparison to a mean level of 7.5 nM/L (95% CI = 2.8–12.1) for the 88 mesothelioma patients. The SMRP levels were increased in 52% of the MM patients and 5% of asbestos-exposed individuals.

In another series, Scherpereel et al. [141] reported blood SMRP levels in 74 mesothelioma patients, 35 patients with secondary carcinomas in the pleura and 28 cases of benign pleural abnormalities associated with asbestos exposure (BPA). They [141] found that serum SMRP levels were significantly higher for epithelioid MMs than for biphasic or sarcomatoid MMs. They [141] also found that the median value for patients with pleural MM was 2.05 ± 2.5 nM/L, in comparison to a level of about 1.0 ± 1.8 nM/L for the metastatic carcinoma group, and in the BPA cases the level was approximately 0.55 ± 0.6 nM/L. Scherpereel et al. [141] commented that serum SMRP levels had a poor capacity for discrimination between pleural MM and secondary carcinoma, related to high

SMRP levels in some of the carcinoma patients. They [141] commented further that pleural biopsy tissue remained the "gold standard" for the diagnosis of pleural MM, and in 2007 Scherpereel and Lee [140] added the comment that the "… proposed markers [SMRP, osteopontin and megakaryocyte potentiating factor] have insufficient accuracy to replace cytohistology as the gold standard for diagnosis for mesothelioma."

In a large-scale prospective study of serum SMRP concentrations among 538 asbestos-exposed subjects attending the Dust Diseases Board in Sydney, Australia, Park et al. [122] found a mean SMRP levels of 0.8 ± 0.45 nM in 223 healthy asbestos-exposed individuals; 15 had elevated SMRP levels (2.8%); [30] one subject had lung cancer, but none was diagnosed with MM (individuals with SMRP levels ≥ 2.5 nM were investigated further by CT scanning and positron-emission tomography). Subjects with pleural plaques had a slightly higher mean concentration of SMRP than those without – a finding thought to be explicable by low-grade pleural inflammation related to the plaques [122]. Park et al. [122] concluded that a high false-positive was observed for SMRP levels and that it seems "… unlikely to prove useful for screening for MM."

In 2009, Creaney et al. [30] reviewed the usefulness of blood SMRP levels for detection of MM, in comparison to osteopontin and megakaryocyte potentiating factor, and they concluded that at present soluble mesothelin remains the best biomarker for MM, but is beset with "… a lack of sensitivity for early-stage disease and for all malignant mesothelioma histologies …."

In 2007, Creaney et al. [32] had also reported mesothelin levels in effusion fluids from 52 patients with pleural MM, as opposed to 56 patients with cancers other than mesothelioma and 84 with benign pleural effusions. Significantly greater pleural fluid concentrations of mesothelin were found in the MM patients than in either of the other two groups, with a specificity of 98% and a sensitivity of 67% for the MM group in comparison to those with non-neoplastic effusions. In seven of ten cases, mesothelin levels were elevated before the diagnosis of MM was made (by 0.75–10 months); four out of eight such cases had elevated mesothelin concentrations in the effusion fluid but not in the serum. The highest mesothelin levels were found in peritoneal fluid in patients with ovarian carcinoma. Significant differences in the mean mesothelin values in pleural effusion fluid were found for epithelial (47 ± 1.0 nM), biphasic (30 ± 0.8), and sarcomatoid (4.5 ± 1.4) MMs; for pleural sarcomatoid MMs the mesothelin concentrations were not significantly different from those in patients with nonmalignant effusions. MM patients with high concentrations of mesothelin in effusion fluid had a median survival of 14 months, as opposed to 8 months for those with low mesothelin levels – probably reflecting MMs with an epithelial component as opposed to sarcomatoid mesotheliomas.

Therefore, the following conclusions can be drawn:

- Blood SMRP levels are elevated in most cases of epithelioid MMs, but other cancers can also be associated with elevated serum SMRP concentrations, including lung and, in particular, ovarian cancers, as well as apparently benign disorders.
- The SMRP levels appear to be greatest for advanced-stage epithelioid MMs, with suboptimal sensitivity for the detection of early-stage MM.
- Epithelioid MMs are associated with higher SMRP levels in serum and effusion fluid than biphasic or sarcomatoid MMs; for sarcomatoid MMs, the mean effusion fluid SMRP levels appear to be no greater than for benign effusions.

- For patients with proven MM, low concentrations of SMRP in blood or effusion fluid appear to represent a marker for a poor prognosis, presumably correlating with the histological subtype and corresponding to predominantly sarcomatoid MMs.
- As indicated in the 2007 BTS statement on MM [22], its diagnosis remains an essentially clinicopathological exercise.
- Serum SMRP levels cannot replace cytologic or biopsy diagnosis of MM, except in unusual circumstances (e.g., a frail elderly patient whose physical condition contraindicates biopsy, or for whom past biopsies have been nondiagnostic, but who has high serum SMRP levels, such as levels >15 nM/L).
- Serial assays of serum SMRP levels may find a role as an indicator of prognosis for MM and as a means to assess its progress or response to treatment.

10.3.4
Serum Osteopontin (OPN) Levels

The significance of serum osteopontin (OPN) levels as a marker for MM is more problematic and doubtful than testing for serum SMRP concentrations [140], with a reported sensitivity of about 47% for the detection of MM [33]. An acidic glycoprotein normally synthesized by osteoblasts – like angiopoietin-1 (ANG-1) also produced by osteoblasts – OPN (SPP1) [72] is said to be a "constraining factor" [57] on hemopoietic stem cell proliferation in the bone marrow. Elevated blood OPN levels have been recorded in patients with MM [124], but elevated levels have also been recorded in a variety of other disorders that include carcinomas of the head and neck region [41,173] and cervix [173], as well as lung [45], ovarian [7], gastric [185], and hepatocellular carcinomas [79]. Elevated OPN levels have also been found in patients with inflammatory bowel disease [106].

Therefore, it appears that serum OPN levels have poor sensitivity and specificity for the detection of MM [49,51,52], but serial serum OPN assays may find a role in assessment of the progress of MM and its response to treatment [24,50,130,140].

10.3.5
Megakaryocyte Potentiating Factor (MKPF)

As discussed in the preceding section on SMRP, MKPF appears to be closely related to SMRP [97,133,139]. It lacks specificity for the detection of MM [140], with poor sensitivity for the detection of non-epithelioid MMs [49], and Creaney et al. [33] found that it had a sensitivity of only 34%. Iwahori et al. [73] found that MKPF was of greater diagnostic value for MM than SMRP and that these two markers had about equal specificity. Even so, assays of serum MKPF appear to have no advantage over SMRP for the detection of MM; like SMRP and OPN, serial measurements of MKPF may be of value in assessment of the progress of MM and its response to treatment [113,130,140], perhaps in conjunction with those other markers and CA125.

10.3.6
CA125

Immunohistochemical investigation of tissue sections for CA125 has no value in the discrimination between MM and adenocarcinomas developing at various anatomic sites, such as those arising in the ovary, lung, and breast [5,10,87,195]. For example, Bateman et al. [10] found that 15/17 cases of MM labeled for CA125 (88%) in comparison to 7/14 cases of adenocarcinomas metastatic to lung and pleura (50%). Attanoos et al. [5] recorded positive immunostaining for CA125 in 19/20 ovarian papillary serous adenocarcinomas (95%) and 2/3 primary peritoneal serous adenocarcinomas, in comparison to 8/32 peritoneal MMs (all in females). In a Japanese study on 90 epithelioid

MMs and 51 adenocarcinomas of lung, Kushitani et al. [87] found that 85% of the MMs and 80% of the adenocarcinomas were positive for CA125. In a further study on effusion fluids, Zhu and Michael [195] found positive staining of all 20 metastatic ovarian carcinomas for CA125, in comparison to 8/13 adenocarcinomas of lung (62%) and 6/13 cases of metastatic breast carcinoma (46%).

However, there is evidence that assays of serum CA125 levels are useful and sensitive for the assessment of the progression of MM and, therefore, its prognosis or for its response to treatment. Hedman et al. [58] found that serum CA125 concentrations increased as the disease progressed, whereas stable disease was accompanied by a decrease in CA125 levels. In a Turkish study on 11 peritoneal MMs, Kebapci et al. [78] found that the mean serum CA125 level was 230 U/mL, within a range of 19–1,000 U/mL (this study gave a normal reference range of 1.2–32 U/mL). In a later study from Italy on 60 cases of peritoneal MM, Baratti et al. [8] recorded a baseline sensitivity of 53% for serum CA125 in the MM patients: in patients who underwent debulking surgery the serum CA125 concentration fell in 21/22 patients who had elevated baseline levels, but it stayed high in all 9 patients with grossly persistent MM, and elevated CA125 levels developed in all 12 patients who developed progressive disease after the surgery and other treatment.

Therefore, there is reasonable evidence that serum CA125 levels represent a sensitive but nonspecific marker for MM, and that serial measurements of the serum levels are a useful means for monitoring the progression of MM or its response to therapeutic measures, especially when the results are correlated with other serum markers as discussed above.

10.3.7
Summary

The serum biomarkers discussed above have the advantage that they represent even less invasive studies than thoracentesis or serosal-surface biopsies, but they are beset with problems of specificity for MM and insensitivity for early-stage disease and non-epithelioid subtypes of MM. At present they cannot replace conventional cytological and biopsy diagnosis of MM, except as probability markers in unusual circumstances, for example, when biopsy is contraindicated. However, either individually or in combination, assays for these proteins may be useful for the monitoring of diagnosed MMs and for the assessment of responsiveness (or lack of it) to treatment strategies. As newer treatments are introduced for MM they may assume increasing importance to assess the effectiveness of such treatment, especially in clinical trials.

10.4
Aquaporins and Malignant Mesothelioma

Over recent years, it has been shown that the transport of water across cells is not explicable by simple diffusion driven by osmotic gradients, but instead is regulated and facilitated by a superfamily of membrane-related proteins known as the aquaporins (AQPs) [80,84]. The AQPs appear to represent an ancient group of proteins that developed at an early stage of evolution and they have been found not only in mammals, but also in amphibia, insects, plants, and microorganisms [18,82]. At least 13 AQPs have been identified (AQP0 to AQP12) [70], which show differential expression in various mammalian tissues [80,91,166,169,172]. As examples, AQP1 is expressed in the endothelial cells that line small blood vessels and it mediates proximal tubule fluid reabsorption in the kidney, the secretion of aqueous humor in the eye, and also cerebrospinal fluid, and lung water homeostasis [80]. AQP2 mediates vasopressin-dependent renal collecting duct water permeability [18,80] and AQP4 is abundant in brain [80], whereas AQP5 influences fluid secretion in salivary and lacrimal glands and is abundant

in alveolar epithelium of the lung [80,166]. The importance of AQPs is demonstrated by the fact that water permeability driven by osmosis between the gas-exchange membranes of the lung is reduced by a factor of 10 if AQP1 or AQP5 are deleted, and it is reduced even more when AQP1 and AQP4 or AQP1 and AQP5 are deleted together [171]. In this context, the function of AQPs has been investigated using AQP-knockout mice, and Verkman et al. [166,167,171,172] have developed and studied transgenic mice that lack AQPs 1, 3, 4, and 5. Various phenotype abnormalities were found in the null mice: in the kidney, deletion of AQP1 or AQP3 resulted in polyuria, but AQP4 deletion resulted in a mild concentrating defect only. Deletion of AQP5 caused defective saliva production. In the brain, deletion of AQP4 conferred protection from brain swelling induced by acute water intoxication.

The lung expresses several AQPs: [19,171] AQP1 is found in vascular endothelium, whereas AQP3 appears to be localized to the epithelium lining large air passages and AQP4 in large and small airway lining cells. AQP5 has been found in alveolar epithelium. AQP1 has also been demonstrated in the mesothelium of the pleura and peritoneum in both experimental models [75,76,81,95,112,193], and for humans [36,47,88,93,155]. Song et al. [154] found that achievement of osmotic equilibrium for pleural fluid took place rapidly in wild-type mice (50% equilibration in <2 min) but was slowed in AQP1 null mice (to less than 25%).

More recently, the study of AQPs has moved from the realm of normal physiology to that of pathology [3,82,91], although the study of AQPs in various disease processes is still in its infancy. AQP2 is the vasopressin-regulated water channel implicated in some hereditary and acquired renal diseases affecting urine-concentrating ability [167]: AQP11-null mice die from uremia as a result of polycystic kidneys [70], whereas AQP2-null humans suffer from hereditary non-X-linked nephrogenic diabetes insipidus [170]. AQP4 appears to play an important role in cerebral edema [4,15,46,117,

118,120,135,136,158], and antibodies to AQP4 are implicated in the pathogenesis of neuromyelitis optica [74,107,108,125,126,138,156,157, 159,160,163,175,176].

In addition, there is evidence that AQP expression can influence the pathogenesis, growth, and metastatic potential of tumor cells that express AQP water channels (in both stromal vascular endothelium and/or the neoplastic cells themselves, in a variety of tumors) [25,38,65,103,115,116,137] and AQP1 appears to be related to angiogenesis in tumors [28]. For example, Hoque et al. [65] found that AQP1 as assessed by immunohistochemical staining – in several types of primary lung tumors that included 16 squamous cell carcinomas, 21 adenocarcinomas, and 7 so-called bronchioloalveolar carcinomas (BACs) – was overexpressed in 62% (13/21) and in 75% (6/8) of cases of adenocarcinoma and BAC, respectively, whereas all cases of squamous cell carcinoma and normal lung tissue were negative. The authors [65]

concluded that: "Forced expression of full-length AQP1 cDNA in NIH-3T3 cells induced many phenotypic changes characteristic of transformation … although further details on the molecular function of AQP1 related to tumorigenesis remain to be elucidated, our results suggest a potential role of AQP1 as a novel therapeutic target for the management of lung cancer."

Others have also suggested that AQPs may represent a target for treatment by AQP inhibitors/blockaders that have been identified [53,66–68,94,119,161,168,187,190,191,194], by way of target inhibition of AQPs themselves or growth factors such as vascular endothelial growth factor (VEGF) that appear to be closely associated with mesothelial-related growth.

We have recently carried out preliminary investigation of AQPs in pleural MM, based upon two observations: (1) as indicated above, AQP1 is expressed in the pleura and peritoneum, not only in the endothelium lining

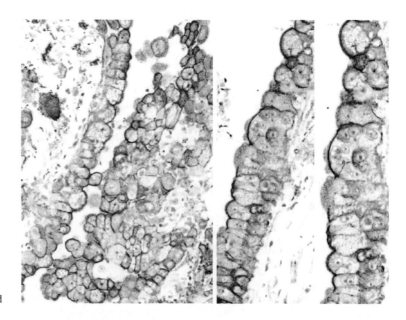

Fig. 10.7 AQP1 expression in an invasive MM of epithelioid type, predominantly membrane-related

submesothelial blood vessels but also in the mesothelium itself and (2) even early-stage MMs, with apparently minimal tumor bulk, usually present with a pleural effusion that may be massive. Therefore, we postulated that pleural MMs may be accompanied by overexpression of AQP1 or the acquisition of other AQPs. Our preliminary immunohistochemical studies have identified consistent strong membranous expression of AQP1 with apical prominence by the tumor cells (labeling in stromal blood vessels is also seen) in epithelioid MMs (Fig. 10.7), with weaker and inconsistent expression of AQP9. Interestingly, so far we have found little or no labeling in sarcomatoid mesotheliomas or the sarcomatoid component of biphasic tumors. At present it is unclear whether this reflects approximately "normal" (or even subnormal) AQP1 expression per unit cell, within an expanded cell population, or whether it represents overexpression by individual tumor cells.

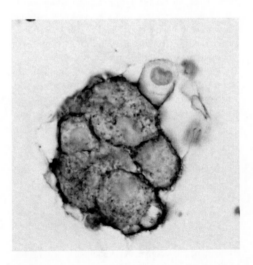

Fig. 10.8 AQP1 expression in a pleural effusion fluid of MM of epithelioid type. Similar distribution in labelling as in the histological section (Fig. 10.7) is seen. Preliminary studies suggest that labelling may be more prominent in malignant lesions versus RMPs, but further studies are needed to confirm that impression

However, in pleural effusion fluids, it appears that in malignant mesothelial cells this pattern is also seen (Fig. 10.8). Further work will be required to investigate the potential uses of this new marker.

References

1. Acurio A, Arif Q, Gattuso P et al (2008) The value of immunohistochemical markers in differentiating benign from malignant mesothelial lesions. Mod Pathol 21(1S):334A
2. Afify A, Zhou H, Howell L, Paulino AF (2005) Diagnostic utility of GLUT-1 expression in the cytologic evaluation of serous fluids. Acta Cytol 49(3):621–626
3. Agre P, Kozono D (2003) Aquaporin water channels: molecular mechanisms for human diseases. FEBS Lett 555(1):72–78
4. Amiry-Moghaddam M, Frydenlund DS, Ottersen OP (2004) Anchoring of aquaporin-4 in brain: molecular mechanisms and implications for the physiology and pathophysiology of water transport. Neuroscience 129(4):999–1010
5. Attanoos RL, Webb R, Dojcinov SD, Gibbs AR (2002) Value of mesothelial and epithelial antibodies in distinguishing diffuse peritoneal mesothelioma in females from serous papillary carcinoma of the ovary and peritoneum. Histopathology 40(3):237–244
6. Attanoos RL, Griffin A, Gibbs AR (2003) The use of immunohistochemistry in distinguishing reactive from neoplastic mesothelium: a novel use for desmin and comparative evaluation with epithelial membrane antigen, p53, platelet-derived growth factor-receptor, P-glycoprotein and Bcl-2. Histopathology 43(3):231–238
7. Bao LH, Sakaguchi H, Fujimoto J, Tamaya T (2007) Osteopontin in metastatic lesions as a prognostic marker in ovarian cancers. J Biomed Sci 14(3):373–381
8. Baratti D, Kusamura S, Martinetti A et al (2007) Circulating CA125 in patients with peritoneal mesothelioma treated with cytoreductive surgery and intraperitoneal hyperthermic perfusion. Ann Surg Oncol 14(11):500–508
9. Baruch AC, Wang H, Staerkel GA et al (2007) Immunocytochemical study of the expression

of mesothelin in fine-needle aspiration biopsy specimens of pancreatic adenocarcinoma. Diagn Cytopathol 35(3):143–147

10. Bateman AC, Al-Talib RK, Newman T et al (1997) Immunohistochemical phenotype of malignant mesothelioma: predictive value of CA125 and HBME-1. Histopathology 30(1):49–56

11. Battifora H, McCaughey W (1995) Tumors of the serosal membranes, Third series, AFIP Atlas of Tumor Pathology. American Registry of Pathology, Washington, DC

12. Ben-Ezra JM, Kornstein MJ, Grimes MM, Krystal G (1994) Small cell carcinomas of the lung express the Bcl-2 protein. Am J Pathol 145(5):1036–1040

13. Bergeret A, De Terrasson FG (1999) Social impact of screening and of medical surveillance on people exposed to asbestos. Rev Mal Respir 16(6pt2):1327–1331

14. Beyer HL, Geschwindt RD, Glover CL et al (2007) MESOMARK: a potential test for malignant pleural mesothelioma. Clin Chem 53(4):666–672

15. Bloch O, Papadopoulos MC, Manley GT, Verkman AS (2005) Aquaporin-4 gene deletion in mice increases focal edema associated with staphylococcal brain abscess. J Neurochem 95(1):254–262

16. Bolen JW, Hammar SP, McNutt MA (1986) Reactive and neoplastic serosal tissue: a light-microscopic, ultrastructural, and immunocytochemical study. Am J Surg Pathol 10(1):34–47

17. Bolen JW, Hammar SP, McNutt MA (1987) Serosal tissue: reactive tissue as a model for understanding mesotheliomas. Ultrastruct Pathol 11(2–3):251–262

18. Borgnia M, Nielsen S, Engel A, Agre P (1999) Cellular and molecular biology of the aquaporin water channels. Annu Rev Biochem 68: 425–458

19. Borok Z, Verkman AS (2002) Lung edema clearance: 20 years of progress: invited review: role of aquaporin water channels in fluid transport in lung and airways. J Appl Physiol 93(6): 2199–2206

20. Brambilla E, Cagle PT, Churg AM, Colby TV, Gibbs AR, Hammar SP, Hasleton PS, Henderson DW, Inai K, Praet M, Roggli VL, Travis WD, Vignaud JM (2006) International Mesothelioma Panel. In: Galateau-Sallé F (ed) Pathology of malignant mesothelioma. Springer, London

21. Brauer C, Baandrup U, Jacobsen P et al (2009) Screening for asbestos-related conditions. Ugeskr Laeger 171:433–436

22. British Thoracic Society Standards of Care Committee (2007) BTS statement on malignant mesothelioma in the UK, 2007. Thorax 62(Suppl 2):ii1–ii19

23. Cagle PT, Brown RW, Lebovitz RM (1994) P53 immunostaining in the differentiation of reactive processes from malignancy in pleural biopsy specimens. Hum Pathol 25(5):443–448

24. Ceresoli GL, Chiti A, Zucali PA et al (2007) Assessment of tumor response in malignant pleural mesothelioma. Cancer Treat Rev 33(6):533–541

25. Chen Y, Tachibana O, Oda M et al (2006) Increased expression of aquaporin 1 in human hemangioblastomas and its correlation with cyst formation. J Neurooncol 80(3):219–225

26. Churg A, Colby TV, Cagle P et al (2000) The separation of benign and malignant mesothelial proliferations. Am J Surg Pathol 24:1183–1200

27. Churg A, Cagle PT, Roggli VL (2006) Tumors of the serosal membranes. American Registry of Pathology/Armed Forces Institute of Pathology, Washington, DC

28. Clapp C, de la EG Martinez (2006) Aquaporin-1: a novel promoter of tumor angiogenesis. Trends Endocrinol Metab 17(1):1–2

29. Creaney J, Robinson BW (2005) Detection of malignant mesothelioma in asbestos-exposed individuals: the potential role of soluble mesothelin-related protein. Hematol Oncol Clin North Am 19:1025–1040

30. Creaney J, Robinson BW (2009) Serum and pleural fluid biomarkers for mesothelioma. Curr Opin Pulm Med 15(6):366–370

31. Creaney J, Christansen H, Lake R et al (2006) Soluble mesothelin related protein in mesothelioma. J Thorac Oncol 1(1):172–174

32. Creaney J, Yeoman D, Naumoff L et al (2007) Soluble mesothelin in effusions: a useful tool for the diagnosis of malignant mesothelioma. Thorax 62(7):569–576

33. Creaney J, Yeoman D, Demelker Y et al (2008) Comparison of osteopontin, megakaryocyte potentiating factor, and mesothelin proteins as markers in the serum of patients with malignant mesothelioma. J Thorac Oncol 3(8):851–857

34. Cury PM, Butcher DN, Corrin B, Nicholson AG (1999) The use of histological and immunohistochemical markers to distinguish pleural malignant mesothelioma and in situ mesothelioma

from reactive mesothelial hyperplasia and reactive pleural fibrosis. J Pathol 189(2):251–257

35. Das M, Muhlenbruch G, Mahnken AH et al (2007) Asbestos Surveillance Program Aachen (ASPA): initial results from baseline screening for lung cancer in asbestos-exposed high-risk individuals using low-dose multidetector-row CT. Eur Radiol 17(5):1193–1199

36. Devuyst O, Ni J (2006) Aquaporin-1 in the peritoneal membrane: implications for water transport across capillaries and peritoneal dialysis. Biochim Biophys Acta 1758(8):1078–1084

37. Diederich S, Wormanns D, Heindel W (2003) Lung cancer screening with low-dose CT. Eur J Radiol 45(1):2–7

38. Endo M, Jain RK, Witwer B, Brown D (1999) Water channel (aquaporin 1) expression and distribution in mammary carcinomas and glioblastomas. Microvasc Res 58(2):89–98

39. Esposito V, Baldi A, De Luca A et al (1997) P53 immunostaining in differential diagnosis of pleural mesothelial proliferations. Anticancer Res 17(18):733–736

40. Esteban JM, Yokota S, Husain S, Battifora H (1990) Immunocytochemical profile of benign and carcinomatous effusions: a practical approach to difficult diagnosis. Am J Clin Pathol 94(6):698–705

41. Eto M, Kodama S, Nomi N et al (2007) Clinical significance of elevated osteopontin levels in head and neck cancer patients. Auris Nasus Larynx 34(3):343–346

42. Falleni M, Pellegrini C, Marchetti A et al (2005) Quantitative evaluation of the apoptosis regulating genes Survivin, Bcl-2 and Bax in inflammatory and malignant pleural lesions. Lung Cancer 48(2):211–216

43. Fasola G, Belvedere O, Aita M et al (2007) Low-dose computed tomography screening for lung cancer and pleural mesothelioma in an asbestos-exposed population: baseline results of a prospective, nonrandomized feasibility trial – an Alpe-adria Thoracic Oncology Multidisciplinary Group Study (ATOM 002). Oncologist 12(10):1215–1224

44. Fleming MV, Guinee DG Jr, Chu WS et al (1998) Bcl-2 immunohistochemistry in a surgical series of non-small cell lung cancer patients. Hum Pathol 29(1):60–64

45. Frey AB, Wali A, Pass H, Lonardo F (2007) Osteopontin is linked to p65 and MMP-9 expression in pulmonary adenocarcinoma but not in malignant pleural mesothelioma. Histopathology 50(6):720–726

46. Geeson F, Saadoun S, Papadopoulos M et al (2002) Aquaporin-4 water channel expression in human vasogenic brain oedema. J Anat 200(5):523

47. Goffin E, Combet S, Jamar F et al (1999) Expression of aquaporin-1 in a long-term peritoneal dialysis patient with impaired transcellular water transport. Am J Kidney Dis 33(2):383–388

48. Gordon GJ, Mani M, Maulik G et al (2008) Preclinical studies of the proteasome inhibitor bortezomib in malignant pleural mesothelioma. Cancer Chemother Pharmacol 61(4):549–558

49. Greillier L, Baas P, Welch JJ et al (2008) Biomarkers for malignant pleural mesothelioma: current status. Mol Diagn Ther 12(8):375–390

50. Grigoriu BD, Scherpereel A, Devos P et al (2007) Utility of osteopontin and serum mesothelin in malignant pleural mesothelioma diagnosis and prognosis assessment. Clin Cancer Res 13:2928–2935

51. Grigoriu BD, Gregoire M, Chahine B, Scherpereel A (2008) New diagnostic markers for malignant pleural mesothelioma. Bull Cancer 95(2):177–184

52. Grigoriu BD, Grigoriu C, Chahine B et al (2009) Clinical utility of diagnostic markers for malignant pleural mesothelioma. Monaldi Arch Chest Dis 71(1):31–38

53. Haddoub R, Rutzler M, Robin A, Flitsch SL (2009) Design, synthesis and assaying of potential aquaporin inhibitors. Handb Exp Pharmacol 385–402

54. Hammar SP, Henderson DW, Klebe S, Dodson RF (2008) Neoplasms of the pleura. In: Tomashefski JFJ (ed) Dail and Hammar's Pulmonary pathology, chap 43, vol 2, 3rd edn. Springer, New York, pp 558–734

55. Hassan R, Laszik ZG, Lerner M et al (2005) Mesothelin is overexpressed in pancreatobiliary adenocarcinomas but not in normal pancreas and chronic pancreatitis. Am J Clin Pathol 124(6):838–845

56. Hassan R, Remaley AT, Sampson ML et al (2006) Detection and quantitation of serum mesothelin, a tumor parker for patients with mesothelioma and ovarian cancer. Clin Cancer Res 12(2):447–453

57. Haylock DN, Nilsson SK (2006) Osteopontin: a bridge between bone and blood. Br J Haematol 134(5):467–474

58. Hedman M, Arnberg H, Wernlund J et al (2003) Tissue polypeptide antigen (TPA), hyaluronan and CA 125 as serum markers in malignant mesothelioma. Anticancer Res 23(1B):531–536

59. Henderson DW, Shilkin KB, Whitaker D et al (1992) The pathology of mesothelioma, including immunohistology and ultrastructure. In: Henderson DW, Shilkin KB, Langlois SL, Whitaker D (eds) Malignant mesothelioma. Hemisphere, New York, pp 69–139

60. Henderson DW, Comin CE, Hammar SP et al (1997) Malignant mesothelioma of the pleura: current surgical pathology. In: Corrin B (ed) Pathology of lung tumors. Churchill Livingstone, New York, pp 241–280

61. Henderson DW, Shilkin KB, Whitaker D (1998) Reactive mesothelial hyperplasia vs mesothelioma, including mesothelioma in situ: a brief review. Am J Clin Pathol 110(3):397–404

62. Henschke CI, Yankelevitz DF (2000) Screening for lung cancer. J Thorac Imaging 15(1):21–27

63. Henschke CI, McCauley DI, Yankelevitz DF et al (1999) Early Lung Cancer Action Project: overall design and findings from baseline screening. Lancet 354(173):99–105

64. Ho M, Bera TK, Willingham MC et al (2007) Mesothelin expression in human lung cancer. Clin Cancer Res 13(5):1571–1575

65. Hoque MO, Soria JC, Woo J et al (2006) Aquaporin 1 is overexpressed in lung cancer and stimulates NIH-3T3 cell proliferation and anchorage-independent growth. Am J Pathol 168(4):1345–1353

66. Huber VJ, Tsujita M, Yamazaki M et al (2007) Identification of arylsulfonamides as Aquaporin 4 inhibitors. Bioorg Med Chem Lett 17(5): 1270–1273

67. Huber VJ, Tsujita M, Kwee IL, Nakada T (2009) Inhibition of aquaporin 4 by antiepileptic drugs. Bioorg Med Chem 17(1):418–424

68. Huber VJ, Tsujita M, Nakada T (2009) Identification of aquaporin 4 inhibitors using in vitro and in silico methods. Bioorg Med Chem 17(1):411–417

69. Husain AN, Colby TV, Ordonez NG et al (2009) Guidelines for pathologic diagnosis of malignant mesothelioma: a consensus statement from the International Mesothelioma Interest Group. Arch Pathol Lab Med 133(8):1317–1331

70. Ishibashi K, Hara S, Kondo S (2009) Aquaporin water channels in mammals. Clin Exp Nephrol 13(2):107–117

71. Isik R, Metintas M, Gibbs AR et al (2001) P53, p21 and metallothionein immunoreactivities in patients with malignant pleural mesothelioma: correlations with the epidemiological features and prognosis of mesotheliomas with environmental asbestos exposure. Respir Med 95(7):588–593

72. Ivanov SV, Ivanova AV, Goparaju CM et al (2009) Tumorigenic properties of alternative osteopontin isoforms in mesothelioma. Biochem Biophys Res Commun 382(3):514–518

73. Iwahori K, Osaki T, Serada S et al (2008) Megakaryocyte potentiating factor as a tumor marker of malignant pleural mesothelioma: evaluation in comparison with mesothelin. Lung Cancer 62(1):45–54

74. Jarius S, Paul F, Franciotta D et al (2008) Mechanisms of disease: aquaporin-4 antibodies in neuromyelitis optica. Nat Clin Pract Neurol 4(4):202–214

75. Jiang JJ, Bai CX, Hong QY et al (2003) Effect of aquaporin-1 deletion on pleural fluid transport. Acta Pharmacol Sin 24(4):301–305

76. Jiang J, Hu J, Bai C (2003) Role of aquaporin and sodium channel in pleural water movement. Respir Physiol Neurobiol 139(1):83–88

77. Kato Y, Tsuta K, Seki K et al (2007) Immunohistochemical detection of GLUT-1 can discriminate between reactive mesothelium and malignant mesothelioma. Mod Pathol 20(2): 215–220

78. Kebapci M, Vardarell E, Adapinar B, Acikalin M (2003) CT findings and serum ca CA125 levels in malignant peritoneal mesothelioma: report of 11 new cases and review of the literature. Eur Radiol 13(12):2620–2626

79. Kim J, Ki SS, Lee SD et al (2006) Elevated levels of osteopontin levels in patients with hepatocellular carcinoma. Am J Gastroenterol 101(9):2051–2059

80. King LS, Agre P (1996) Pathophysiology of the aquaporin water channels. Annu Rev Physiol 58:619–648

81. King LS, Nielsen S, Agre P (1996) Aquaporin-1 water channel protein in lung: ontogeny, steroid-induced expression, and distribution in rat. J Clin Invest 97(10):2183–2191

82. King LS, Kozono D, Agre P (2004) From structure to disease: the evolving tale of aquaporin biology. Nat Rev Mol Cell Biol 5():687–698

83. King J, Thatcher N, Pickering C, Hasleton P (2006) Sensitivity and specificity of immunohistochemical antibodies used to distinguish

between benign and malignant pleural disease: a systematic review of published reports. Histopathology 49(6):561–568

84. Knepper MA (1994) The aquaporin family of molecular water channels. Proc Natl Acad Sci USA 91(14):6255–6258

85. Koskinen K, Rinne JP, Zitting A et al (1996) Screening for asbestos-induced diseases in Finland. Am J Ind Med 30(3):241–251

86. Koskinen K, Pukkala E, Reijula K, Karjalainen A (2003) Incidence of cancer among the participants of the Finnish Asbestos Screening Campaign. Scand J Work Environ Health 29(1):64–70

87. Kushitani K, Takeshima Y, Amatya VJ et al (2007) Immunohistochemical marker panels for distinguishing between epithelioid mesothelioma and lung adenocarcinoma. Pathol Int 57(4):190–199

88. Lai KN, Li FK, Lan HY et al (2001) Expression of aquaporin-1 in human peritoneal mesothelial cells and its upregulation by glucose in vitro. J Am Soc Nephrol 12(5):1036–1045

89. Lantuejoul S, Laverriere MH, Sturm N et al (2000) NCAM (neural cell adhesion molecules) expression in malignant mesotheliomas. Hum Pathol 31(4):415–421

90. Lauritzen AF (1987) Distinction between cells in serous effusions using a panel of antibodies. Virchows Arch A 411(3):299–304

91. Lee MD, King LS, Agre P (1997) The aquaporin family of water channel proteins in clinical medicine. Medicine (Baltimore) 76(3):141–156

92. Leung AN, Muller NL, Miller RR (1990) CT in differential diagnosis of diffuse pleural disease. AJR Am J Roentgenol 154(3):487–492

93. Liakopoulos V, Zarogiannis S, Eleftheriadis T, Stefanidis I (2006) Aquaporin-1 and sodium transport in the peritoneal membrane – need for more research? Kidney Int 70 (9):1663, author reply – 4

94. Liakopoulos V, Zarogiannis S, Hatzoglou C et al (2006) Inhibition by mercuric chloride of aquaporin-1 in the parietal sheep peritoneum: an electrophysiologic study. Adv Perit Dial 22:7–10

95. Liang Q, Xu SR, Liu W et al (2005) Expressions of aquaporin-1 on peritonea in hepatic cirrhotic rats with ascites [Chin]. Zhonghua Yi Xue Za Zhi 85(15):1027–1030

96. Lyons-Boudreaux V, Mody DR, Zhai J, Coffey D (2008) Cytologic malignancy versus benignancy: how useful are the "newer" markers in body fluid cytology? Arch Pathol Lab Med 132(1):23–28

97. Maeda M, Hino O (2006) Molecular tumor markers for asbestos-related mesothelioma: serum diagnostic markers. Pathol Int 56(11):649–654

98. Mangano WE, Cagle PT, Churg A et al (1998) The diagnosis of desmoplastic malignant mesothelioma and its distinction from fibrous pleurisy: a histologic and immunohistochemical analysis of 31 cases including p53 immunostaining. Am J Clin Pathol 110(2):191–199

99. Mason MR, Bedrossian CW, Fahey CA (1987) Value of immunocytochemistry in the study of malignant effusions. Diagn Cytopathol 3(3):215–221

100. Mastrangelo G, Ballarin MN, Bellini E et al (2008) Feasibility of a screening programme for lung cancer in former asbestos workers. Occup Med (Lond) 58(3):175–180

101. Mayall FG, Goddard H, Gibbs AR (1993) The frequency of p53 immunostaining in asbestos-associated mesotheliomas and non-asbestos-associated mesotheliomas. Histopathology 22(4):383–386

102. Mayall F, Heryet A, Manga D, Kriegeskotten A (1997) P53 immunostaining is a highly specific and moderately sensitive marker of malignancy in serous fluid cytology. Cytopathology 8(1):9–12

103. Mazal PR, Susani M, Wrba F, Haitel A (2005) Diagnostic significance of aquaporin-1 in liver tumors. Hum Pathol 36(11):1226–1231

104. Metintas M, Ucgun I, Elbek O et al (2002) Computed tomography features in malignant pleural mesothelioma and other commonly seen pleural diseases. Eur J Radiol 41(1):1–9

105. Miettinen M, Sarlomo-Rikala M (2003) Expression of calretinin, thrombomodulin, keratin 5, and mesothelin in lung carcinomas of different types: an immunohistochemical analysis of 596 tumors in comparison with epithelioid mesotheliomas of the pleura. Am J Surg Pathol 27(2):150–158

106. Mishima R, Takeshima F, Sawai T et al (2007) High plasma osteopontin levels in patients with inflammatory bowel disease. J Clin Gastroenterol 41(2):167–172

107. Misu T, Fujihara K, Nakamura M et al (2006) Loss of aquaporin-4 in active perivascular lesions in neuromyelitis optica: a case report. Tohoku J Exp Med 209(3):269–275

108. Misu T, Fujihara K, Itoyama Y (2008) Neuromyelitis optica and anti-aquaporin 4

antibody – an overview. Brain Nerve 60(5):
527–537

109. Mullick SS, Green LK, Ramzy I et al (1996)
P53 gene product in pleural effusions. Practical
use in distinguishing benign from malignant
cells. Acta Cytol 40(5):855–860

110. Narasimhan SR, Yang L, Gerwin BI,
Broaddus VC (1998) Resistance of pleural
mesothelioma cell lines to apoptosis: relation
to expression of Bcl-2 and Bax. Am J Physiol
275(1pt1):L165–L171

111. Navratil E, Gaulard P, Kanavaros P et al
(1995) Expression of the bcl-2 protein in B cell
lymphomas arising from mucosa associated
lymphoid tissue. J Clin Pathol 48(1):18–21

112. Nishino T, Devuyst O (2008) Clinical application of aquaporin research: aquaporin-1 in the
peritoneal membrane. Pflugers Arch 456(4):
721–727

113. Onda M, Nagata S, Ho M et al (2006)
Megakaryocyte potentiation factor cleaved
from mesothelin precursor is a useful tumor
marker in the serum of patients with mesothelioma. Clin Cancer Res 12(14):4225–4231

114. Ordonez NG (2003) Value of mesothelin
immunostaining in the diagnosis of mesothelioma. Mod Pathol 16(3):192–197

115. Oshio K, Binder DK, Bollen A et al (2003)
Aquaporin-1 expression in human glial tumors
suggests a potential novel therapeutic target
for tumor-associated edema. Acta Neurochir
Suppl 86:499–502

116. Oshio K, Binder DK, Liang Y et al (2005)
Expression of the aquaporin-1 water channel
in human glial tumors. Neurosurgery 56(2):
375–381

117. Papadopoulos MC, Verkman AS (2005)
Aquaporin-4 gene disruption in mice reduces
brain swelling and mortality in pneumococcal
meningitis. J Biol Chem 280(14):13906–13912

118. Papadopoulos MC, Verkman AS (2007)
Aquaporin-4 and brain edema. Pediatr Nephrol
22(6):778–784

119. Papadopoulos MC, Verkman AS (2008)
Potential utility of aquaporin modulators for
therapy of brain disorders. Prog Brain Res
170:589–601

120. Papadopoulos MC, Manley GT, Krishna S,
Verkman AS (2004) Aquaporin-4 facilitates
reabsorption of excess fluid in vasogenic brain
edema. FASEB J 18(11):1291–1293

121. Papp T, Schipper H, Pemsel H et al (2001)
Mutational analysis of N-ras, p53, p16INK4a,
p14ARF and CDK4 genes in primary human

malignant mesotheliomas. Int J Oncol 18(2):
425–433

122. Park EK, Sandrini A, Yates DH et al (2008)
Soluble mesothelin-related protein in an
asbestos-exposed population: the dust diseases
board cohort study: the Dust Diseases Board
cohort study. Am J Respir Crit Care Med
178(8):832–837

123. Pass HI, Carbone M (2009) Current status of
screening for malignant pleural mesothelioma.
Semin Thorac Cardiovasc Surg 21(2):97–104

124. Pass HI, Lott D, Lonardo F et al (2005)
Asbestos exposure, pleural mesothelioma, and
serum osteopontin levels. N Engl J Med
353(15):1564–1573

125. Pittock SJ, Lennon VA (2008) Aquaporin-4
autoantibodies in a paraneoplastic context.
Arch Neurol 65(5):629–632

126. Pittock SJ, Weinshenker BG, Lucchinetti CF
et al (2006) Neuromyelitis optica brain lesions
localized at sites of high aquaporin 4 expression. Arch Neurol 63(7):964–968

127. Qiao YL, Tockman MS, Li L et al (1997) A
case-cohort study of an early biomarker of
lung cancer in a screening cohort of Yunnan
tin miners in China. Cancer Epidemiol
Biomarkers Prev 6(11):893–900

128. Ramael M, Lemmens G, Eerdekens C et al
(1992) Immunoreactivity for p53 protein in
malignant mesothelioma and non-neoplastic
mesothelium. J Pathol 168(4):371–375

129. Ramael M, van den Bossche J, Buysse C et al
(1992) Immunoreactivity for P-170 glycoprotein in malignant mesothelioma and in non-
neoplastic mesothelium of the pleura using the
murine monoclonal antibody JSB-1. J Pathol
167(1):5–8

130. Ray M, Kindler HL (2009) Malignant pleural
mesothelioma: an update on biomarkers and
treatment. Chest 136:888–896

131. Robinson BW, Creaney J, Lake R et al (2003)
Mesothelin-family proteins and diagnosis of
mesothelioma. Lancet 362(9396):1612–1616

132. Robinson BW, Creaney J, Lake R et al (2005)
Soluble mesothelin-related protein: a blood
test for mesothelioma. Lung Cancer 49(Suppl
1):S109–S111

133. Rump A, Morikawa Y, Tanaka M et al (2004)
Binding of ovarian cancer antigen CA125/
MUC16 to mesothelin mediates cell adhesion.
J Biol Chem 279(10):9190–9198

134. Saad RS, Cho P, Liu YL, Silverman JF (2005)
The value of epithelial membrane antigen expression in separating benign mesothelial prolifera-

tion from malignant mesothelioma: a comparative study. Diagn Cytopathol 32(3):156–159

135. Saadoun S, Papadopoulos MC (2009) Aquaporin-4 in brain and spinal cord oedema. Neuroscience 161(3):764–772

136. Saadoun S, Papadopoulos M, Bell B et al (2002) The aquaporin-4 water channel and brain tumour oedema. J Anat 200(5):528

137. Saadoun S, Papadopoulos MC, Davies DC et al (2002) Increased aquaporin 1 water channel expression in human brain tumours. Br J Cancer 87(6):621–623

138. Saikali P, Cayrol R, Vincent T (2009) Anti-aquaporin-4 auto-antibodies orchestrate the pathogenesis in neuromyelitis optica. Autoimmun Rev 9(2):132–135

139. Sapede C, Gauvrit A, Barbieux I et al (2008) Aberrant splicing and protease involvement in mesothelin release from epithelioid mesothelioma cells. Cancer Sci 99(3):590–594

140. Scherpereel A, Lee YC (2007) Biomarkers for mesothelioma. Curr Opin Pulm Med 13(4):339–443

141. Scherpereel A, Grigoriu B, Conti M et al (2006) Soluble mesothelin-related peptides in the diagnosis of malignant pleural mesothelioma. Am J Respir Crit Care Med 173(10):1155–1160

142. Scherpereel A, Astoul P, Baas P et al (2009) Guidelines of the European Respiratory Society and the European Society of Thoracic Surgeons for management of Malignant Pleural Mesothelioma. Eur Respir J 35(3):479–495

143. Schneider J, Presek P, Braun A et al (1999) P53 protein, EGF receptor, and anti-p53 antibodies in serum from patients with occupationally derived lung cancer. Br J Cancer 80(12):1987–1994

144. Segal A, Whitaker D, Henderson D, Shilkin K (2002) Pathology of mesothelioma. In: Robinson BWS, Chahinian AP (eds) Mesothelioma. Martin Dunitz, London, pp 143–184

145. Segers K, Ramael M, Singh SK et al (1994) Immunoreactivity for bcl-2 protein in malignant mesothelioma and non-neoplastic mesothelium. Virchows Arch 424(6):631–634

146. Segers K, Kumar-Singh S, Weyler J et al (1996) Glutathione S-transferase expression in malignant mesothelioma and non-neoplastic mesothelium: an immunohistochemical study. J Cancer Res Clin Oncol 122(10):619–624

147. Shen J, Pinkus GS, Deshpande V, Cibas ES (2009) Usefulness of EMA, GLUT-1, and XIAP for the cytologic diagnosis of malignant

mesothelioma in body cavity fluids. Am J Clin Pathol 131(4):516–523

148. Shiomi K, Miyamoto H, Segawa T et al (2006) Novel ELISA system for detection of N-ERC/mesothelin in the sera of mesothelioma patients. Cancer Sci 97(6):928–932

149. Shiomi K, Hagiwara Y, Sonoue K et al (2008) Sensitive and specific new enzyme-linked immunosorbent assay for N-ERC/mesothelin increases its potential as a useful serum tumor marker for mesothelioma. Clin Cancer Res 14(5):1431–1437

150. Silverman JF, Nance K, Phillips B, Norris HT (1987) The use of immunoperoxidase panels for the cytologic diagnosis of malignancy in serous effusions. Diagn Cytopathol 3(2):134–140

151. Simon F, Johnen G, Krismann M, Muller KM (2005) Chromosomal alterations in early stages of malignant mesotheliomas. Virchows Arch 447(4):762–767

152. Soini Y, Jarvinen K, Kaarteenaho-Wiik R, Kinnula V (2001) The expression of P-glycoprotein and multidrug resistance proteins 1 and 2 (MRP1 and MRP2) in human malignant mesothelioma. Ann Oncol 12(9):1239–1245

153. Sone S, Takashima S, Li F et al (1998) Mass screening for lung cancer with mobile spiral computed tomography scanner. Lancet 351(9111):1242–1245

154. Song Y, Yang B, Matthay MA et al (2000) Role of aquaporin water channels in pleural fluid dynamics. Am J Physiol Cell Physiol 279(6):C1744–C1750

155. Szeto CC, Lai KB, Chow KM et al (2005) The relationship between peritoneal transport characteristics and messenger RNA expression of aquaporin in the peritoneal dialysis effluent of CAPD patients. J Nephrol 18(2):197–203

156. Takagi M, Tanaka K, Suzuki T et al (2009) Anti-aquaporin-4 antibody-positive optic neuritis. Acta Ophthalmol 87(5):562–566

157. Takahashi T, Fujihara K, Nakashima I et al (2006) Establishment of a new sensitive assay for anti-human aquaporin-4 antibody in neuromyelitis optica. Tohoku J Exp Med 210(4):307–313

158. Tan WL, Wong JH, Liew D, Ng IH (2004) Aquaporin-4 is correlated with peri-tumoural oedema in meningiomas. Ann Acad Med Singapore 33(5 Suppl):S87–S89

159. Tanaka K (2008) Anti-aquaporin 4-antibody detection system. Nippon Rinsho 66(6):1093–1097

160. Tani T, Sakimura K, Tsujita M et al (2009) Identification of binding sites for anti-aqua-

porin 4 antibodies in patients with neuromyelitis optica. J Neuroimmunol 211(1-2):110–113

161. Tanimura Y, Hiroaki Y, Fujiyoshi Y (2009) Acetazolamide reversibly inhibits water conduction by aquaporin-4. J Struct Biol 166(1): 16–21

162. Tiitola M, Kivisaari L, Huuskonen MS et al (2002) Computed tomography screening for lung cancer in asbestos-exposed workers. Lung Cancer 35(1):17–22

163. Uzawa A, Mori M, Iwai Y et al (2009) Association of anti-aquaporin-4 antibody-positive neuromyelitis optica with myasthenia gravis. J Neurol Sci 287(1-2):105–107

164. van der Kwast TH, Versnel MA, Delahaye M et al (1988) Expression of epithelial membrane antigen on malignant mesothelioma cells: an immunocytochemical and immunoelectron microscopic study. Acta Cytol 32(2):169–174

165. van Meerbeeck JP, Hillerdal G (2008) Screening for mesothelioma: more harm than good? Am J Respir Crit Care Med 178(8): 781–782

166. Verkman AS (1998) Role of aquaporin water channels in kidney and lung. Am J Med Sci 316(5):310–320

167. Verkman AS (1999) Lessons on renal physiology from transgenic mice lacking aquaporin water channels. J Am Soc Nephrol 10(5): 1126–1135

168. Verkman AS (2001) Applications of aquaporin inhibitors. Drug News Perspect 14(7):412–420

169. Verkman AS (2002) Physiological importance of aquaporin water channels. Ann Med 34(3): 192–200

170. Verkman AS (2002) Renal concentrating and diluting function in deficiency of specific aquaporin genes. Exp Nephrol 10(4):235–240

171. Verkman AS, Matthay MA, Song Y (2000) Aquaporin water channels and lung physiology. Am J Physiol Lung Cell Mol Physiol 278(5):L867–L879

172. Verkman AS, Yang B, Song Y et al (2000) Role of water channels in fluid transport studied by phenotype analysis of aquaporin knockout mice. Exp Physiol 85. Spec No: 233S–241S

173. Vordermark D, Said HM, Katzer A et al (2006) Plasma osteopontin levels in patients with head and neck cancer and cervix cancer are critically dependent on the choice of ELISA system. BMC Cancer 15(6):207–212

174. Walts AE, Said JW, Shintaku IP (1987) Epithelial membrane antigen in the cytodiagnosis of effusions and aspirates: immunocytochemical and ultrastructural localization in benign and malignant cells. Diagn Cytopathol 3(1):41–49

175. Waters P, Vincent A (2008) Detection of anti-aquaporin-4 antibodies in neuromyelitis optica: current status of the assays. Int MS J 15(3):99–105

176. Waters P, Jarius S, Littleton E et al (2008) Aquaporin-4 antibodies in neuromyelitis optica and longitudinally extensive transverse myelitis. Arch Neurol 65(7):913–919

177. Whitaker D (1983) The mesothelium of the rat and its response to injury. Ph.D. thesis, The University of Western Australia, Perth

178. Whitaker D, Papadimitriou JM (1985) Mesothelial healing: morphological and kinetic investigations. J Pathol 145(2):159–175

179. Whitaker D, Sterrett G, Shilkin K (1989) Early diagnosis of malignant mesothelioma: the contribution of effusion and fine needle aspiration cytology and ancillary techniques. In: Peters GA, Peters BJ (eds) Asbestos disease update March 1989. A special supplement to the sourcebook on Asbestos diseases: medical, legal, and engineering aspects. Garland Law Publishing, New York, pp 73–112

180. Whitaker D, Henderson DW, Shilkin KB (1992) The concept of mesothelioma in situ: implications for diagnosis and histogenesis. Semin Diagn Pathol 9(2):151–161

181. Whitaker D, Manning LS, Robinson BW, Shilkin KB (1992) The pathobiology of the mesothelium. In: Henderson DW, Shilkin KB, Langlois SL, Whitaker D (eds) Malignant mesothelioma. Hemisphere, New York, pp 25–68

182. Whitaker D, Shilkin KB, Sterrett GF (1992) Cytological appearances of malignant mesothelioma. In: Henderson DW, Shilkin KB, Langlois SL, Whitaker D (eds) Malignant mesothelioma. Hemisphere, New York, pp 167–182

183. Wolanski KD, Whitaker D, Shilkin KB, Henderson DW (1998) The use of epithelial membrane antigen and silver-stained nucleolar organizer regions testing in the differential diagnosis of mesothelioma from benign reactive mesotheliosis. Cancer 82(3):583–590

184. Wu M, Yuan S, Szporn AH et al (2005) Immunocytochemical detection of XIAP in body cavity effusions and washes. Mod Pathol 18(12):1618–1622

185. Wu CY, Wu MS, Chiang EP et al (2006) Elevated plasma osteopontin associated with gastric carcinoma development, invasion and survival. Gut 56(5):782–789

186. Wu M, Sun Y, Li G et al (2007) Immuno-histochemical detection of XIAP in mesothe-lium and mesothelial lesions. Am J Clin Pathol 128(5):783–787

187. Xiang Y, Ma B, Li T et al (2004) Acetazolamide inhibits aquaporin-1 protein expression and angiogenesis. Acta Pharmacol Sin 25(6): 812–816

188. Yaziji H, Battifora H, Barry TS et al (2006) Evaluation of 12 antibodies for distinguishing epithelioid mesothelioma from adenocarci-noma: identification of a three-antibody immu-nohistochemical panel with maximal sensitivity and specificity. Mod Pathol 19(4):514–523

189. Yen MJ, Hsu C-Y, Mao T-L et al (2006) Diffuse mesothelin expression correlates with prolonged patient survival in ovarian serous carcinoma. Clin Cancer Res 12(3pt1):827–831

190. Yool AJ, Brokl OH, Pannabecker TL et al (2002) Tetraethylammonium block of water flux in Aquaporin-1 channels expressed in kidney thin limbs of Henle's loop and a kid-ney-derived cell line. BMC Physiol 2:4

191. Yukutake Y, Hirano Y, Suematsu M, Yasui M (2009) Rapid and reversible inhibition of aquaporin-4 by zinc. Biochemistry 48(51): 12059–12061

192. Zalay Z, Nemeth L, Sugar J (1992) Screening and pathological diagnosis of asbestosis and mesothelioma: a review. J Environ Pathol Toxicol Oncol 11(5-6):317–321

193. Zhang W, Xie CM, Li ZP (2007) Expression of aquaporin-1 in rat pleural mesothelial cells and its specific inhibition by RNA inter-ference in vitro. Chin Med J (Engl) 120(24): 2278–2283

194. Zheng YY, Lan YP, Tang HF, Zhu SM (2008) Propofol pretreatment attenuates aquaporin-4 over-expression and alleviates cerebral edema after transient focal brain ischemia reperfusion in rats. Anesth Analg 107(6):2009–2016

195. Zhu W, Michael CW (2007) WT1, monoclo-nal CEA, TTF1, and CA125 antibodies in the differential diagnosis of lung, breast, and ovar-ian adenocarcinomas in serous effusions. Diagn Cytopathol 35(6):370–375